Evidence-Based Practice
Intellectual Disabilities

Evidence-Based Practice and Intellectual Disabilities

Edited by

Peter Sturmey and Robert Didden

WILEY Blackwell

This edition first published 2014
© 2014 John Wiley & Sons, Ltd.

Registered Office
John Wiley & Sons, Ltd., The Atrium, Southern Gate, Chichester, West Sussex, PO19 8SQ, UK

Editorial Offices
350 Main Street, Malden, MA 02148–5020, USA
9600 Garsington Road, Oxford, OX4 2DQ, UK
The Atrium, Southern Gate, Chichester, West Sussex, PO19 8SQ, UK

For details of our global editorial offices, for customer services, and for information about how to apply for permission to reuse the copyright material in this book please see our website at www.wiley.com/wiley-blackwell.

The right of Peter Sturmey and Robert Didden to be identified as the authors of the editorial material in this work has been asserted in accordance with the UK Copyright, Designs and Patents Act 1988.

Library of Congress Cataloging-in-Publication Data
Sturmey, Peter.
Evidence-based practice and intellectual disabilities / Peter Sturmey, Robert Didden.
    pages   cm
  Includes bibliographical references and index.
ISBN 978-0-470-71068-5 (hardback) – ISBN 978-0-470-71069-2 (paper)   1. People with mental disabilities–Psychology.   2. Evidence-based social work.   I. Didden, Robert.   II. Title.
  HV3004.S858 2014
  362.3′53–dc23
                                          2013042692
A catalogue record for this book is available from the British Library.

Cover image: © causeandeffectAU / iStockphoto
Cover design by Nicki Averill Design & Illustration

Set in 10.5/13pt Minion by SPi Publisher Services, Pondicherry, India
Printed in Malaysia by Ho Printing (M) Sdn Bhd

1   2014

Contents

Contributors

Amanda B. Bosch is Assistant Professor and Coordinator, Low Incidence Disabilities and Autism (LIDA) Program, Sam Houston State University. She received her PhD in Behavior Analysis from the University of Florida. Her research interests include assessment and treatment of stereotypy and empirically validated versus scientifically untested treatments for autism.

Wiebe Braam is a physician for people with intellectual disability and affiliated with the 's Heeren Loo care center. He specializes in the treatment of sleep problems in individuals with intellectual disabilities. His clinical and research interest is in the role of melatonin in sleep disorders and autism.

Leopold Curfs is Director of the Governor Kremers Centre at the Academic Hospital Maastricht and Maastricht University. He was rewarded with the Governor Kremers professorship at the Faculty of Health, Medicine and Life Sciences of Maastricht University, a Research Chair in Intellectual Disability at the Maastricht University Medical Centre.

Robert Didden is Professor of Intellectual Disabilities, Learning, and Behavior at the Behavioural Science Institute of the Radboud University Nijmegen and a Psychologist affiliated with Trajectum, a center for the treatment of severe behavioral and/or mental health problems in individuals with mild intellectual disability.

Klaus Drieschner is Senior Researcher of Trajectum, a large treatment facility for individuals with mild intellectual disability and severe problem behavior, including offenders. His current research concerns treatment effectiveness, routine outcome monitoring, inpatient aggression, and test construction. Earlier, he published on treatment motivation, treatment engagement, and nonverbal therapy.

Douglas G. Field is Chief of Pediatric Gastroenterology and the Vice Chair of Pediatric Outreach at the Penn State Hershey Medical Center and Professor of ediatrics at the Penn State College of Medicine. His clinical and research interests involve working with children with feeding problems.

Olive Healy is Lecturer in Psychology at the National University of Ireland and Program Director of the structured PhD in Applied Behavior Analysis and lectures on the MSc program. She has over 15 years of experience in the treatment of developmental disorders.

Giulio E. Lancioni is Professor in the Department of Psychology, University of Bari, Italy. His research interests include development and assessment of assistive technologies, training of social and occupational skills, and evaluation of strategies for examining preference and choice with individuals with severe/profound intellectual and multiple disabilities.

Russell Lang is Assistant Professor of Special Education. She has published over 100 research papers and multiple book chapters concerning the education and treatment of children with autism and other developmental disabilities. His primary research interest is in the treatment of problematic and challenging behaviors in individuals with autism spectrum disorders.

William R. Lindsay is Professor of Psychology at the University of Abertay and Honorary Professor at Bangor University and Deakin University. He has published over 300 articles and chapters and given many presentations on cognitive therapy and offenders. He has published five books on offenders and Cognitive Behavior Therapy for people with intellectual disability (ID).

Sinéad Lydon is a PhD candidate in Applied Behavior Analysis at the National University of Ireland, Galway. Her doctoral research, funded by the Irish Research Council, investigates the contribution of psychophysiological measurement to the understanding, assessment, and treatment of challenging behavior in Autism Spectrum Disorder.

Anneke Maas is a Lecturer in the Bachelor's and Master's Program in Special Education at Radboud University Nijmegen, the Netherlands, and behavioral consultant at the outpatient sleep clinic of 's Heeren Loo Advisium in Wekerom. She will soon defend her PhD thesis entitled "Sleep problems in individuals with genetic disorders associated with intellectual disability" at Maastricht University, the Netherlands.

Clodagh Murray completed her PhD in Applied Behavior Analysis at the National University of Ireland, Galway, with research focusing on increasing variability in children with autism spectrum disorders (ASD). She has extensive experience in delivering behavioral interventions and is currently course coordinator of the PostGraduate Diploma in Behavior Analysis at Trinity College Dublin.

Nicole Neil is Adjunct Lecturer and Doctoral Student, Department of Psychology, Queens College, City University of New York. She earned her Master's in Applied Disability Studies at Brock University, Canada. Her current research interests include applied behavior analysis and repetitive behavior and increasing communication in children with Down syndrome.

Mark F. O'Reilly is the Mollie Villeret Davis Professor in Learning Disabilities. His research focuses on functional assessment and treatment of severe challenging behavior, interventions to promote generalization and maintenance of skills, and examining how behavioral interventions must adapt to be respectful and supportive of diversity.

John T. Rapp is Associate Professor of Psychology, Auburn University. He received his doctoral degree in Behavior Analysis from the University of Florida in 2003. His current research interests include the assessment and treatment of automatically reinforced behavior such as stereotypy, research methods, and compliance.

Joel E. Ringdahl is Assistant Professor in the Behavior Analysis and Therapy Program in the Rehabilitation Institute, Southern Illinois University. He received his PhD in Psychology from Louisiana State University. His research interests include functional analysis and treatment of severe behavior problems exhibited by individuals with developmental disabilities.

Laura J. Seiverling is a Licensed Psychologist and Board Certified Behavior Analyst at the Cindy and Tod Johnson Center for Pediatric Feeding Disorders at St Mary's Hospital for Children in Bayside, NY. She specializes in treating children with autism spectrum disorder who have food selectivity.

Jeff Sigafoos received his PhD in Educational Psychology from the University of Minnesota in 1990. He is currently a Professor in the School of Educational Psychology at Victoria University of Wellington in New Zealand. His research focuses on communication intervention for individuals with developmental disabilities.

Marcel Smits is a Neurologist and Head of the Center for Sleep–Wake Disturbances and Chronobiology of the Gelderse Vallei Hospital in Ede. He is also a member of the Governor Kremers Dutch Expertise Centre for sleep disturbances in individuals with intellectual disabilities. He supervises several PhD studies on biological clock sleep disturbances.

Peter Sturmey is Professor of Psychology at Queens College and the Graduate Center, City College of New York. He publishes widely on developmental disabilities. His interests include evidence-based practice, autism, clinical case formulation, staff and parent training, restrictive behavioral interventions, and behavior analytic approaches to psychopathology.

Tricia Vause obtained her PhD in Clinical Psychology. She is an Associate Professor in the Department of Child and Youth Studies and is cross-appointed to the Centre for Applied Disability Studies at Brock University, Ontario, Canada. She has over 17 years of experience in working with persons with developmental disabilities and is a board certified behavior analyst (BCBA-D).

Timothy R. Vollmer is Professor of Psychology, University of Florida. He received his PhD in psychology from the University of Florida and has held positions at Louisiana State University and the University of Pennsylvania before returning to the University of Florida in 1998. He specializes in the assessment and treatment of behavior disorders.

Keith E. Williams is the Director of the Feeding Program at the Penn State Hershey Medical Center and a Professor of Pediatrics at the Penn State College of Medicine. He is the coauthor of over 50 books, articles, and book chapters on feeding problems in children.

Preface

Aim of This Volume

It is now well-established that people with intellectual disabilities (IDs) have an increased risk for developing behavioral and/or mental health problems including aggressive and self-injurious behavior and anxiety and depression. Such problems usually have adverse consequences for them and their relatives, staff members, and others who are involved in their care and treatment. The body of knowledge on prevalence rates and risk factors for behavioral and/or mental health problems in individuals with IDs has grown, and the number of scientific studies on the effectiveness of treatment for such problems has increased during the last decades. This may be explained in part by the increased focus on evidence-based practice in the field of IDs from funding agents and governments as well as the expansion of evidence-based practice outside of medicine.

Despite the increasing body of scientific knowledge, many children and adults with IDs and/or autism receive ineffective treatment, no treatment at all, or are even subjected to harmful therapies. Individuals with IDs have the same rights to high standards of treatment as other people; however, professionals may be unaware of the literature concerning evidence-based practice, misinformed about treatment effectiveness, indifferent or hostile to scientific approaches to treatment or unable to use it in practice, or they may lack appropriate training in providing effective therapies to people with IDs.

The aim of this volume is to provide an overview of the evidence base of psychological therapies for specific disorders and challenging behaviors often encountered in this target group. For each of these disorders/behaviors, psychological treatments are evaluated using the Chambless and Hollon (1998) criteria for evidence-based practice. In addition, each chapter includes a selective review on studies on prevalence rates and risk factors. Each chapter finishes with clinical guidelines for professional caregivers and therapists.

We hope that this volume informs professional caregivers and therapists about the state of the art of effective treatments, which may help them provide more effective treatment to individuals with IDs. This volume may also be a useful resource for students who undergo training in the use of psychological treatments and for managers, agencies, and funding bodies when designing and funding services for individuals with intellectual and developmental disabilities.

Overview of the Volume

This book is divided into two parts. Part I, "Foundational Issues and Overview," consists of four chapters by the first editor, which sets the stage for Part II, "Specific Disorders and Challenging Behaviors." Chapter 1, "Evidence-Based Practice: An Overview," defines evidence-based practice (EBP) and reviews the rationale and methods for using EBP. It also describes a few controversies related to EBP in passing. The next two chapters, "Adaptive Behavior" and "Maladaptive Behavior," summarize the results of approximately 100 meta-analyses of treatment related to IDs and/or autism. The final chapter in Part I asks the contentious question "But Is It Worth It?" and reviews the economic data on treatment efficacy. It finds several plausible examples of treatments that may pay society back for the investment in treatment.

Both aggression and self-injury are some of the most challenging and often treatment-responsive problems for individuals with ID and/or autism. Thus, Part II, "Specific Disorders and Challenging Behaviors," begins with a review of treatment of aggressive behavior from Olive Healy, Sinéad Lydon, and Clodagh Murray and of self-injurious behavior from Jeff Sigafoos, Mark F. O'Reilly, Giulio E. Lancioni, Russell Lang, and Robert Didden. Stereotypic behavior is stigmatizing and interferes with learning and adaptive behavior. Thus, Timothy R. Vollmer, Amanda B. Bosch, Joel E. Ringdahl, and John T. Rapp provide a review of this problem. Recently, greater attention has been given to feeding problems, such as overselectivity and food refusal. Keith E. Williams, Laura J. Seiverling, and Douglas G. Field review the treatment of feeding problems. Chapter 9, "Sleep Problems," by Robert Didden, Wiebe Braam, Anneke Maas, Marcel Smits, Peter Sturmey, Jeff Sigafoos, and Leopold Curfs, reviews a variety of treatments including melatonin and behavioral interventions for sleep problems in people with IDs and/or autism.

Anxiety and depression are often referred to as the *common colds* of mental health. There is good evidence that teenagers and adults with ID and/or autism, like the rest of us, experience these problems frequently. Hence, Chapter 10 by Peter Sturmey, William R. Lindsay, Tricia Vause, and Nicole Neil and Chapter 11 by Peter Sturmey and Robert Didden review the evidence-based practice concerning the treatment of anxiety and depression, respectively. Offenders with ID represent a special challenge to society, and their treatment is especially important to prevent harm to future potential victims. Thus, the final chapter, "Offenders with Developmental

Disabilities," by Peter Sturmey and Klaus Drieschner reviews the limited data available on this difficult question.

Future Directions

From this volume, it is evident that various types of skills deficits and behavioral problems and disorders may be treated effectively primarily using behavioral treatments and some nonbehavioral ones, such as melatonin. The chapters propose guidelines implementing these evidence-based treatments in clinical practice.

Although implementing treatments that have been shown to be effective under controlled research circumstances may or may not always be easy to implement in regular settings, it is our contention that there is now sufficient evidence to begin dissemination of evidence-based practice to professionals working in diverse settings as generic and mainstream mental health settings, medium and high-security settings, organizations providing early intervention, and care centers. Dissemination requires selection of socially important targets that can be effectively and economically treated by local practitioners. Such an endeavor requires readily accessible and easy to use treatment manuals and related materials and protocols to train and support local practitioners in evidence-based practices. Thus, future research should evaluate how to disseminate these evidence-based practices to professionals working with clients with intellectual disabilities in typical settings.

Future research should also address five other issues. First, little attention continues to be given to treatment generalization in behavioral interventions, and this issue has been almost completely ignored by other approaches. Second, although therapies may be effective in short-term demonstrations, little is known about long-term effectiveness and benefits. Third, little is known about cost benefits of many commonly used treatments, and future research should address that important issue. The third step is to analyze for whom this treatment works best, how to increase treatment compliance and reduce dropout, and which elements contribute to its effectiveness. Future studies should be conducted exploring which variables predict treatment outcome. Behavioral treatments address this by using functional assessment and analysis to predict effective and contraindicated treatments and the effects of treatment integrity and staff and parent training on outcome and treatment integrity. In the treatment of offenders, this question is addressed by consideration of criminogenic needs in case formulation. Future research should also explore other methods, especially those that identify independent variables amenable to change. Fourth, the field of evidence-based practice in intellectual disabilities is rapidly evolving, and new approaches are being developed such as eye movement desensitization reprocessing for trauma and trauma-related problems, dialectical behavior therapy for challenging behaviors, intensive interaction, new psychopharmacological agents, new diets, and new technology, such as IPODs. Future research should continue to evaluate new therapies as they evolve. A final issue is the contribution to treatment outcome of the relationship between client and therapist to treatment outcome.

Reference

Chambless, D., & Hollon, S. (1998). Defining empirically supported therapies. *Journal of Consulting and Clinical Psychology, 66,* 7–18.

Acknowledgments

We would like to thank all our authors for their patience in writing and often rewriting their chapters. We would also like to thank Bill Lindsay and John Taylor for significant input in developing the chapter on offenders with intellectual disabilities.

Part I

Foundational Issues and Overview

1

Evidence-Based Practice
An Introduction

Peter Sturmey

Evidence-Based Practice

Questions concerning evidence-based practice (EBP) permeate services for people with developmental disabilities. A parent must decide whether or not to participate in early intervention for their child with autism and stay at home instead of working. A teacher selects certain target behaviors and teaching strategies for a child and decides not to teach other skills and not to use other teaching strategies. An agency for adults with disabilities decides whether to operate traditional, center-based services or to implement a new job coaching service. A city, state, or government agency decides whether or not to fund early intervention or to place some individuals in specialized, expensive, out-of-district services.

EBP is reflected in many educational and clinical decisions by individual teams. Consider the following example. A team of professionals in special education attempt to treat food refusal in a child with autism for 6 months using sensory integration therapy. Not only did the child continue to refuse food, but the child continued to lose weight. When outside therapists proposed using escape extinction (see Chapter 8) as an EBP, the educators oppose such treatment on the grounds that it does not address the sensory needs of the child and will not work or they refuse to treat the problem by "conditioning" or "behavior modification" which they think is "inhuman" or "disrespectful." After 2 weeks of escape extinction, the child now ate a wide range of foods and gained weight; resources are no longer wasted on ineffective therapy and useless discussion of ineffective treatment.

EBP is not some academic question. If we are concerned with personally significant outcomes and avoidance of harm for individuals with developmental

Evidence-Based Practice and Intellectual Disabilities, First Edition.
Edited by Peter Sturmey and Robert Didden.
© 2014 John Wiley & Sons, Ltd. Published 2014 by John Wiley & Sons, Ltd.

disabilities, it is one that we all face. This chapter outlines some of the issues in the application of EBP to services for people with intellectual disabilities (ID), autism, and other developmental disabilities. The next section examines the general and operational definitions of EBP. The next sections examine the ethical and economic rationales for EBP and the methods associated with EBP, such as systematic reviews and meta-analyses. The final section reviews some of the application of EBP to ID, autism, and other developmental disabilities.

What Is Evidence-Based Practice?

Some definitions

Some general definitions
The definition of EBP is anticipated in Paul's (1967) famous questions: "What treatment, by whom, is most effective for this individual with that specific problem, and which set of circumstances?" (p. 111) which—nearly 50 years ago—raised the issue of not only what kinds of psychological therapy are effective but also how a practitioner should apply or not apply the results of therapy outcome research to specific clients with specific problems. Paul's question is echoed in Sackett, Richardson, Rosenberg, and Haynes' (1997) definition of EBP as "the integration of best research evidence with clinical expertise and patient values" (p. 1). This definition is cited very often and is the basis for similar definitions, such as those by the Institute of Medicine (2001) and the American Psychological Association's (APA) Presidential Task Force on EBP (2006).

Table 1.1 lists a number of definitions of EBP. An examination of these definitions shows that they are aspirational rather than operational, as they do not describe the methods by which we might determine and apply best research evidence clearly. For example, the meaning of the words such as "most effective," "integrate," "clinical

Table 1.1   Some Definitions of EBP

1. "… the integration of best research evidence with clinical expertise and patient values" (Sackett et al., 1997, p. 1)
2. "Evidence-based practice in psychology (EBPP) is the integration of the best available research with clinical expertise in the context of patient characteristics, culture, and preferences" (APA, 2006, p. 273) (http://www.apa.org/practice/resources/evidence/evidence-based-statement.pdf)
3. "… a decision-making process that integrates the best available evidence with family and professional wisdom and values" (Buysse & Wesley, 2006, p. 12)
4. EBP early childhood intervention practices are "informed by research, in which the characteristics and consequences of environmental variables are empirically established and the relationship directly informs what a practitioner can do to produce a desired outcome" (Dunst, Trivette, & Cutspec, 2002, p. 3)

expertise," "wisdom" and "values," and "informed by research" is not specified in these definitions, although some sources, such as Straus, Glasziou, Richardson, and Haynes (2011), do describe specific procedures that practitioners can use to determine what is EBP and how to use it effectively with specific particular clients. Some definitions give greater emphasis to science and EBP, such as Sackett et al.'s (1997) and Dunst et al.'s definitions. Other definitions, such as Buysse and Wesley's, appear to give equal weight to clinical experience and wisdom and only reference "best available evidence" rather than research or empirically validated treatments. Some definitions emphasize that evidence must be current and the "best available evidence" but also that this evidence must be integrated into clinical decision making. Finally, all of these definitions state that evidence and experience must be "integrated," but these definitions do not specify what constitutes integration or how it can be achieved.

These definitions illustrate the tension between the role of science and personal and professional experience should have in determining what an appropriate treatment is for a specific person. They also reflect the tension between personal and professional autonomy and choice over selection of treatment versus restriction of choice and autonomy implied by restriction of practice to only EBP by funding agencies and professional organizations. For example, the explicit aim of some meta-analyses is to determine the standards of practice in developmental disabilities (Scotti, Evans, Meyer, & Walker, 1991). Professional practice is also restricted by treatment algorithms and practice guidelines. For example, National Institute for Clinical Excellence's (NICE) (2012) guidelines for adults with autism baldly state, "Do not provide facilitated communication" (p. 24). They also guide professionals as how to conduct certain treatments. For example, when conducting social learning programs for adults with autism, the guidelines state that they should "typically include: ... modeling ... peer feedback (for group-based programs) or individual feedback (for individually delivered programs) ... discussion and decision-making ... explicit rules ... [and] ... suggested strategies for dealing with difficult social situations." A clinician who does not follow such evidence-based, professional practice guidelines would have to justify deviations from them or use of alternate approaches and might encounter censure during peer review or any legal proceedings if a client or someone else is harmed. A final important observation on these definitions is that they go beyond merely generating lists of treatment that meet the criteria for EBP. EBP also requires the application and adaption of research findings to the actual effective delivery of the best intervention to real-world clients in real-world settings by local practitioners to achieve actual client outcomes for the specific client at hand.

Operational definitions
As well as these general definitions of EBP, there are also operational definitions of EBP. Here, we can discern two kinds of approaches. The first is to determine if a specific treatment is an EBP. For example, Chambless and Hollon (1998) operationally defined an EBP in two ways. When discussing randomized controlled trails (RCTs),

they write that "Only when a treatment has been found efficacious in at least two studies by independent research teams do we consider its efficacy to have been established and label it an efficacious treatment. If there is only one study supporting a treatment's efficacy, or if all of the research has been conducted by one team, we consider the findings promising but would label such treatments as possibly efficacious, pending replication" (p. 10), and later, when discussing small N experiments, they wrote that "We consider a treatment to be possibly efficacious if it has proved beneficial to at least three participants in research by a single group. Multiple replications (at least three each) by two or more independent research groups are required before we consider a treatment's efficacy as established (each in the absence of conflicting data)."

The second approach is to determine what an EBP is for a specific client and a specific presenting problem. Straus et al. (2011) described a five-step procedure that a practitioner should use to identify an EBP for a specific clinical situation. Step 1 was to convert an unmet information need into an answerable question. Step 2 was to find the best evidence available to answer that question. Step 3 was to appraise the evidence critically as to its validity, effect size (ES), and applicability to the situation at hand. The fourth step was to integrate the results of step 3 with practitioner expertise and the client's biology, values, and circumstances. Finally, step 5 was to implement the EBP with the particular client and evaluate both the effectiveness and efficiency of that intervention. NICE's (2012) description of the six steps of EBP is a modification of these guidelines. This approach to defining EBP is closer to clinical practice and fulfills the function of taking a clinical problem and translating research on treatment outcome to application with a specific client.

These two approaches illustrate different procedures because they reflect two different kinds of questions. The first kind of question is a research question relating to the current status of scientific evidence generally for a treatment, a problem, or the application of a treatment or range of treatments to a problem. For example, we might ask a very broad question such as "What is the most effective treatment for challenging behavior?" or we might ask more focused questions such as "Does functional analysis produce more effective treatments than functional assessment for the treatment of aggression in preschool children with autism?" or "What are the effects of PECS training on requesting, spoken language and challenging behavior?" These questions result in identification of specific treatments as EBPs and may generate lists of approved and nonapproved treatments or treatments rank ordered in various ways. For example, treatments may be ranked by degree of empirical support, ES, risk of harm, cost, etc., or some combination of these. For example, Chambless and Hollon's (1998) criteria classified therapies as "possibly efficacious" or "efficacious." The second kind of question related to how a practitioner can apply the available evidence to a specific client and, thus, is closer to answering Paul's (1967) question. For example, here, we might ask, "What is the best treatment of self-injury for this teenager with Lesch–Nyhan syndrome that we can implement and that he and his family will support?"

Other definitions

Chambless and Hollon's (1998) criteria for EBP are often cited, but they are not the only operational definition of EBP. For example, Chambless and Hollon noted that their own criteria differed from those of the Division 12 task force (1998) which defined EBPs as having *specificity*; that is, for the Division 12 task force (1998), an EBP had to be superior to sugar pill or psychological placebo and another psychological treatment to be considered an EBP. In contrast, Chambless and Hollon only required superiority to a wait list control, arguing that "if a treatment works, for whatever reason, and if this effect can be replicated by multiple independent groups, then the treatment is likely to be of value clinically, and a good case can be made for its use" (p. 10). Other systematic reviews and meta-analysis, such as those by NICE, among others, have restricted evidence to exclude evidence from small N experiments. Thus, NICE's (2012) clinical guideline on adults with autism excluded all small N experiments with adults with autism, leading to conclusions that differ from the conclusions in other meta-analyses and systematic reviews of small N experiments of interventions with adults with ASD (Bishop-Fitzpatrick, Minshew, & Eack, 2013; Chowdhury & Benson, 2010; Palmen, Didden, & Lang, 2010). For example, whereas NICE (2012) did not discuss the use of behavioral interventions, Palmen et al.'s (2010) systematic review identified 20 small N experiments with 116 participants which evaluated social, academic, vocational, and domestic skills. They concluded that "behavioral interventions can be successfully used to improve adaptive skills in young adults with high functioning ASD" (pp. 614–615).

Similar differences in definitions of EBPs can also be seen in definitions of EBPs using small N experiments. For example, when defining EBP in special education, Horner et al. (2005) proposed that "A practice may be considered evidence based when (a) a minimum of five single-subject studies that meet minimally acceptable methodological criteria and document experimental control have been published in peer-reviewed journals, (b) the studies are conducted by at least three different researchers across at least three different geographical locations, and (c) the five or more studies include a total of at least 20 participants" (p. 176). These criteria are more stringent than Chambless and Hollon's, and, thus, a treatment might meet criteria as an EBP using one set of criteria, but not when using another set.

Some definitions of EBP distinguish multiple levels of evidence. For example, Rusch and Frances' (2000) *Expert consensus guidelines for treatment of psychiatric and behavioral problems in mental retardation* distinguished three levels of evidence. First-line treatments were "options that the panel feels are usually appropriate as initial treatment for a given situation" (pp. 162–163). Second-line treatments "are reasonable choices for clients/patients who cannot tolerate or do not respond to the first line choices" (p. 163), and third-line treatments "are usually inappropriate or used only when preferred treatments have not been effective" (p. 163). They defined these levels of treatment operationally as scores on a 9-point Likert scale as rated by an expert panel where first line was defined as at least 50% of the panel rating the treatment as a 9 and second-line treatment's entire confidence limits had to be greater than 6.5. A third-line treatment was one in which a portion of the confidence limit fell below 3.5.

Some approaches to EBP propose treatment algorithms and stepped-care approaches which recommend different treatment intensities—often with increasing costs—as one proceeds from at-risk populations (primary or secondary prevention) to severe, chronic treatment-nonresponsive problems (clinical treatment). For example, Rusch and Frances' (2000) guidelines identified first-, second-, and third-line treatments, suggesting that practitioners should use these guidelines to sequence treatment options. In the literature on offenders, treatments are sometimes developed according to responsivity–need–risk model in which clients with higher risk for offending receive more intensive treatments.

Rationale

There are a number of reasons why we should be interested in EBP. These can be grouped under two categories: professional and personal ethics (Schreck & Miller, 2010) and economics and efficiency.

Professional and personal ethics

Standards of professional and personal ethics require practitioners to adhere to the principles of beneficence and nonmalfeasance, namely, doing good and avoiding harm to the client. In addition, therapists should be competent to treat their clients effectively, select treatments based on scientific evidence (where available), appraise the likely effects of all alternate therapies, have specific treatment objectives, and cooperate to reduce conflicts with other professionals (Schreck & Miller, 2010). Finally, clinicians should be honest with their clients, which includes giving their clients an honest appraisal of the likely response to treatment, benefits, and risks of harm, including unknown risks of harm for unevaluated therapies (APA, 2010). Service funders too have ethical obligations to maximize client benefit and the funders by investing resources in treatments that are effective and in an equitable fashion. Thus, professional ethics for practitioners and administrators points in the direction of implementing EBPs to increase client gains, avoid client harms, and use limited resources wisely.

Psychotherapy economics and personal ethics intersect. Individual therapists and services implicitly and explicitly make choices over limited resources every moment at work. (These choices may be influenced by other factors such as funding and number of treatment sessions allocated by supervisors or state-approved plans.) They choose how much time to spend with each client, when to take on new clients, and when to leave others on waiting lists or when to seek out new clients. They allocate clients to high-cost individualized treatment by professionals or choose to allocate them to cheaper therapies delivered in groups by other therapists, perhaps with more limited therapeutic skills. They choose between investing time in continuing education, thereby reducing client treatment, with the possible benefit to clients in the future if the therapists become more competent in treating important, common, treatment-responsive problems. They engage in administrative, research, and other activities and with no immediate client outcome, but with the possibility of distant client benefits. None of us can escape the economic implications for psychotherapy practice!

Psychological treatments sometimes harm clients
It is tempting to believe that psychological treatments do not harm clients, but this is untrue. Lilienfield (2007) lists several harmful psychological treatments including one related to developmental disabilities. These included facilitated communication, which has the potential to result in false accusations of child abuse against family members.

A second recent comes from the use of psychotherapy and autism in France. The BBC (Schofield, 2012, http://www.bbc.co.uk/news/magazine-17583123) reported that in France psychoanalysis and psychiatry dominates the treatment of autism. This model maintains Bettelheim's psychoanalytic model that autism is caused by so-called refrigerator mothers (Bettelheim, 1967). Consequently, the treatments offered include wrapping the child in cold sheets to reconnect them with their partially clothed bodies ("packing"). This may result in children crying and struggling and has been implemented without parental knowledge for extended periods of time in some cases (Cheng, 2012). Other psychoanalytic treatments for autism include psychoanalysis for the family. In France, only approximately 20% of children with autism receive education, and of these, many receive only part-time education. Schofield suggested that psychoanalysis results in denial of education and effective treatment, very high rates of family divorce, and single mothers left alone to manage their child with autism without help. Currently, there is no evidence that any of these psychoanalytic treatments are effective, although psychoanalysts offer uncorroborated anecdotal reports of "spectacular" results. According to Cheng, Marie Dominique Amy, president of French psychotherapy and psychiatry association, claimed that after packing, "Amy said she had seen autistic children start talking, writing and drawing after the sessions." There are no empirical studies supporting these claims.

Failure to provide effective treatment
There is a much more insidious and ubiquitous form of harm: failure to provide effective treatment. We often observe high-need clients who receive no treatment, who receive unnecessarily extensive assessments, or who are referred to other services that do not materialize for months or sometimes a year. A more subtle problem is that services do indeed respond to individuals with high needs but do so by preventing the opportunity to engage in challenging behavior. For example, a high-need individual might be placed on one-on-one staffing, separated from a group, or from materials or other people so they cannot engage in challenging behavior. This strategy may be legitimate as a first, short-term strategy to prevent harm, but, as a long-term strategy, it denies effective treatment to the person

resulting in both a restricted lifestyle and harm to the individual and others because the challenging behavior goes untreated.

After a choking incident, for example, an individual with life-threatening pica might be placed on one-on-one staffing, and all objects that they might ingest might be removed. Such strategies avoid client harm in the short term, but this individual might benefit from a number of effective, nonaversive EBPs such as noncontingent reinforcement and environmental enrichment based on functional assessment and analyses (McAdam, Beidbord, Dahl, & Williams, 2012) (see meta-analyses of pica treatment by Hagopian, Rooker, & Rolider, 2001; McAdam et al., 2012; McAdam, Sherman, Sahaddon, & Napolitano, 2004). If, however, the individual does not receive effective, evidence-based interventions, then the individual will continue to live in a highly restrictive environment indefinitely and will not receive effective treatment to increase appropriate behavior and decrease pica. Thus, in such circumstances, this individual may be kept safe for many months until they are then engage in life-threatening pica again.

The *Right to Effective Treatment* statement (Van Houten et al., 1988) addresses the issue of access to effective treatment. Some aspects of this statement—such as access to a responsive environment and services whose overriding goal is personal welfare—are noncontroversial, even if many services struggle to do these things. The right to the most effective treatment procedures available, however, is most controversial because (a) the statement labeled some nonaversive interventions as unacceptable due to the lack of treatment effect or treatment that produces change too slowly and (b) it opened the door to "quicker acting, but temporary more restrictive procedures" (p. 383) (see Table 1.2 for a summary of Van Houten et al.). This issue continues to be recognized in contemporary statements on restraint and restraint reduction in which calls for judgments concerning the risk to benefit ratio, including the risks of ineffective treatment and the harm and distress that accrues the person from not treating and treating ineffectively and the possibility that a more intensive intervention that reduces harm and results in better client outcomes (Applied Behavior Analysis International, 2010).

Some saw the *Right to Effective Treatment* statement (Van Houten et al., 1988) as an open door for the use of aversive treatments, such as contingent electric shock, an issue that still resonates today. Thus, the *Right to Effective Treatment* statement and other events in the 1980s stimulated the growth of organization such as TASH and the Positive Behavior Support movement to promote effective, nonaversive treatments.

Economics and efficiency

The cost of services has always been an important consideration in determining services available to people with developmental disabilities. Economic analysis of mental health services generally (Knapp & McDaid, 2012) assumes that mental health systems should alleviate symptoms, promote quality of life, support caregivers, and improve life chances but notes that this is done within the context of

Table 1.2 A Summary of the Right to Effective Treatment Statement
(Van Houten et al., 1988)

Right	Examples
1. Therapeutic environment	Physical and social environment is safe, humane, and responsive and has an acceptable standard of living. The individual has access to therapeutic and leisure services and leisure and enjoyable materials. Activities and materials should respect client choices and be age appropriate. There should be frequent positive interactions to ensure enjoyment, learning, and independence with the fewest restrictions necessary to ensure individual safety and development
2. Personal welfare	Behavioral treatment to promote functional skills and independence, immediate, and long-term welfare with active individual or proxy participation. Risk and professional performance is overseen by human rights and peer review committees to impose community and professional standards
3. Treatment by a competent behavior analyst	Person delivering services must have academic training and clinical competence. For complex problems, a doctoral-level behavior analyst is needed to ensure appropriate assessment, treatment, training to service providers, consultation, and follow-up
4. Programs that teach functional skills	Services have the goal to increasing individuals' effective functioning to teach adaptive behavior, behavior to terminate aversive stimulation, reduction in behavior that is dangerous and restricts access to independence and social acceptability, and behavior that is beneficial to society. All individuals should be treated as capable of learning. This may include temporary exposure to discomfort and risk
5. Behavioral assessment and ongoing evaluation	A diagnostic assessment and a behavioral assessment that includes interviews, direct observation, and incorporation of behavior assessment information into a treatment plan. Ongoing evaluation using objective, public data
6. Most effective treatment available	Effective and scientifically validated treatment. Individual and public educated concerning most effective treatment. Restrictive procedures are unacceptable unless shown to be safe and effective. Nonrestrictive interventions are unacceptable when more effective, faster-acting alternatives are available

limited resources that must be allocated carefully to how the resources are used to achieve client outcomes. For many products, such as groceries, consumers are routinely exposed to purchasing the product and can readily judge the cost and quality of the product. Mental health services are not like groceries because people purchase them infrequently, it is difficult to judge their quality, and they often come with perceived stigma. Additionally, often the consumer themselves do not directly purchase them; rather, a third party such as a family member, guardian, or service provider purchases those products on behalf of the consumers. In some cases, such as offenders, courts impose services and treatment on clients. Resources for mental health come from prepayment systems, such as taxes, salary-based contributions, voluntary health insurance schemes (also known as private health insurance), and out-of-pocket expenses used to purchase services on the basis of efficiency, that is, achieving the maximum relevant outcome for the price, and equity, that is, fairness of the distribution of outcomes, access, and payment across individuals and society.

Cost-effectiveness analysis is one approach to economic evaluation of human services which asks two questions: "Does it work?" but also "Is it worth it?" Cost data include staff salaries in prevention, treatment, and other services; facility costs, such as cleaning; overheads, such as personal; and capital costs, such as buildings. Effectiveness can be measured by using common metrics, such as changes in standard measures of depression. Effectiveness can also be measured using quality-adjusted life years (QALYs), a measure of years of perfect quality of life and the cost of increasing the number of QALYs due to treatment. Some cost-effectiveness evaluations use monetary values by comparing the total costs and benefits of two or more treatment options, including no or minimal treatment.

Decisions to implement EBPs are made both individual and societal levels. For example, a practitioner might decide to increase the number of sessions given to one client and reduce the number of sessions to another. Alternatively, an agency, government, or insurance provider might decide to stop funding early intervention and provide sensory integration therapy within a certain agency. (Chapter 4 discusses this issue in more detail.)

Methods Used in Evidence-Based Practice

Evidence-based approaches are characterized by systematic reviews and meta-analyses. These approaches use (a) explicit statement of research questions; (b) efforts to make procedures such as literature searches transparent by describing search strategies, inclusion, and exclusion criteria; (c) in the case of meta-analysis, objective methods of measuring, combining, and disaggregating treatment ESs; (d) clear rules for describing the strength and quality of evidence; and (e) dissemination and evaluation of EBPs to practice through professional training and support and service design or application to individual cases. The next sections review each of these five aspects of EBP.

Formulating a research or clinical question

Why does someone conduct a systematic review or meta-analysis? Why does a practitioner ask a question concerning the application of EBP to a particular case? What question are we trying to answer?

Schlosser, Wendt, and Sigafoos (2007) noted that the purpose of systematic reviews and meta-analyses is sometimes unstated or unclear. For example, if a paper states that its purpose is to "summarize" or "review" the literature on a particular treatment or problem, it can readily become unfocussed and the research question does not guide the authors how to search the literature. To solve this problem, Schlosser et al. recommended stating research questions using this three-part format: subject (the participants), verb (the intervention), and object (an outcome). Thus, a better question than the original research question would be: "In adolescents with mild ID, what are the effects of job coaching, on chances of employment in integrated settings, income, and comprehensive treatment costs?"

Clinicians also face the challenge of formulating clear, answerable questions when attempting to identify the best treatment for a specific client using EBP (Straus et al., 2011), but how should a clinician formulate such as question? For example, consider a clinician working with a 50-year-old woman with mild ID and a diagnosis of borderline personality disorder who presents challenges to the staff because she refuses to comply with preventative medical treatment for poor circulation in her legs. If the problem goes untreated, there is a possibility that she may have infections, ulceration, or even amputation, but when the staff ask her to engage in any rehabilitation, she curses at them, scratches her legs, destroys the equipment, and throws things at the staff. What question should the clinician ask? They might ask "well what do I do?" which might be a general cry for help from someone in a difficult situation who does not know the best course of action. They could ask questions about the best treatment for noncompliance in adults with mild ID, or they could ask what the best treatment for borderline personality disorder is. (In the end, since the clinician could find no literature specifically on the treatment of borderline personality disorder in adults with mild ID, the clinician simplified the question and searched for EBPs for borderline personality disorder. She went on to modify those procedures for someone with mild ID.)

Systematic searches

To address the issues of bias or incompleteness of literature included in traditional narrative reviews, systematic reviews and meta-analyses attempt to describe their search strategies completely and with transparency. Search strategies may include online searches; searching of reference sections of articles retained from the searches and/or from review articles, book chapters, etc.; searching of citations of articles; online searching of journal contents; contacting authors and/or leading researchers; and hand searches of journals. Online searches may vary along a number of dimensions including (a) the number of databases searched; (b) the variety of databases search, for example, whether the databases include primarily psychological, educational, special education, medical, rehabilitation, theses, or other content areas; (c) the range of years searched; (d) the choice of disability-related and other search terms and whether supplementary searches are conducted after the initial search; (e) the inclusion/exclusion criteria; and (f) whether or not and how raters are trained to search the resulting abstracts and the reliability and validity of their searching. Most emphasis has been placed on the reliability and transparency or reporting searches, but validity has received less attention.

For example, some systematic reviews include flow diagrams showing the numbers of papers located and retained various stages of the searches, and some report the reliability of doing so by having more than one person to conduct the search. Some searches also report an explicit procedure to resolve whether to include papers where raters disagree on inclusion.

Searches also vary in terms of their difficulty. For example, searching for a very specific intervention in a very specific population, such as the effects of Active Support on staff and client behavior (Hamelin & Sturmey, 2013), is relatively easy because there is a unique string to use ("Active Support") and a small literature with relatively few authors. Thus, it is relatively easy to conduct a complete search. On the other hand, broad searches, such as psychosocial treatments for internalizing behavior disorders, would be quite difficult to do because the literature is large and dispersed across many sources, and there are many synonyms for both "psychosocial treatments" and "internalizing disorders." Thus, such a search would probably effortful and expensive and also impossible to conduct a complete search.

The issue of validity is illustrated by Duggan, Morris, and Adams (1997) who evaluated the accuracy and completeness of online search strategies. First, they hand searched the *Journal of Intellectual Disability Research* from 1957 to 1994 and identified 56 RCTs in that journal. None used the word "randomized" in the title, and a mere nine used it in the abstract. Of 37 RCTs published between 1974 and 1994, 3 and 37 were in Psychlit and MEDLINE, respectively, although MEDLINE contained one incorrect abstract. When they evaluated online searches of the journal to identify RCTs, all searches identified only a few of the RCTs, perhaps reflecting problems with poor-quality indexing and keywords. Duggan et al. show that online searches alone may result in incomplete samples of the literature and researchers should supplement them with other search methods, such as hand searchers of references sections and journal content pages.

Meta-analysis

One characteristic EBP methodology is meta-analysis, a family of statistical procedures that calculate numerical measures of ESs and combine data from multiple studies. Meta-analyses use these data to estimate the average ES for relevant questions, such as the average ES for a particular clinical problem and treatment, or more focused questions, such as the average ES for specific treatments for specific problems. As a field develops, important questions may change from "Does any treatment work for this problem?" to "Does this specific treatment work for this problem?" to "Does this specific treatment work for this problem in this specific population?" to "What is the relative effectiveness of one treatment over another?" to "How does this new treatment compare to existing, standard treatment treatments?" Which question is relevant depends on the extent of the literature in a particular field. For example, within the field of treatment of depression, there are over 200 RCTs permitting answers of some focused specific questions (Cuijpers et al., 2012). For borderline personality disorder, there are few RCTs that have evaluated only two treatments (Sneed, Ferteck, Kanellopoulos, & Culag-Reinlieb, 2012) permitting answers to only general questions as to treatment effectiveness and the relative effectiveness of only two psychosocial treatments. Finally, for somatization disorder, a recent review identified no adequate RCTs or small N experiments; thus, there was no experimental evidence available to guide practice (Allen & Woolfolk, 2012).

Meta-analysis methods have been developed for both RCTs and small N experiments. There are a wide range of ES measures. For RCTs, the most commonly used measure is Cohen's d, which expresses the differences between the means of experimental and control groups as a z-score, usually using the standard deviations of the pretreatment scores in both groups. In meta-analyses of small N experiments, the most commonly used metric is the proportion of nonoverlapping data points between treatment and baseline, although many other ES measures exist for small N experiments.

Meta-analysis was originally applied to experimental psychology in the late 1950s (Glass, 2000). In response to critiques of the effectiveness of psychotherapy (Eysenck, 1957) and the limitations of unsystematic narrative review, meta-analysis was rapidly adopted as a tool to evaluate psychotherapy outcome research (Smith & Glass, 1977). Meta-analysis is now widely in many fields. Many professional bodies and government agencies now use systematic reviews and meta-analysis to ensure that clients have access to the most effective and efficient therapies and are protected from harmful treatments. Consequently, they have appointed expert panels and even funded government agencies, such as NICE in the United Kingdom, to use EBP methods to direct professional practice and government funding. Such initiatives produce the lists of therapies that are deemed to meet criteria for EBP such as those from NICE, Cochrane reviews, and the APAs and pronouncements from professional bodies, as to therapies that are evaluated and shown to be effective, ineffective, or harmful and unevaluated therapies. Such pronouncements often grade therapies in terms of the strength of the evidence to support conclusions.

The results of meta-analyses, especially those from government and professional bodies, are often translated into practice guidelines. These guidelines indicate which treatments should be preferred and which should be avoided and in which order practitioners should implement treatments. Often, practice guidelines, sometimes referred to as stepped-care approaches, begin by recommending simple, cheap, preventative effective treatments, if they are available. Next, they may move onto more expensive but more effective treatments, perhaps delivered in groups by non-clinical staff or nonspecialist therapists. The last stage of guidelines may be specialist therapies that are costly, delivered by highly trained individual therapists for relatively treatment-resistant problems. Sometimes, practice guidelines may include relatively expensive treatments that have limited effectiveness because other better alternatives have already been attempted (see NICE, 2012, for examples of practice guidelines for adults with ASD based on systematic reviews and meta-analyses).

Quality of evidence

A most vexing question is that of quality of evidence. If the study quality is low that may reduce our confidence that change occurred and/or that the treatment caused the change and thus mean that we cannot conclude that treatment is an EBP. EBP criteria give preeminence to experiments because they enhance the probability that observed changes were due to treatment and not to other factors such as to the effects of the treatment and not to chance, passage of time, the possibility that assessment alone resulted in change, or inadvertent confounding of different types of clients with treatment conditions (Campbell, 1969; Kazdin, 2010). Nonexperimental studies, such as narrative case studies, AB single case reports, pre–post group designs, and group designs without randomization, are usually seen as poor-quality studies. A series of nonexperiments—no matter how many or diffi-cult it may be to conduct experiments—can never exclude factors other than treatment as explanations of change.

Quality of randomized controlled trials

For many, RCTs are the "gold standard" of evidence, but not all RCTs are well designed, and we cannot always be confident in the conclusion that the treatment caused the change in some important outcome. The list of requirements for a well-designed RCT is long, making it expensive and effortful to conduct a well-conducted RCT; perhaps no study can meet all requirements.

CONSORT standards   One of the most recent sets of codified standards is the 2012 CONSORT standards (Moher, Schulz, Altman, & the CONSORT Group, 2010). One of the important aims of CONSORT standards is transparency. The authors should report all relevant information including a flow diagram for all participants who entered the RCT including the numbers (a) assessed for eligibility, (b) excluded from treatment with reasons for exclusion, (c) randomized to each intervention, (d) who did not receive the assigned intervention and the reasons, (e) lost to follow-up and the reasons the number of participants who discontinued intervention and the reasons, and (f) included and excluded in analysis and the reasons. When an RCT reports all these numbers, it is to evaluate the quality of the RCT and judge the effects of recruitment and inclusion on external validity, the effects of attrition, and statistical analyses on internal validity.

The 2010 CONSORT standards generated 25 standards for reporting an RCT and set of standards for the abstract of an RCT. Moher et al. (2010) also justified and illustrated each standard. For example, there are four standards (numbers 8a, 8b, 9, and 10) related to randomization. Standard 8b described that the report should describe the type of randomization and details of any restriction used during randomization so that it is unclear if the authors truly randomized participants. For example, if an author states that they randomized participants to two groups, it is unclear how they did that; however, if they state that they block randomized consecutive groups of three participants using a constrained randomization sequence generated by Stat 9.0 (StataCorp, College Station, TX), then it is clear what they did and the threats to internal validity are lessened. The reader is referred to Moher et al. for a complete listing of CONSORT standards.

Grading of recommendations assessment, development, and evaluation Guyatt et al. (2010) aim to provide "a highly structured, transparent, and informative system for rating quality of evidence" (p. 996). GRADE rates the quality of evidence of studies that are included in a meta-analysis by rating the quality of the RCT, consistency of findings across RCTs, if the available evidence is directly related to the question at hand, the degree of precision that the data allow, and any publication bias. An important consideration in GRADE is rating of the significance of the dependent variable, since some dependent variables, such as mortality, are more important than other outcome variables, such as flatulence. The degree of precision refers to the magnitude of treatment effect and the sample sizes. Thus, if treatment effects are very large in several RCTs with large samples, we can be confident that the treatment is robustly effective, and if the dependent variable is important, then we can attach greater social significance to the findings.

Researchers rarely considered the social significance of the dependent variable in meta-analyses in developmental disabilities, but this may be very important. For example, in considering the effectiveness of interventions for anger and aggression, we might place different degrees of significance to different outcomes, such as acquisition of adaptive skill, aggression, injuries to others, and quality of life. An example of the application of GRADE to treatment and developmental disabilities is NICE's (2012) guidelines for the treatment of adults with autism.

Quality of small N experiments
As with RCTs, small N experiments vary widely in their quality and their ability to let us confidently conclude that the treatment caused the change in some socially important behavior. Horner et al. (2005) defined the quality of small N experiments as follows: "Single-subject research documents a practice as evidence-based when (a) the practice is operationally defined; (b) the context in which the practice is to be used is defined; (c) the practice is implemented with fidelity; (d) results from single-subject research document the practice to be functionally related to change in dependent measures; and (e) the experimental effects are replicated across a sufficient number of studies, researchers and participants to allow confidence in the findings." They then went on to define each of these five criteria in further detail.

The National Center on Autism's *National Standards Project* on EBP and autism also developed a quality checklist, the *Scientific Merit Rating Scale* (SMRS), for the quality of small N experiments. The SMRS has five domains: "(a) research design,

(b) measurement of the dependent variable, (c) measurement of the independent variable or procedural integrity, (d) participant ascertainment, and (e) generalization" (p. 16). The SMRS generates a 6-point rating from 0 to 5 of study quality with operational definitions of each level of evidence for each of the five domains listed earlier. Consider a study with an SMRS rating of 3. In terms of research design, such a study would have at least two comparisons of control and treatment conditions, at least 3 data points per condition, and at least two participants, and some data loss would be possible. In terms of measurement of the dependent variable, there might be no calibration data to ascertain the absolute accuracy of the data, interobserver agreement (IOA) might be better than 80% or a kappa greater than .4, IOA might be collected for at least 20% of the data, and data might only be collected in the treatment condition. With respect to measurement of the independent variable, treatment accuracy might be at least 80%, implementation data might be taken in 20% of parts of sessions, and no treatment fidelity IOA might be reported. In terms of participant ascertainment, diagnoses might be confirmed by an independent professional, or the study might use blind evaluation using at least one psychometric instrument, or an independent qualified diagnostician might use DSM criteria. Finally, treatment generalization might either use objective data with some maintenance or collect generalization data across at least some settings, stimuli, or persons. The National Standards Project (National Autism Center, 2009) developed a coding manual to assist in the coding of the quality of the studies, and they trained reviewers to a criterion of at least 80% IOA. After initial training on one small *N* article, they also collected IOA on coding on one article by each reviewer and coding IOA remained above 80%. The National Autism Center (2009) developed a *strength of evidence* classification system which judged the strength of evidence across available studies with four level of strength of evidence including a final category to distinguish ineffective from harmful treatments (see Table 1.3).

Strategies for handling study quality

Studies that may enter into systematic reviews and meta-analyses vary in their quality. To address this, systematic reviews and meta-analyses have commonly used two strategies for handling study quality. The first is to apply relatively stringent inclusion criteria during the literature search phase. For example, a systematic review of group designs might only include RCTs and exclude pre–post designs. Similarly, a systematic review of small *N* experiments might exclude AB designs since they are not experiments or require a certain number of baseline and intervention data points. Although it is possible to set the bar higher—for example, by insisting that only papers with treatment integrity or follow-up data are included— few systematic reviews and meta-analyses have done so, probably because in many cases there would be little literature left to review.

The second strategy is to include studies of varying quality and report ESs broken down by study quality. For example, a meta-analysis might report ES for experiments and nonexperiments or for "low"- and "high"-quality studies as measured on a quality checklist. If both low- and high-quality studies agree on the ES, one may be

Table 1.3 A Summary of the Four Levels of Evidence from the National Standards Project

Level of evidence	Definition
Established	1. Two group designs or four small *N* experiments with at least 12 participants with no conflicting results or at least three group experiments or six small *N* experiments with a minimum of 18 participants with no more than one study reporting conflicting results 2. Had SMRS scores of 3 or greater 3. Reported beneficial treatment effects for specific targets 4. These results may be supplemented by other lower-quality studies
Emerging	1. One group design or two small *N* experiments with a minimum of six participants with no conflicting results 2. SMRS scores of 2 3. Beneficial treatment effects on one dependent variable for a specific target 4. These studies may be supplemented by those with higher or lower SMRS scores
Unestablished	1. May or may not be based on research 2. Had beneficial effects reported on very poorly controlled studies with SMRS scores of 0 or 1 3. Have claims based on testimonials, opinions, or speculation 4. Were ineffective, unknown, or adverse treatment effects based on poorly controlled studies
Ineffective/harmful	1. Had two group designs or four small *N* experiments with at least 12 participants with no conflicting results or at least three group experiments or six small *N* experiments with a minimum of 18 participants with no more than one study reporting conflicting results 2. SMRS scores of at least 3 3. No beneficial treatment effects for one dependent measure for a specific target behavior or had adverse treatment effect reports on dependent variable

Adapted from National Autism Center. (2009). *National standards project*. Randolph, MA: Author.

more confident on the magnitude of the ES than otherwise; however, if low-quality studies produce larger ESs than poor-quality studies, one might be more conservative and only use the estimates of ES from good-quality studies.

Some systematic reviews and meta-analyses use the scores on quality checklists to split studies into "high"- and "low"-quality studies. This may not be a good idea, as some checklists give an equal or greater number of points to how an abstract is written as to whether or not the RCT randomized adequately. The former is nice, but does not threaten the ability to conclude if the treatment caused the change, but the latter is an essential feature of an RCT that is probably fatal to the ability to answer this question. Some systematic reviews and meta-analyses have addressed this problem by defining "high"-quality studies as those that have all of several features (e.g., reporting ES separately for small N experiments with reliability, experimental control, treatment integrity, generalization, and social validity data).

Small N experiments: in or out?

There is a considerable disagreement over the relative status of RCTs and small N experiments. In fact, many authors refer to RCTs as the "gold standard" of evidence. This is unsurprising as the conventions of group designs are the foundation of evaluation of drugs and, by extension, other medical procedures. Psychology's adoption of the group design, hypothesis testing, and statistical testing as the foundation of knowledge in experimental psychology places high value on RCTs. The convention in hypothetico-deductive psychological science is that hypotheses flow from extant theories, which are tested in experiments and theories are confirmed or modified, dependent upon the results of experiments (Chiesa, 1994). Indeed, some have referred to RCT position in behavioral science as hegemonistic (Keenan & Dillenberger, 2011).

Some authors and organizations such as the NICE and Cochrane reviews explicitly exclude small N experiments from consideration. Thus, several reviews of EBP and developmental disabilities have concluded that early intensive behavioral intervention is not an EBP (e.g., Maginnis, 2008). Others downgrade evidence from small N experiments by describing them incorrectly as "case studies" or "prescientific studies." Others have suggested that the external validity from small N experiments is problematic due to the small number of participants, which is true unless researchers conduct direct and systematic replications, which has in fact occurred in many areas.

Others have criticized RCTs and defended small N experiments equally vociferously. Chiesa (1994) has pointed out the basic flaws in the logic of RCTs in which experimenters conduct a group design to infer causality between the independent and dependent variables and make this inference based on statistically significant changes in group mean scores. Inspection of individual scores, however, may reveal that only some—perhaps only a few—participants did indeed change; many may remain unchanged; some may get worse and some get worse because of the treatment. Given that many participants do not change and some changed for the worse, it is illogical to conclude that the treatment caused the improvement, since for some portion of the participants, the improvement did not occur.

Most experimental psychologists and those involved in psychological therapy outcome research ignore these conceptual objections, but there are also procedural problems. Namely, part of the rationale for RCTs is that the experimenter defines a population, the experiment is conducted on a random sample from that population, and the results from that sample are then generalized to the population. Of course, almost all experiments do not define the population and for that and for other practical reasons cannot randomly sample from the undefined population. Thus, even if we ignore Chiesa's logical objections to RCTs, we cannot ignore the impracticality of conducting RCTs in the manner in which they are supposed to be conducted and the limits to generalization from RCTs which are not based on random samples.

Another important question for EBP is to predict the best treatment for specific individuals (Chiesa, 1994; Keenan & Dillenberger, 2011). This indeed is the question that clients and therapists ask: They do not ask if the average person will benefit from this treatment. They ask if *this specific person here and now* will benefit from this treatment for this problem. Since the mean score of the treatment group in an RCT predicts individual response to treatment so poorly, RCTs offer limited guidance on treatment selection for individual clients.

Other issues

Grouping treatments

When conducting systematic reviews and meta-analyses, how should the authors label treatments? Is it a video modeling and behavioral antecedent procedure or a social learning intervention?

One approach to grouping therapies is to do so empirically. Smith and Glass (1977) used multidimensional scaling to group therapies into four "superclasses": behavioral, psychoanalytic, Gestalt–Rogerian, and rational emotional therapy/transactional analysis. To date, there are no such examples related to developmental disabilities, but such data might be interesting. Such "superclasses" of therapies are crude and omit distinctions that are very important to some researchers and practitioners. For example, some might make a very clear distinction between behavior analysis, behavior modification, PBS, and cognitive behavioral therapy (CBT); others might readily lump them together. Reporting agreement of coding of papers into therapy types addresses only the reliability but not the validity of coding.

One good example of this is the status of client self-talk. Suppose client learns to say "Stop! Walk away and relax" (loud or privately) when someone irritates them and, once they have done so and they do indeed relax, say to themselves "That was good. I am relaxed now. That was the adult thing to do." What kind of therapy is this? It is tempting to call it cognitive therapy since it involved verbal self-instruction and self-praise. Behavior analysis, however, also contains an account of self-control in which a person learns to modify their own behavior by emitting one behavior, the controlling response, to influence the future probability of another response, the controlled behavior. This behavioral model places emphasis on the variables that influence the emission of the controlled response, such as its establishing operations, discriminative stimuli, and consequences (Skinner, 1953). Cognitive therapists view such procedures as evidence of covert private behavior and changes in alleged cognitive structures, whereas behaviorists see such procedures as examples of self-control (Skiner, 1953; Sturmey, 2006a, 2006b). Thus, both parties might agree if the procedure is effective but would disagree on the status given to the observed behavior, the model of causality for the observed change in behavior, and the type of therapy.

A final aspect of this problem is that when there are combinations of procedures, such as CBT, different authors place different emphasis or infer efficacy for only one component of the package (Ward-Horner & Sturmey, 2012). For example, CBT for depression is an EBP for depression which includes behavioral activation and cognitive restructuring, but behavioral activation alone produces similar ESs to the CBT package (Cuijpers et al., 2012; Sturmey, 2009a), suggesting that behavioral activation alone is the effective component of CBT for depression. Similar concerns have been raised over the debate over the effectiveness of CBT with people with developmental disabilities in areas such as CBT and anger management, where it is unclear what the contribution is from nonbehavioral components (Sturmey, 2006a, 2006b, 2006c; Travis & Sturmey, 2013), although there is not agreement among professionals on this point.

Flatulence or mortality?

If two treatments have the same ES, are they equally valuable? Perhaps not. Treatments that have a modest reduction in mortality are probably more socially and personally significant than those that reduce flatulence. Thus, a significant but neglected problem is evaluating the social or clinical significance of dependent variable(s).

Meta-analyses emphasize the magnitude of ESs, not the importance of the outcomes. This problem is apparent in the literature on developmental disabilities. For example, Chapter 2 reviews the meta-analyses of skills training interventions, some of which relate broad impact on the rate of development and the possibility of returning children with ASD to typical functioning and not consuming special education, mental health, or residential services. Other meta-analyses relate to more narrow dependent variables, such as learning to shop or use technology. Such outcomes may be personally significant but may often be personally and financially less valuable than interventions that have broad impact on development and which may lead to removal of diagnoses such as autism. This problem is also evident in Chapter 12 of this volume on offenders, which only found data from experiments on short-term immediate behavioral outcomes, but no did not find data from experiments on reoffending, although such data are available from nonexperiments. Thus, the evaluation of individual systematic reviews and meta-analyses requires consideration of the value of the dependent variables used in the experiments that go into the meta-analyses.

Application and dissemination

Recall that the aim of EBP is for practitioners to apply the best treatment to actual clients effectively to achieve socially significant outcomes for each client. This can be done at the level of individual cases or entire services. There are few examples of the former with individuals with developmental disabilities, although Schlosser and Raghavendra (2004) illustrated how to formulate a clinical question for an individual case and use systematic reviews and meta-analyses to answer the questions about treatment options (see Chapter 2). Additionally, Straus et al. (2011) developed a useful manual for the application of evidence-based approaches to medical problems, which can be used successfully to identify effective EBPs to use with individuals with ID or autism.

There are several examples of disseminating EBPs. Perhaps the best known is Britain's Improving Access to Psychological Therapies Project to disseminate EBPs for anxiety and depression in the British National Health Services. Following NICE systematic reviews and meta-analyses that identified CBT as an EBP for depression and anxiety, NICE developed treatment guidelines, and an economic analysis indicated the possibility that CBT would result in significant cost savings (Layard, Clark, Knapp, & Mayraz, 2006). Thus, NICE identified a common, treatment-responsive problem which could be treated effectively with manualized treatment by many commonly available and trainable therapists that would result in large-scale personal benefits and economic benefits for society. Subsequent demonstration projects showed that large-scale implementation is possible (Clark, 2011) but required considerable effort to train and maintain therapist consistency in implementing CBT and systematic monitoring of client outcomes. Foa, Gillihan, and Bryant (2013) describe multiple projects to disseminate prolonged exposure therapy for PTSD in multiple locations across the world and the adaptations they made to numerous local contexts.

Perhaps the closest to such large-scale dissemination in developmental disabilities is Willner et al.'s (2013) recent evaluation of cognitive behavioral anger management. The trial was a multisite trial which involved multiple local therapists and 179 individuals with ID and anger management problems randomly assigned to CBT or treatment as usual. Based primarily on staff ratings, the treatment group had less anger-related problems and more use of coping skills following treatment. Interestingly, this trial did measure treatment integrity and individual attendance at therapy, both of which were highly variable and sometimes low. It indicates that it is possible to implement CBT for individuals with ID using local care staff and a treatment manual over multiple sites but also suggests that such an approach needs to be improved with greater attention to therapist training, treatment integrity, client attendance, and perhaps other interventions for nonresponders.

Evidence-Based Practice and Developmental Disabilities

EBP has until recently been relatively neglected. This has led some to opine that there is no evidence but only compassion available to guide practice (King, 2005). Others have suggested that there is insufficient evidence to guide treatment of mental health problems in adults with disabilities (Hastings, Hatton, Lindsay, & Taylor, 2013) or that there is insufficient evidence to prefer one therapy over another (Emerson, 2006)—the so-called Dodo Bird hypothesis. These claims contrast with numerous systematic reviews and meta-analyses (see Chapters 2 and 3) identifying

EBPs and some economic analyses demonstrating the economic benefits of some interventions with people with ID/autism (see Chapter 4).

Why is there controversy? First, many common practices have little or no support, including sensory integration therapy, TEACCH, social stories, psychotherapy, and counseling. Practitioners and advocates for these treatments and people who genuinely believe that such treatments are effective are naturally put on the defensive by claims of lack of evidence. Second, there is a disagreement over the status of RCTs and small N experiments. As this book demonstrates, the majority of evidence comes from small N experiments. Sometimes, small N experiments are described incorrectly as "prescientific" or "case studies." Sometimes, they are criticized because of the small number of participants and hence the apparent lack of generality, but such criticism fails to take note of the role of direct and systematic replication in making generalization (Sidman, 1960). Sometimes, they are criticized because of the small number of studies that report generalization and maintenance data. While it is true that only about a third of small N experiments do so, almost no group designs evaluating the nonbehavioral treatments report any data on generalization, treatment integrity, or social validity. So, for those who do not accept small N experiments as experiments, there is indeed not much evidence left when they are eliminated from consideration. Fourth, almost all evidence comes from studies of children and adolescents with some but much less evidence to guide practice. Thus, some who work with adults may dismiss the evidence from children and adolescents as being irrelevant. Fifth, different professionals and researchers define the same problem in different way (Sturmey, 2009b). Why did this client throw the chair across the room? A behaviorist would say she emitted aggressive operant behavior that in the past had been reinforced by removal of irritating people. A cognitive behavioral therapist might say she has inappropriate beliefs and her labeling of the situation as threatening caused her to throw the chair. An SIT therapist might say she was hypersensitive to noise, and a psychiatrist might say she has an underlying depression. Hence, each ideological camp may dismiss evidence from each other's perspective, because it does not address the "real" problem: The cognitive therapist can dismiss the evidence for behavioral treatment because it treats aggression, not anger; the psychiatrist can dismiss it because it does not treat the real problem of depression; etc. Finally, professional training in ID is often of poor quality. It barely prepares or fails to pre-pare new professionals on how to treat people with disabilities effectively and is often ambiguous about the status of EBP. Hence, new professionals are left at sea as how to acquire critical skills. In the process, many fail to learn important skills or learn ineffective or harmful ones.

A Challenge Revisited

At the beginning of this chapter, we considered an example of challenges to practitioners and services. The example of food refusal could have gone differently for the individual concerned. The educators could have been trained effectively in special education to use EBPs before becoming special education teachers. Given that food refusal is a relatively rare problem, it may be unlikely that they would have been skilled in that specific problem. If they were well trained in EBP, however, they could have applied functional assessment to the problem and derived an effective treatment from first principles. Alternatively, they could have recognized early on that they did not have expertise in this problem and could have sought effective consultation and training. Perhaps their school could have given them better support and supervision to promote effective professional skills to ensure they focused on child outcomes and being open to using outside consultants effectively, rather than defending ineffective and somewhat harmful treatment. Such an approach would have achieved child outcomes early and avoided harm to the child, answering the ethical imperative for EBP, and precious resources would not have been invested in ineffective treatment, answering the economic imperative for EBP.

References

Allen, L. A., & Woolfolk, R. L. (2012). Somatoform and factitious disorders. In P. Sturmey & M. Hersen (Eds.), *Handbook of evidence-based practice in clinical psychology: Vol. 2. Adults* (pp. 365–394). Hoboken, NJ: Wiley.

American Psychological Association. (2010). *Ethical principles of psychologists and code of conduct*. Washington, DC: Author.

APA Presidential Task Force on Evidence-Based Practice. (2006). Evidence-based practice in psychology. *The American Psychologist, 61*, 271–285.

Applied Behavior Analysis International. (2010). *Statement on restraint and seclusion, 2010*. Retrieved August 16, 2013, from http://www.abainternational.org/abai/policies-and-positions/restraint-and-seclusion,-2010.aspx (accessed on October 11, 2013).

Bettelheim, B. (1967). *The empty fortress: Infantile autism and the birth of the self*. New York: The Free Press.

Bishop-Fitzpatrick, L., Minshew, N. J., & Eack, S. M. (2013). A systematic review of psychosocial interventions for adults with autism spectrum disorders. *Journal of Autism and Developmental Disabilities, 43*, 687–694.

Buysse, V., & Wesley, P. W. (2006). *Evidence-based practice in the early childhood field*. Washington, DC: Zero to Three.

Campbell, D. T. (1969). Reforms as experiments. *American Psychologist, 24*, 409–429.

Chambless, D. L., & Hollon, S. D. (1998). Defining empirically supported therapies. *Journal of Consulting and Clinical Psychology, 66*, 7–18.

Cheng, M. (2012). *French autistic kids mostly get psychotherapy*. Retrieved August 12, 2013, from http://usatoday30.usatoday.com/news/health/story/2012-05-18/France-autism-psychotherapy/55056318/1 (accessed on October 11, 2013).

Chiesa, M. (1994). *Radical behaviorism: The philosophy and the science*. Boston: Authors Cooperative.

Chowdhury, M., & Benson, B. A. (2010). Use of differential reinforcement to reduce behavior problems in adults with intellectual disabilities: A methodological review. *Research in Developmental Disabilities, 32*, 383–394.

Clark, D. M. (2011). Implementing NICE guidelines for the psychological treatment of depression and anxiety disorders: The IAPT experience. *International Review of Psychiatry, 23,* 318–327.

Cuijpers, P., Van Straten, A., Driessen, E., Van Oppen, P., Bockting, C., & Anderson, G. (2012). Depression and dysthymic disorders. In P. Sturmey & M. Hersen (Eds.), *Handbook of evidence-based practice in clinical psychology: Vol. 2. Adults* (pp. 243–284). Hoboken, NJ: Wiley.

Duggan, L. M., Morris, M., & Adams, C. M. (1997). Prevalence study of the randomized controlled trials in the *Journal of Intellectual Disability Research*: 1957–1994. *Journal of Intellectual Disability Research, 41,* 232–237.

Dunst, C. J., Trivette, C. M., & Cutspec, P. A. (2002). *Toward an operational definition of evidence-based practices.* Ashville, NC: Winterberry Press.

Emerson, E. (2006). The need for credible evidence: Comments on 'On some recent claims for the efficacy of cognitive therapy for people with Intellectual Disabilities'. *Journal of Applied Research in Intellectual Disabilities, 19,* 121–123.

Eysenck, H. J. (1957). The effects of psychotherapy: An evaluation. *Journal of Consulting Psychology, 16,* 319–324.

Foa, E. B., Gillihan, S. J., & Bryant, R. A. (2013). Challenges and successes in dissemination of evidence-based treatments for posttraumatic stress: Lessons learned from prolonged exposure therapy. *Psychological Science in the Public Interest, 14,* 65–111.

Glass, G. V. (2000). *Meta-analysis at 25.* Retrieved August 19, 2013, from http://www.gvglass.info/papers/meta25.html (accessed on October 11, 2013).

Guyatt, G. H., Oxman, A. D., Vist, G. E., Kunz, R., Falck-Ytter, Y., Alonso-Coello, P., et al. (2010). GRADE: An emerging consensus on rating quality of evidence and strength of recommendations. *British Medical Journal, 336,* 924–926.

Hagopian, L. P., Rooker, G. W., & Rolider, N. U. (2011). Identifying empirically supported treatments for pica in individuals with intellectual disabilities. *Research in Developmental Disabilities, 32,* 2114–2120.

Hamelin, J., & Sturmey, P. (2013). Psychological treatment: What does the evidence tell us? To appear. In E. Tsakanikos & J. McCarthy (Eds.), *Handbook of psychopathology in intellectual disabilities.* New York: Springer.

Hastings, R. P., Hatton, C., Lindsay, W. R., & Taylor, J. L. (2013). Psychological therapies for adults with intellectual disabilities: Future directions for research and practice. In J. L. Taylor, W. R. Lindsay, R. P. Hastings, & C. Hatton (Eds.), *Psychological therapies for adults with intellectual disabilities* (pp. 266–276). Chichester, UK: Wiley.

Horner, R. H., Carr, E. G., Halle, J., McGee, G., Odom S., & Wolery, M. (2005). The use of single-subject research to identify evidence-based practice in special education. *Exceptional Children, 71,* 165–179.

Institute of Medicine. (2001). *Crossing the quality chasm: A new health system for the 21st century.* Washington, DC: National Academy Press.

Kazdin, A. E. (2010). *Single-case research designs: Methods for clinical and applied settings* (2nd ed.). New York: Oxford University Press.

Keenan, M., & Dillenberger, K. (2011). When all you have is a hammer…: RCTs and hegemony in science. *Research on Autism Spectrum Disorders, 5,* 1–13.

King, R. (2005) Proceeding with compassion while awaiting the evidence. Psychotherapy and individuals with mental retardation. *Mental Retardation, 43,* 448–450.

Knapp, M., & McDaid, D. (2012). Economics of evidence-based practice and mental health. In P. Sturmey & M. Hersen (Eds.), *Handbook of evidence-based practice in clinical psychology: Vol. 1. Children and adolescents* (pp. 71–94). Hoboken, NJ: Wiley.

Layard, R., Clark, D., Knapp, M., & Mayraz, G. (2006). Cost-benefit analysis of psychological therapy. *National Institute Economic Review, 202,* 90–98.

Lilienfield, S. O. (2007). Psychological treatments that cause harm. *Perspectives on Psychological Science, 2,* 53–70.

Maginnis, K. (2008). *Independent review of autism services.* Retrieved August 19, 2013, from http://www.dhsspsni.gov.uk/independent_review_of_autism_services_final_report.pdf (accessed on October 11, 2013).

McAdam, D., Breidbord, J., Dahl, A., & Williams, D. E. (2012). Pica. In M. Hersen & P. Sturmey (Eds.), *Handbook of evidence-based practice in clinical psychology: Vol. 1. Children and adolescents (pp. 323–338).* New York: Wiley.

McAdam, D. B., Sherman, J. A., Sheldon, J. B., & Napolitano, D. A. (2004). Behavioral interventions to reduce the pica of persons with developmental disabilities. *Behavior Modification, 28,* 45–72.

Moher, D., Schulz, K. F., Altman, D. G., & the CONSORT Group. (2010). CONSORT 2010. Statement: Updated guidelines for reporting parallel group randomised trials. *BMC Medicine, 8,* 18.

National Autism Center. (2009). *National standards project.* Randolph, MA: Author.

National Institute for Clinical Excellence. (2012). *Autism. The NICE guideline on recognition, referral diagnosis and management of adults on the autism spectrum.* Leicester, UK: The British Psychological Society and The Royal College of Psychiatrists.

Palmen, A., Didden, R., & Lang, R. (2010). A systematic review of behavioral intervention research on adaptive skill building in high-functioning young adults with autism spectrum disorder. *Research in Autism Spectrum Disorders, 6,* 602–617.

Paul, G. L. (1967). Strategy of outcome research in psychotherapy. *Journal of Consulting Psychology, 31,* 109–118.

Rusch, A. J., & Frances, A. (Eds.). (2000). Expert consensus guidelines for treatment of psychiatric and behavioral problems in mental retardation. *American Journal on Mental Retardation, 105,* 159–228.

Sackett, D. L., Richardson, S. W., Rosenberg, W. R., & Haynes, R. B. (1997). Evidence-based medicine; how to practice and teach EBM. London: Churchill- Livingstone.

Schlosser, R. W., & Raghavendra, P. (2004). Evidence based practice in augmentative and alternative communication. *Augmentative and Alternative Communication, 20,* 1–21.

Schlosser, R. W., Wendt, O., & Sigafoos, J. (2007). Not all systematic reviews are created equal: Considerations for appraisal. *Evidence-Based Communication Assessment and Intervention, 1,* 138–150.

Schofield, H. (2012). France's autism treatment 'shame'. Retrieved August 12, 2013, from http://www.bbc.co.uk/news/magazine-17583123 (accessed on October 11, 2013).

Schreck, K. A., & Millar, V. A. (2010). How to behave ethically in a world of fads. *Behavioral; Interventions, 25,* 307–324.

Scotti, J. R., Evans, I. M., Meyer, L. H., & Walker, P. (1991). A meta-analysis of intervention research with problem behavior: Treatment validity and standards of practice. *American Journal on Mental Retardation, 96,* 233–256.

Sidman, M. (1960). *Tactics of scientific research: Evaluating experimental data in psychology.* New York: Basic Books.

Skinner, B. F. (1953). *Science and human behavior*. New York: Pearson.

Smith, M. L., & Glass, G. V. (1977). Meta-analysis of psychotherapy outcome studies. *American Psychologist, 32,* 372–360.

Sneed, J. R., Ferteck, E. A., Kanellopoulos, D., & Culag-Reinlieb, M. E. (2012). Borderline personality disorder. In P. Sturmey & M. Hersen (Eds.), *Handbook of evidence-based practice in clinical psychology: Vol. 2. Adults* (pp. 507–530). Hoboken, NJ: Wiley.

Straus, S., Glasziou, P., Richardson, W. S., & Haynes, R. B. (2011). *Evidence-based medicine. How to practice it* (4th ed.). London: Churchill Livingston.

Sturmey, P. (2006a). Against psychotherapy with people who have mental retardation: In response to the responses. *Mental Retardation, 44,* 71–74.

Sturmey, P. (2006b). On some recent claims for the efficacy of cognitive therapy for people with intellectual disabilities. *Journal of Applied Research in Intellectual Disabilities, 19,* 109–118.

Sturmey, P. (2006c). In response to Lindsay and Emerson. *Journal of Applied Research in Intellectual Disabilities, 19,* 125–129.

Sturmey, P. (2009a). Behavioral activation is an evidence-based treatment of depression. *Behavior Modification, 33,* 818–829.

Sturmey, P. (2009b). *Varieties of case formulation*. Chichester, UK: Wiley.

Travis, R., & Sturmey, P. (2013). Using behavioural skills training to treat aggression in adults with mild intellectual disability in a forensic setting. *Journal of Applied Research in Intellectual Disabilities, 26,* 481–488.

Van Houten, R., Axelrod, S., Bailey, J. S., Favell, J. E., Foxx, R. M., Iwata, B. A., et al. (1988). The right to effective behavioral treatment. *Journal of Applied Behavior Analysis, 11,* 111–114.

Ward-Horner, J. C., & Sturmey, P. (2012). Component analysis of behavior skills training in functional analysis. *Behavioral Interventions, 27,* 75–92.

Willner, P., Rose, J., Jahoda, A., Stenfert Kroese, B., Felce, D., Cohen, D., et al. (2013). Group-based cognitive-behavioural anger management for people with mild to moderate intellectual disabilities: Cluster randomized controlled trial. *British Journal of Psychiatry, 203,* 288–296.

2

Adaptive Behavior

Peter Sturmey

Until recently, some authors claimed that there was insufficient evidence for the effectiveness of any psychosocial treatments for people with developmental disabilities, and all practitioners could do was to proceed "with compassion while awaiting the evidence" (King, 2005). For some, King's point is well taken, since there are fewer published randomized controlled trials (RCTs) of psychosocial treatments in developmental disabilities than with other populations that have been published/ conducted. But this argument ignores both those RCTs that do exist and the hundreds of small N experiments that also provide evidence on the effectiveness of psychosocial treatments. But this situation is now changed. There are at over 100 meta-analyses of psychosocial treatments for people with developmental disabilities and a similar number of systematic reviews (see Hamelin & Sturmey, 2013; Maffei-Almodovar & Sturmey, 2013, and Sturmey, 2012 for partial reviews).

This and the subsequent chapters review meta-analyses of treatment effectiveness of psychosocial treatments for children and adults with developmental disabilities, including ID and autism spectrum disorders (ASD). The material reviewed in this chapter on adaptive behavior (AB) and the next chapter on maladaptive behavior excluded individual RCTs and small N experiments, editorials, and other commentaries; meta-analyses of treatment of other disabilities, such as ADHD, traumatic brain injury, learning disabilities; systematic reviews without meta-analyses; conference papers and abstracts; expert panels; government and insurance company technical reports; book chapters; psychopharmacology; dietary and other nutritional and healthcare interventions, including iodine supplementation, secretin, acupuncture, and healthcare checks; reviews of methodology; and reviews

Evidence-Based Practice and Intellectual Disabilities, First Edition.
Edited by Peter Sturmey and Robert Didden.
© 2014 John Wiley & Sons, Ltd. Published 2014 by John Wiley & Sons, Ltd.

of interventions in other populations, unless they reported effect sizes (ESs) separately for people with developmental disabilities. Only articles published up to May 2013 were included. Two meta-analyses of deinstitutionalization were included. The meta-analyses were organized into six broad areas. The current chapter reviewed two kinds of interventions: (a) treatments that aimed to increase AB broadly, including early intervention (EI) for children with ID or at risk for ID and EIBI for children with ASD, and (b) interventions to increase specific AB, such as social skills, communication skills, or specific academic performances, such as reading and math. The next chapter reviews four kinds of intervention: (a) interventions for maladaptive behaviors, broadly defined; (b) interventions for specific maladaptive behavior, such as aggression, SIB, and pica; (c) specific intervention methods, such as noncontingent reinforcement; and (d) interventions for specific populations, such as adults with ASD. Some meta-analyses could have been classified in more than one category. For example, a meta-analysis of social skills training with adolescents with ASD could be classified under specific AB (social skills) or population (autism). This review grouped meta-analyses hierarchically, that is, meta-analyses were placed in the earliest category possible. Thus, the meta-analysis of social skills for adolescents with autism was classified under social skills, not under population (autism).

General Adaptive Behavior

Early intervention

Early intervention (EI) refers to a very wide range of procedures including skills training, teaching interaction, play, language stimulation, and other skills to parents, teaching parents jobs skills, etc. EI may also take place in the home, in centers, or in combinations of settings and may be conducted by family members, staff, or both. EI varies widely in intensity, both in number of hours per week and number of weeks per year and in the theoretical orientation of the program. Finally, EI varies significantly with respect to participants. For example, EI may take place for children who are at risk for disabilities, children with mild disabilities, and children with established disabilities with known causes, such as Down syndrome. The goals of EI may include acceleration of the rate of development, as shown through changes in IQ/developmental quotient or other broad measures of development, and changed in specific developmental domains, such as language or academic performance. The rationales for EI include ameliorating current existing or preventing future disability, giving children a developmental advantage when they go to school, and potential benefits to parents, such as reduction in stress or burden or care. EI also has the potential for large savings through avoidance or deferment of service use and reduction of costs related to avoided greater disability, although such benefits have to be positively demonstrated, rather than assumed (see Chapter 4).

Meta-analyses of group designs

There were three meta-analyses of group designs evaluating EI and four meta-analyses of small N experiments. The first comes from White (1985) who compiled a database of over 2,500 EI documents which include approximately 300 empirical studies of EI for children who were economically disadvantaged and children with established handicaps. Additionally, White, Buch, and Castro (1985) reviewed 52 previous EI reviews to generate hypotheses, conducted computer-based searches, and wrote letters to colleagues to identify potential studies. Studies were coded using a 90-item checklist with at least 85% agreement among coders. When studies reported multiple outcomes in the same domain and/or time period, the authors only calculated an ES for each domain/time period to reduce effects of individual studies reporting multiple outcomes. These authors also reported ESs separately when ESs were calculated directly from individual studies, such as those that directly compared different intensities of interventions. There were 2,266 ESs from 326 studies. Of 1,131 ESs from experiments, 906 were from disadvantaged children, 215 were from children with handicaps, and 85 were from children with medical risks. Studies were published from 1937 to 1984, and 70% were published after 1970. Forty percent of the outcomes were IQ, and 60% of the ESs were measured immediately after intervention. Only 11% of ESs were measured more than 36 months after EI, all for disadvantaged children rather than children with established disabilities.

For disadvantaged children, the immediate benefit of EI was approximately 0.5 standard deviations. This represented an 8-point gain in IQ, a change from 30th to 50th percentile for motor functioning. For reading, this represented a change from the 10th to 22nd percentile or a 10-month gain in reading at the second grade. There was little evidence for the effects of type of program, and the effects rapidly washed out such that there was little evidence of the effects of EI 36 months after EI. For children with established handicaps, there was much less data of which only 16% of studies were of good quality with no studies with more than 12-month follow-up data. The best estimate of the immediate effects of EI is approximately 0.4 from good quality studies (20 ESs, 11 studies) and 0.72 for all studies (179 ESs, 65 studies).

White (1985) also reported small magnitude effects of mediating variables. The first mediating variable was parental involvement. For disadvantaged children, the ESs for parent involvement were 0.52 (683 ESs) and 0.42 (200 ESs) for all studies. ES were 0.40 (171 ESs) and 0.51 (54 ESs) for studies with minor or no parental involvement or major or exclusive parental involvement, respectively. For children with handicaps, the ESs from all studies were 0.72 (137 ESs) and 0.59 (70 ESs). ESs were 0.38 (17 ES) and 0.43 (6 ESs) for studies with minor or no parental involvement or major or exclusive parental involvement, respectively. For within study comparisons of parental involvement, ESs were approximately 0, although one study reported an ES of 0.18. Thus, there was little evidence for any large effect of parent involvement in EI. White noted that most outcomes were IQ, and almost no studies directly measured parental involvement. The second mediating variable was child age at which EI began. There was little evidence that age at which intervention began made any large difference. ESs were very similar at all ages at which intervention began.

Casto and Mastropieri (1986) reported a meta-analysis of 74 EI studies for preschoolers with existing handicaps. They searched four databases and previous reviews and wrote to prominent EI researchers. The studies must have included preschoolers aged 0–5 years and tested any form of EI. The authors used a standard, 98-item coding system for all studies and reported 87% agreement on coding. They also reported checking all ED calculations independently. There were 215 ESs. Most (44%) children had ID or combinations of handicaps (29%). Studies were published from 1937, but most were published after 1970. The most common measure was IQ, as well as measures of language, motor, social–emotional, and self-help skills. The authors reported data separately for all studies and only good quality studies. The ES was the standardized mean difference between the experimental and control groups for experiment and between pre- and postdata for pre–post studies.

The overall ES for the immediate effects of EI was moderately large for all studies (mean $d = 0.68$, 215 ESs) but notably smaller for good quality studies (mean $d = 0.40$, 23 ESs). ESs varied as a function of the dependent variable: The ESs were 0.85, 0.58, 0.67, 0.61, 0.39, and 0.43 for IQ, social, language, motor, academic, and other measures, respectively. The authors reported five other findings. First, ESs were moderately large when parents were both involved a lot (adjusted mean ES = 0.59) and involved little or not at all (adjusted mean ES = 0.72). Second, ES was not a function of age at the start of intervention, failing to support the commonly held belief that starting EI at an early age is better than starting EI at a later age. Third, there was no effect of degree of program structure on ES. Finally, ES was greatest for more intense EI. Thus, adjusted ESs were 0.45, 0.63, and 0.88 for <50, 50–100, and >500 hr of intervention per year, respectively. ESs were 0.59 and 0.71, and unadjusted ESs were 0.80 for <2, 2–10, and >10 hr/week. Finally, ESs declined rapidly at follow-up: ESs for good quality studies were 0.43 (20 ESs) and 0.13 (3 ESs) immediately after EI and at 1–12 months follow-up, and there was a general lack of follow-up data for any kind from almost all studies. Thus, there was little empirical support for even short-term post-EI effects and no evidence for long-term effects of EI.

The third meta-analysis of EI group studies comes from Shonkoff and Hauser-Cram (1987) who used search strategies similar to Casto and Mastropieri (1986). This search identified 31 studies which included children enrolled before the age of 36 months and children whose principal handicap was not their family's economic status and were raised in a family or foster home, but not in an institution. The studies also had to evaluate only one treatment and be of relatively good methodological quality. Thus, they focused on the best quality evidence for children with biological handicaps in EI aged below 3 years. The meta-analysis yielded 91 ESs. Since there was no association between the number of ESs per study and ES magnitude and since there was no difference in ESs between experiments and pre–post studies, their analyses was based on the 91 ESs.

There was a medium ES of EI (mean ES = 0.62, range −0.94 to 2.08). The ES was a function of the dependent variable: The mean ESs were 0.62 (46 ESs), 0.43 (14 ESs), and 1.17 (11 ESs) for IQ/DQ, motor, and language outcomes, respectively. ESs were also a function of the population: The mean ESs were 0.11 (6 ESs), 0.42 (29 ESs), and

0.70 (20 ESs) for ID, developmental delay, and mixed samples, respectively. There was no effect of age of enrollment, except for children with mild impairments who had better outcomes when they were enrolled earlier. More structured programs had larger ESs (ES = 0.92, 29 ESs) than less structured programs (ES = 0.59, 40 ESs). Programs with greater planned parent involvement had larger ESs (ES = 0.70, 74 ESs) than those with limited/no parental involvement (ESs = 0.30, 17 ESs). Finally, programs that targeted parents and infants together had larger ESs (ES = 0.74, 56 ESs) than those that did not (ES = 0.44, 56 ESs). The authors concluded that EI was effective for many children with biological handicaps but noted that the range of outcome measures was limited. They also noted that their results differed from those of Casto and Mastropieri (1986) in that Shonkoff and Hauser-Cram found effects of program structure and parental involvement, whereas Casto and Mastropieri did not. Shonkoff and Hauser-Cram suggested that this might reflect the fact that Casto and Mastropieri's meta-analysis focused on children aged 0–5 years rather than 0–3 years; additionally, it may be possible that the dependent variables used may be more sensitive to change in younger than in older children.

Meta-analyses of small N experiments
There is a series of four related meta-analyses of EI using small N experiments. The first comes from Mastropieri and Scruggs (1985) who conducted a meta-analysis of EI for socially withdrawn children that included a substantial proportion of children with disabilities. They identified a group of 44 small N experiments from a larger pool of EI studies (see preceding text). They then selected studies that described participants as handicapped or socially withdrawn and were aged less than 66 months at the onset of intervention, evaluated specific behavioral procedures, and displayed the data graphically. Eighteen experiments with 19 dependent variables met inclusion criteria. They then coded studies using a standard set of criteria. Coding reliability was 94% among four trained raters. Measures included both percentage of nonoverlapping data (PND) and an *ad hoc* 3-point rating of overall effectiveness. There was an average of three participants per experiment. Thirty-nine percent, 22%, 22%, 11%, and 6% were children with behavior disorders, "mental retardation," who were socially isolated, autistic, and "mild handicaps," respectively. Of 32% of participants with IQ data, the mean IQ was 55 (SD = 15).

Seventy-five percent of 12 "effective" studies and 14% of 7 "partially effective" studies used reinforcement of child behavior. When confederate peer interaction was directly reinforced, the median PND was 100% (range 24–100%, 20 ESs), but when confederate peer interaction was not reinforced, the median PND was only 67% (range 0–94%, 11 ESs). When target children's social initiations or responses were directly reinforced, PNDs were uniformly high (100% [3 ESs] and 96% [2 ESs], respectively). In contrast, the PND was low (36%, 15 ESs) when target participants initiations were not reinforced, but was high when initiations were reinforced (PND = 94%, 19 ESs). The authors also evaluated the effects of prompting and rein- forcement during modeling and found much larger ESs when modeling was combined with prompting and reinforcement (PND = 100%, 5 ESs) than when it was used alone (mean PND = 44%, 10 ESs). The authors concluded that reinforcement of child behavior was highly effective at increasing social behavior in both target and confederate children. ESs for generalization data were small (median PND = 33%, rage 3–70%) but were larger immediately following intervention in the same setting (median PND = 62%, range 50–70%, 5 ESs) than in different settings or after delayed intervals (median PND = 14.5%, range 3–60%, 8 ESs). The experiments were also limited in that only 11 studies reported interobserver agreement.

Scruggs, Mastropieri, and McEwen (1988) conducted the third meta-analysis of small N experiments which focused on interventions for physical, motor, and nutritional functioning related to EI. This meta-analysis identified 14 studies with 21 children with 42 outcomes. Reliability of coding was 97%. It included 9 nonexperiments using AB designs, 10 reversal designs, and 22 multiple baseline designs. Interventions included reinforcement, "tender loving care, modeling, prompting and reinforcement and adaptive equipment." There were six studies on feeding and rumination and five on motor interventions. The median PNDs were 100% (range 66.7–100%), 100% (range 66.7–100%), and 33.3% (range 0–100%) for training, maintenance, and generalization, respectively. ESs were unaffected by gender, setting, and target behavior. Interventions that planned generalization had larger ESs (median PND = 100%) than those that did not (median PND = 33.3%). ESs were also a function of type of intervention ($p < .032$): ESs for no reinforcement were 33.3% (range 0–100%, 15 ESs); for social reinforcement were 80.4% (range 67–94%, 2 ESs); for combined reinforcement and punishment were 90% (range 77–100%, 4 ESs); for tangible, nonedible reinforcement were 100% (range 67–100%, 12 ESs); for edible reinforcement were 100% (range 92–100%, 6 ESs); and for punishment were 100% (range 100–100%, 3 ESs). The authors concluded that (a) treatments were in general successful; (b) the studies were limited due to the use of AB designs in some studies; (c) there was a lack of studies comparing treatments; (d) planned generalization was superior to "train and hope"; and (e) reinforcement was superior to lack of reinforcement.

Finally, Scruggs, Mastropieri, Forness, and Kavale (1988) conducted a meta-analysis of 20 small N published and unpublished experiments and nonexperiments. There were 44 participants evaluating early language intervention which were published between 1968 and 1986. There were 128 ESs (approximately 5.5 per study).

Overall, ESs were relatively large. For example, PNDs were 86% and 93% for children aged under 48 months and over 48 months, respectively. Treatments included reinforcement only, direct instruction (a form of prompting and reinforcement), time delay, mand-model (a program to teach requesting with planned generalization from one-to-one teaching to the natural environment), total communication (combined verbal and sign communication), and other treatments including vestibular stimulation and structured music activities. The meta-analysis did not detect any statistically significant differences in ESs between treatment types. Likewise, ESs were not a function of age, gender, intervener (teacher vs. parent vs. researcher vs. peer), type of dependent variable, and type of reinforcement. ESs, however, were larger in schools (median PND = 94.6%, range 0–100%, 39 studies) than homes (median PND = 83.3, range 0–100%, 23 ESs) and institutions (median PND = 63.2%, range 2–95%, 23 ESs).

ESs were larger for training (median PND = 83%, range 0–100%, 69 ESs) and maintenance (median PND = 1–100%, range 0–100%, 28 ESs) than generalization (median PND = 62%, range 0–100%, 31 ESs). Generalization ESs were large for generalization across settings (median PND = 97%, range 0–100%, 14 ESs) and behavior or person (median PND = 94%, range 0–100%, 6 ESs) and close to 0 for generalization across stimuli (median PND = 17%, range 0–100%, 9 ESs) and stimuli and settings (median PND = 0% range 0–47%, 4 ESs). There was a very large effect of planning generalization (median PND = 97%, range 0–100%, 18 ESs) versus train and hope (median PND = 2%, range 0–89%, 13 ESs). The authors concluded that the evidence supports the effectiveness of behavioral principals in EI language interventions and that study characteristics such as participant, setting, and change agent were relatively unimportant.

Scruggs, Mastropieri, and McEwen (1988) commented on the combined outcome of these four meta-analyses of small *N* experiments. They noted that in EI that (a) behavioral treatments were generally effective; (b) different change agents can be effective in using behavioral interventions; (c) positive reinforcements, especially tangible and to a lesser extent social reinforcers, have been validated; and (d) this literature demonstrated the external validity of a behavioral intervention through replication across different target behaviors and participants. They also noted five unanswered questions: (a) there was little information about target population characteristics, (b) family demographic variables, (c) long-term effects of EI, (d) the extent to which generalization can be facilitated, and (e) specific program features such as optimal age, intensity, curriculum, and the effective components of behavioral packages.

Early intensive for autism spectrum disorders

Table 2.1 summarizes 10 meta-analyses of EIBI and other forms of EI for children with ASD. Levy, Kim, and Olive's (2006) literature synthesis calculated ESs for individual studies, but was excluded as it did not synthesize these data into a meta-analysis. These meta-analyses, published between 1999 and 2012, illustrate the progressive development, refinement, and greater degree of acuity and differentiation of conclusions that have been made over time as more data has accumulated. For example, Smith (1999) only reported changes in IQ scores based on 12 studies of which none were RCTs. Later meta-analyses reported data on up to 18 studies, and the number of participants increased to over 300 in some meta-analyses, thereby allowing greater confidence in any conclusions due to multiple independent replications and more accurate estimation of ESs. Subsequent studies have also reported data on multiple outcomes measures including nonverbal IQ, AB composite, expressive and receptive language (see Table 2.1) as well as school placement, psychopathology, and changes in diagnosis (Reichow & Wolery, 2009). Finally, later studies reported more sophisticated statistical analyses, such as indices of reliable change, number needed to treat (NNT) and data on large samples of individual children (Eldevik et al., 2010), and sequential meta-analyses demonstrating the

Table 2.1 The Characteristics of These Meta-Analyses, Their Findings, and Main Conclusions Related to the Effectiveness of EI

Reference	Study characteristics	Main findings	Conclusions
Smith (1999)	1. Twelve studies (9 ABA, 1 TEACCH, 2 Colorado Health Sciences) 2. 0 RCTs 3. Overall *N* could not be calculated 4. Study quality not measured	1. 7–28 points gain in IQ for ABA 2. 3–9 points gain in IQ for TEACCH and Colorado	"… results have been less favorable than reviewers have claimed … Some studies have yielded highly favorable results … others have produced favorable results on some measures but not all … Four others, including one on behavior analytic treatment … and all three studies on other interventions … Found little change …" (p. 41)
Ospina et al. (2008)	1. Thirteen studies (ABA, developmental, and other approaches) 2. Six RCTs 3. *N* = 112 4. Studies quality measured	1. Lovaas superior to special education for AB (WMD = 11), communication and interaction (WMD = 16), overall language (WMD = 13), daily living skills (WMD = 6), expressive language (WMD = 15), IQ (SMD = 0.95), and socialization (WMD = 9.17) 2. Developmental approaches were effective on stereotyped behavior (WMD = −0.40) and time spent in distal social interaction (WMD = 2.85), but effects were not clinically significant 3. There were no differences between Lovaas and special education, developmental approaches, and computer-assisted instruction and on various outcome measures based on a small number of studies 4. There were no effects of TEACCH versus standard care based on measures of imitation skills and eye–hand integration	"Lovaas treatment was superior to special education … two RCTs favored developmental approaches … but the effect size was not clinically significant … Lovaas may improve some core symptoms of autism. … no definitive behavioral or developmental intervention improves all individuals"

Reichow and Wolery (2009)	1. Thirteen studies 2. Two RCTs. 3. $N = 373$ 4. Studies quality measured	1. The mean ES was 0.69 ($p < .0001$) ("large") 2. ES for IQ ranged from −0.19 to 1.58 and 9 of 14 samples had ES > 0.50 3. Based on 10 samples, ES for AB ranged from −0.25 to 0.186 and 5 of 10 samples of an ES > 0.50 4. ESs for expressive and receptive language ranged from 0.23 to 1.72 and 0.45 to 1.79, respectively, and five of six ESs were > 0.50	"EIBI is an effective treatment, on average, for children with autism" (p. 23)
Spreckley and Boyd (2009)	1. Thirteen studies 2. Six RCTs. Four were included in the meta-analysis, of which two were "quasirandomized" 3. $N = 101$ (experimental and controls) 4. Study quality measured	1. There were no differences between children receiving ABA and control children on measures of IQ, AB, and expressive and receptive language	"A[pplied] B[ehavioral] I[ntervention] did not significantly improve the cognitive outcomes of children … There was no additional benefit over standard care for expressive language … receptive language … or adaptive behavior. Currently, there is inadequate evidence that ABI has better outcomes for children with autism" (p. 338)
Makrygianni and Reed (2010)	1. Fourteen studies 2. Number of RCTs not reported, probably because small 3. Number of participants not reported 4. Study quality measured	1. In pre–post studies, ESs for IQ were large for both high-quality (weighted ESs = 0.950) and low-quality studies (weighted ES = 0.909) and for language (0.990 and 0.8897) and medium to large for AB (0.421 and 0.474) for high- and low-quality studies, respectively 2. For comparisons between experimental and control groups, ESs were medium to high for IQ (0.569 and 0.730), language (0.534 and 0.910), and AB (0.971 and 0.656)	"… behavioral programs are effective in improving several developmental aspects in children, and also relative to eclectic to control programs" (p. 577)

(*Continued*)

Table 2.1 (*Continued*)

Reference	Study characteristics	Main findings	Conclusions
Virues-Ortega (2010)	1. Eighteen studies included in meta-analysis 2. Six were RCTs or used "quasirandomized" designs 3. Three hundred and twenty-three experimental and 170 control participants 4. Study quality measured	1. ESs reported for IQ (18 studies), nonverbal IQ (9 studies), receptive (10 studies), expressive (9 studies), and overall language (5 studies), communication (10 studies), daily living skills (10 studies), motor (3 studies), and AB composite (14 studies) 2. Overall ES = 1.19 ($N = 311$, $p < .001$) and 1.31 ($N = 169$, $p < .0001$) for studies with control groups 3. ESs for specific domains for all studies were as follows: nonverbal IQ (0.65), receptive language (1.48), expressive language (1.47), general language (1.07), and AB composite (1.09) 4. ESs were similar when analyses were restricted to studies with control groups and for specific domains of AB	"long-term, comprehensive ABA interventions leads to (positive) medium to large effects in … intellectual functioning, language development, and adaptive behavior … Language-related outcomes were distinctly superior to nonverbal IQ, social functioning and daily living skills" (p. 397)
Eldevik et al. (2010)	1. Sixteen group designs 2. $N = 309$ treatment, 39 comparison interventions, 105 control groups 3. Applied measures of study quality during selection of studies, but did not subsequently measure study quality of those papers in the meta-analysis	1. Children in EIBI were more likely to have a reliable IQ change (29.8%) than those in comparison (2.6%) and control groups (8.7%), and comparable data for AB were 20.6%, 5.7% and 5.1%, respectively (criteria for reliable change were 27 and 21 points for IQ and AB, respectively) 2. NNTs were five and seven, and absolute risk reductions were 23% and 16% for IQ and AB, respectively	"The present analysis provides evidence that intensive behavioral intervention is an evidence-based intervention for children with autism" (p. 400)

Peters-Scheffer, Didden, Korzilius, and Sturmey (2011)	1. Eleven studies 2. One RCT 3. Three hundred and forty-four children with ASD 4. Study quality measured	1. Mean ESs ranged from 4.95 to 15.21 in favor of EIBI 2. Mean differences for full and nonverbal IQ were 11.98 and 11.09 and for receptive and expressive language were 13.94 and 15.21 points, respectively. 3. For AB composite, communication, daily living, and socialization, the differences were 5.92, 10.44, 5.48, and 4.96, respectively 4. Mean Cohen's *d*'s were 2.00, 0.98, 1.10, 2.91, 0.91, 1.32, 0.68, and 1.49 for full IQ, nonverbal IQ, expressive and receptive language, AB, communication, daily living, and social behavior, respectively	"children with ASD participating in EIBI generally outperformed children receiving other treatments or treatment as usual on both IQ and adaptive measures … average differences may be considered to be clinically significant" (pp. 65–67)
Kuppens and Onghena (2012)	1. Fifteen adequate/high-quality studies 2. ?1 RCT 3. $N = 263$ participants 4. Study quality measured	1. Using sequential meta-analysis of group-comparison studies, they found convincing evidence of at least a medium ES for IQ, language, and AB from group-comparison studies 2. Using data from pre–post studies, there was convincing data of a medium ES for IQ, but not for language and AB, despite high statistical power	" … given the convincing evidence for substantial treatment benefit for each outcomes in terms of the group-comparison effectiveness, additional studies on this topic may not be needed" (p. 174)
Strauss et al. (2013)	1. $N = 21$ studies 2. $N = 2$ RCTs 3. $N = 894$ 4. Coded study features and analyzed outcomes by study features and corrected for bias in ES calculations	1. For IQ, 8/12 studies had $g > 0.5$; for language, 2/7 studies had $g > 0.5$; and for AB, 3/8 studies had $g > 0.5$ 2. Outcome was predicted by treatment intensity and parent training but not program duration	1. Comprehensive EIBI programs lead to a modest to large effects on IQ, language, and AB 2. Size of effect depends on treatment integrity and parent training

Note: Data on other analyses, such as mediator analysis were excluded from this table.

cumulative effects of studies as they are published over time in permitting greater degrees of confidence in conclusions (Kuppens & Onghena, 2012).

Examination of Table 2.1 reveals a number of trends. First, earlier meta-analyses were less clear and consistent in their conclusions concerning the effectiveness of EIBI (Ospina et al., 2008; Smith, 1999), perhaps because of the insufficient quantity of data and high-quality studies available at the time of these meta-analyses. Only Spreckley and Boyd (2009) explicitly concluded that EIBI was ineffective; however, Smith, Eisketh, Sallows, and Graupner (2009) pointed out that their analyses were inappropriate because they coded a treatment group as a control group in Sallows and Graupner (2005), thereby reducing the ES. (Examination of the forest plots in Spreckley and Boyd shows that the meta-analysis is based on only three studies per meta-analysis and clearly shows their analysis of the Sallows and Graupner data as an outlier.) All subsequent meta-analyses in Table 2.1 make clear or even strong conclusions concerning the effectiveness of EIBI based on comparisons of pre–post studies and group studies using both wait list controls, less intense EIBI, and treatment as usual. For example, Kuppens and Onghena's (2012) most meta-analyses contrast sharply from others when they concluded that "...given the convincing evidence for substantial treatment benefit for each outcomes in terms of the group-comparison effectiveness, additional studies on this topic may not be needed" (p. 174). Thus, we can be quite confident that EIBI is an evidence-based practice (EBP).

There is also an emerging consensus between nearly all of these meta-analyses on qualifications to this broad conclusion. These meta-analyses have agreed that there are large individual differences between children in response to treatment with some children responding rapidly and making very large gains and others responding slowly or not at all, at least with respect to global outcomes measures, such as IQ and AB composite. Two meta-analyses did not restrict their search strategies to applied behavior analysis (ABA) interventions (Ospina et al., 2008; Smith, 1999), but neither found evidence that other approaches, such as developmental approaches, TEACCH, or special education, were as effective as or more effective than ABA. Again, this conclusion must be tempered because of the lack of experiments that have directly compared two or more treatments (Reichow & Wolery, 2009). These meta-analyses differed substantially in their selection criteria, choice of ES metric, unit of analysis, handling of poor quality studies, statistical analyses used, statistical errors made, research question asked, etc. (Reichow [2011] provided an analysis of five early meta-analyses that amply made this point.) Yet, despite these differences, a broad consensus that EIBI is an EBP is readily apparent. These meta-analyses lumped together many different forms of EIBI, which differ in their intensity, curriculum, mix and sequencing of intervention methods, etc. There may be important differences between different forms of EIBI that result in different ESs which future research should address. Finally, the broad conclusion that EIBI is an EBP does not preclude the possibility that other forms of EI may also be effective. Future research might show this to be true, but at this time, the data on this point are absent.

Deinstitutionalization

One of the rationales offered for deinstitutionalization was that institutional environments were highly restrictive and offered insufficient opportunities for learning, thereby unnecessarily restricting development. Hence, community placement should accelerate acquisition of AB. Two meta-analyses have evaluated the impact of deinstitutionalization on AB (Hamelin, Frijters, Griffiths, Condillac, & Owen, 2011; Lynch, Kellow, & Wilson, 1997). Here we will only consider the most recent of the two.

Hamelin et al. (2011) searched nine databases and found 351 potential articles. Forty-eight were analyzed in more details and 23 met the inclusion criteria. The articles were published between 1976 and 2006 and included 2,083 participants with an average age of 37.9 years (SD = 9.14). Seventeen included participants with all levels of ID, and six included participants with only severe/profound ID. Thirteen used a matched group design, and 10 used repeated measures. There were 15 different measures of AB and 9 different domains of AB. There was an average of 8.25 ESs per study (range 1–32).

The mean value of Cohen's *d* was 0.40 (SD = 0.36, *N* = 138 ESs), a medium positive effect. Studies that had participants with mixed levels of ID had larger ESs (*d* = 0.44, SD = 0.30, 95 ESs) than those with only participants with severe/profound ID (*d* = 0.30 SD = 0.47, 43 ESs). ESs were a function of domain of AB: They were larger for global self-care, social skills, community living, occupational skills, and cognition than communication and physical development skills. ESs were also larger for participants who moved to group homes than those who moved to cluster centers and other community environments. ESs also increased modestly over time. The authors concluded that deinstitutionalization produced a moderate increase in AB. They also noted that even though Lynch et al. (1997) analyzed a different sample of studies and used a different measure of ES, both meta-analyses concurred that deinstitutionalization produced a moderate increase in AB. Hamelin et al. also pointed out that deinstitutionalization was relatively ineffective at improving communication skills and that outcomes depended upon features of the community programs. Thus, community programs should be designed better to address these deficiencies.

Comment

These three literatures—two related to EI and one to deinstitutionalization—all concur that it is possible to intervene to achieve large improvement in broad AB for at least some individuals with developmental disabilities. All share the common feature of a massive environmental design to remove barriers to learning and foster learning.

Specific Adaptive Behaviors

In addition to meta-analyses of interventions to improve broad AB, there have also been many meta-analyses to evaluate interventions to improve specific domains of AB. These include meta-analyses of social skills; language and communication, including alternative and augmentative communication (AAC); peer tutoring to improve academic performance; interventions for reading skills; psychotherapy-related skills such as problem solving and antivictimization programs; purchasing and applied math skills; the effects of exercise on motor and social skills; social stories to address a wide range of specific AB; placement in special education; and teaching the use of technology at work.

Social skills

There were six meta-analyses of social skills training which focused on somewhat different questions and populations. For example, some meta-analyses focused on disabilities broadly defined (Vaughn et al., 2003) or specifically on autism (Bellini, Peters, Benner, & Hopf, 2007; Reichow & Volkmar, 2009; Schneider, Goldstein, & Parker, 2008; Wang & Spillane, 2009; Wang, Parilla, & Cui, 2013) or on young children (Vaughn et al., 2003) or only on peer-mediated strategies (Schneider et al., 2008). Since the questions asked in these meta-analyses were different, each will be reviewed individually.

Vaughn et al. (2003) conducted a meta-analysis of social skills interventions with children aged 3–5 years with a variety of disabilities which used group designs published between 1975 and 1999. There were 23 studies which included both peer reviewed articles, dissertations, and technical reports. There were 12 multiple-group and 12 single-group designs with 699 children with and 203 children without disabilities participating. Two studies of children with autism had mean d's of 0.66–0.87 ("large"), and four studies of children with developmental delays had d's from 0.13 to 0.63 (no effect to "medium"). The authors did not report any quality measure of the studies. Regarding these studies, the authors concluded that "social interventions have yielded positive results" (p. 13).

Bellini et al. (2007) conducted a meta-analysis of 55 small N experiments of school-based social skills interventions for children with autism published between 1986 and 2005 with a total of 157 participants. (They included three AB nonexperiments.) The mean PND was 70% (range 17–100%, 52 studies, "questionable"). PNDs were 80% (range 17–100%, 25 studies) for maintenance and 53% (range 17–100% "low") for generalization. The mean PND was lower for peer-mediated interventions (62%, 10 studies) than for teaching collateral skills (75%, 7 studies), child specific skills (71%, 15 studies), and comprehensive social skills programs (72%, 20 studies). Although there was no difference between individual and group social skills training (72% vs. 69%, 24 and 28 studies, respectively), ESs were larger for individual than group interventions during maintenance (84% vs. 77%, 12 and 13 studies, respectively) and generalization (63% vs. 43%, 8 and 7 studies, respectively).

ESs were larger for classroom-based than pullout interventions for both intervention (76% vs. 62%, 28 and 21 studies, respectively), maintenance (88% vs. 67%, 16 and 9 studies, respectively), and generalization (67% vs. 29%, 8 and 5 studies, respectively). This meta-analysis did not measure study quality. Thus, in contrast to other meta-analyses reviewed here, the authors concluded that "social skills interventions are minimally effective for children with ASD" (p. 159).

Schneider et al. (2008) conducted a meta-analysis of 19 small N experiments published between 1985 and 2007 on peer-mediated interventions in preschool settings. ESs were almost always large: At least one value of Cohen's d was greater than 1.00 in 16 of 19 studies, and weighted φ was 0.72 (18 studies). Most dependent variables were overall social behavior, although some experiments reported data on initiations, responses, sharing, etc. Disaggregation showed that ESs were larger when intervention targeted both children with autism and peers rather than children with autism alone ($\varphi^2 = 56\%$ vs. 38%, respectively.) The authors concluded that "evidence for the efficacy of peer-mediated interventions seems substantial" (p. 159).

Wang and Spillane (2009) conducted a meta-analysis of social skills training for children with autism that focused on the differential effects of different forms of social skills training. There were 36 small N experiments and two group designs published between 1997 and 2008 which involved 147 participants aged 2–17 years. Targeted social skills included maintaining conversation, greetings and requests, and initiating play including turn taking. ESs were a function of treatment type: Video modeling (VM) had a larger ES (mean PND = 84%, range 50–100%, 11 studies) than social stories (67%, range 47–100%, 6 studies) and peer-mediated social skills training (mean PND = 61%, range 35–100%, 9 studies) (also, see section in the following text on social skills training and VM interventions). (Data on other interventions were limited due to the small number of studies.) Study quality was assessed using Mastropieri and Scruggs' (1985–1986) checklist. Twelve studies reported maintenance data (mean PND = 79%, range 38–100%), nine reported data on maintenance (mean PND = 81%, range 40–100%), and nine reported data on follow-up (mean PND = 92%, range 60–100%), but there were insufficient data to report on these features broken down by treatment type. The authors concluded that "While Social Stories, Peer-Mediated, and Video-Modeling interventions all met the criteria for EBP according to Horner et al. (2005), a closer look at PND scores shows that only V[ideo] M[odeling] meets criteria for being evidence-based as well as demonstrating high effectiveness as an intervention strategy" (p. 338).

Reichow and Volkmar (2009) conducted a best evidence synthesis of social skills training for individuals with autism. Best evidence synthesis refers to a form of systematic review and meta-analysis which focuses on best quality studies and organizes the results in a hierarchical fashion, in this case in three levels—participants and research rigor, child age, and different types of intervention. They included 66 studies, of which 10 were group designs and 56 were small N experiments, with 513 individuals with autism published between 2001 and 2008. Thirteen (13%) of studies were of good quality and 53 (87%) were of adequate quality. The authors did not calculate ESs for the small N experiments. Rather, they counted the percentage of successful applications of the independent variable, across behaviors, participants, or both, in each study; however, they did not report aggregated ES data on small N experiments. Of the four group experiments that reported Cohen's d's, the values of Cohen's d were 0.43–0.56, 0.45–1.14, and 3.05 for three experiments, and values of η^2 were 0.22–0.33 in the fourth experiment. The authors made both broad and narrow conclusions. They broadly concluded that "there is much supporting evidence for the treatment of social deficits in autism" (p. 161). Additionally, they concluded that (a) for preschoolers, adolescents, and adults, there were no EBP for social skills; but (b) for school-aged children, social skills groups were an established EBP; and (c) for school-aged children, VM was a promising treatment.

Finally, Wang et al. (2013) conducted a hierarchical linear model meta-analysis of 115 small N experiments with 343 participants published between 1994 and 2012. The mean age was 6.5 years (range 9 months–32 years). The ESs measure was a z-score of the treatment data. The mean ES was 1.40 (confidence interval [CI] = 1.32–1.4, $N = 115$ studies). One hundred and three of 115 studies and 294 of 343 participants had a large ES ($d > .80$). The mean ES was statistically different from 0. The authors assessed the quality of the studies and found most were of high quality (4 or 5 points on a 5-point scale) but many omitted details of participant characteristics. Thus, the authors concluded that "on average S[ocial] S[kills] I[nterventions] for individuals with ASD are effective" (p. 1709).

At first glance, these six meta-analysis studies reached different conclusions and appear perplexing and contradictory: Bellini et al. (2007) concluded that social skills were minimally effective; Reichow and Volkmar (2009) concluded that some social skills training interventions were promising, whereas others were established from some but not all age groups; Wang and Spillane (2009) concluded that VM was highly effective for socials skills training, but other methods were not; yet others' meta-analyses (Schneider et al., 2008; Vaughn et al., 2003; Wang et al., 2013) made fairly broad positive conclusions about the effectiveness of social skills training. A closer examination of these papers, however, suggests that these differences reflect different research questions and the databases searched. For example, one meta-analysis focused on peer-mediated strategies (Schneider et al., 2008) and another focused on preschool children (Vaughn et al.). Additionally, these meta-analyses differed substantially in the years of research that they sampled, with none comprehensively sampling all studies over an extended period of time. Thus, we still await a comprehensive meta-analysis of social skills training. Despite these limitations, there is sufficient agreement across five of the six meta-analyses, which include over 300 participants with over 100 experiments, that social skills training is an EBP.

Language and communication

General language interventions
There were two meta-analyses of interventions for language, one focused specifically on sign language with children with autism (Schwartz & Nye, 2006) and one on

preschool interventions for children with language delays and handicaps (Scruggs Mastropieri, Forness, et al., 1988). Schwartz and Nye (2006) identified seven small *N* and one group experiments on sign language for children aged 4–18 years. The 22 children in the small *N* experiments ranged in age from 4 to 14 years, and the studies were conducted in home, school, and residential settings. Three interventions evaluated signing only, and five interventions evaluated signing plus speech. The mean PND was 80% ("moderate" ES) (range 29–100%), and the ESs were 60% (1 study) for oral communication, 87% for sign language only (5 studies), and 84% for sign plus speech (4 studies). Only three of seven studies reported generalization or follow-up data, and two of these studies found that behavior change occurred during generalization and follow-up. No studies reported treatment fidelity data. The authors concluded that the data offered only "a modicum of support for the use of sign language intervention" (p. 13) for children with autism.

Scruggs, Mastropieri, Forness, and Kavale (1988) conducted a meta-analysis of 20 small *N* studies published between 1968 and 1986 with 44 participants, 36 of whom had developmental delays/autism and 8 of whom had language delays, with 128 ESs. Interventions included reinforcement only, direct instruction, time delay, mand-model, and sign versus speech. The median PND was 83% (range 0–100%, 69 ESs) for intervention, 100% for maintenance (range 0–100%, 28 ESs), and 62% for generalization (range 0–100%, 28 ESs). ES was not a function of participants characteristics, study quality, or dependent variable or intervention method, but ESs were substantially larger for generalization when generalization was planned (median PND = 97%, range 0–100%, *N* = 18) than train and hope (mean PND = 2%, *N* = 13). The authors concluded that this meta-analysis supported the use of behavioral principles in language training.

Augmentative and alternative communication
There has been a large quantity of research on AAC reflected in ten meta-analyses: five meta-analyses of more than one form of ACC and five meta-analyses of Picture Exchange Communication System (PECS). We will first consider the general meta-analysis of AAC and autism published in two related articles (Ganz et al., 2011, 2012); then, we will consider four meta-analyses of specific questions related to promoting generalization (Schlosser & Lee, 2000), application to an individual case (Schlosser & Raghavendra, 2004), and effects of AAC on speech production (Schlosser & Wendt, 2008) and on challenging behavior (Walker & Snell, 2013). Finally, we will consider five meta-analyses on one specific form of AAC: PECS.

General AAC meta-analyses   Ganz et al. (2011) published the most recent and comprehensive meta-analysis of AAC (although also see Schlosser, 2008). Ganz et al. (2011) searched the literature from 1980 to early 2008 and located 24 articles with 58 participants, most (71%) of whom had autism or autism and another developmental disability (12%), which generated 191 ESs. The interventions were divided roughly equally between PECS, speech-generating devices, and other picture-based systems. The overall ES was very large (improvement rate difference

[IRD] = 0.99, CI = 0.98–0.99; Ganz et al., 2012). ESs were moderate to large with mean IRDs being 0.83 (CI = 0.82–0.85), 0.70 (CI = 0.66–0.74), and 0.53 (0.44, 0.62) for ASD, ASD and developmental disability, and multiple disabilities, respectively. ESs were larger for preschool children (IRD = 0.86, CI = 0.85–0.88) than for elementary-aged children (IRD = 0.70, CI = 0.67–0.73) and secondary-aged children (IRD = 0.64, CI = 0.60–0.69).

Ganz et al. (2010) reported that IRDs were a function of target behavior: IRDs were greater for communication skills (0.99, CI = 0.99–0.99) than social skills (IRD = 0.90, CI = 0.84–0.95), academic skills (IRD = 0.79, CI = 0.76–0.82), and challenging behavior (IRD = 0.80, CI = 0.76–0.84). ESs were also a function of AAC type with IRDs being 0.99 (CI = 0.98–0.99), 0.61 (0.57–0.64), and 0.99 (CI = 0.99–1.00) for PECS, other picture-based systems, and speech-generating devices, respectively. These results strongly support the effectiveness and robustness of ACC in nonverbal, minimally verbal, and difficult-to-understand children.

Schlosser and Lee (2000) conducted a meta-analysis of methods to promote generalization and maintenance in AAC. Their search identified 50 studies with 232 ESs published between approximately 1976 and 1995. Approximately 67% of participants were children and approximately 33% were adults. There were 55%, 20%, 9%, 9%, 4%, and 2% of participants classified with multiple disabilities, mental retardation (severe/profound), mental retardation (mild/moderate), autism, mental retardation and autism, and other/combined and physical disabilities, respectively. The authors reported that 45% and 43% of the intervention PNDs were "highly" and "fairly" effective. The corresponding data for generalization were 74% and 11% and 29% and 17% for maintenance. The authors conclude that "AAC interventions are effective in terms of behavior change, generalization, and, although to a lesser degree, maintenance" (p. 221).

An interesting application of meta-analysis to an individual clinical case comes from Schlosser and Raghavendra (2004) who identified an effective treatment for a minimally verbal boy with Down syndrome and ID: His parents wanted to know "What would happen to his development of speech once AAC has been introduced?" To answer this question, the authors identified an unpublished and unobtainable meta-analysis and four relevant studies. The four studies had a PND of 58% (range 10–100%, "questionable"), indicating that AAC might increase the child's vocalizations but was unlikely to inhibit them. This conclusion was tempered by the observation that all four AAC studies used signing and no other forms of AAC. Thus, the experiments could tell the child's parents that AAC might facilitate rather than inhibit their son's speech.

Finally, Schlosser and Wendt (2008) conducted two meta-analyses of AAC on speech production. They located nine small N experiments with 27 participants and two group designs with 98 participants published between 1993 and 2007. Participants in the meta-analysis of small N experiments were aged 81 months (range 37–144), and all but one had no functional speech. Six studies used PECS and three used other forms of AAC. Eighty-one percent of ESs were "ineffective" and only 4 of 21 ESs were "effective." PECS studies teaching requesting had a large ES (mean PND = 95.2%). The authors did not aggregate ES data across the two group designs. They concluded that although there was evidence of effectiveness of AAC on speech production, the

ESs were small to moderate, with some participants not gaining any speech; however, there was no evidence that ACC reduced speech production in any studies.

Meta-analyses of PECS   PECS is a commercially available communication system, which initially teaches requesting and then other more complex communication skills, that has received considerably research attention in recent years. This is reflected in five meta-analyses (Flippin, Reszka, & Watson, 2010; Ganz, Davis, Lund, Goodwyn, & Simpson, 2012; Hart & Banda, 2010; Preston & Carter, 2009; Tincani & Devis, 2011) reflecting the growing number of experiments on PECS and the consequent ability to move from asking broad questions of effectiveness (Preston & Carter) to specific questions concerning specific outcomes such as speech and challenging behavior (Flippin et al., 2010; Hart & Banda, 2010; Tincani & Devis, 2011) and specific populations, such as autism (Ganz et al., 2012; Tincani & Devis, 2011). (Other ACC meta-analyses have also reported ESs for PECS: See preceding text.) These meta-analyses, which were based on approximately 8–16 small N studies, including small N experiments and up to two RCTs, concurred that PECS was effective in teaching simple communication skills, such as manding ("requesting"), and has small and variable effects on speech and challenging behavior. For the purpose of this section, we will only review the data from Ganz et al. because it is the most up-to-date meta-analysis as they used IRD calculations, permitting calculations of CIs for ESs and significance testing.

Ganz et al. (2012) searched multiple databases for publications between 1980 and 2009, and they identified 13 articles with 29 participants with ASD aged 3–17 years. There were 104 IRD calculations. The mean overall effect was IRD = 0.56 (0.49, 0.62), but IRDs were significantly larger for targeted skills (IRD = 0.65, [0.56, 0.73]) than nontargeted skills, such as speech and challenging behavior (IR = 0.45, [0.35, 0.56]). IRDs were 0.61 (0.48, 0.73), 0.73 (0.53, 0.93), and 0.37 (0.22, 0.52) for challenging behavior, socialization, and speech, respectively. These meta-analyses agreed that PECS is an EBP since there is good evidence that children with ID and/or ASD can acquire some simple communication skills through PECS, but that effects on other outcomes are variable and sometimes rather small. These observations on the effectiveness of PECS for challenging behavior were replicated by Walker and Snell (2013) who found that PECS was effective but had had smaller ESs than FCT on treating challenging behavior. Thus, PECS is not a first-line treatment of challenging behavior, but might be a component of a multiple component package for some individuals.

Other specific skills and interventions

Video modeling
Table 2.2 summarizes the main features of five meta-analyses of VM which reported the effects of VM, self video modeling (SVM) (Bellini & Akullian, 2007; Mason et al., 2013; Mason, Ganz, Parker, Burke, & Camargo, 2012), peer modeling (Wang, Ciu, & Parrila, 2011), procedural variations in modeling (Mason, Ganz

Table 2.2 A Table Summarizing Five Meta-Analyses of VM

Reference	Study characteristics	Main findings	Conclusions
Bellini and Akullian, (2007)	1. $N=23$ small N experiments 2. $N=0$ RCTs 3. $N=73$ participants with ASD (aged 3–20 years) 4. Study quality addressed by only including experiments, reporting data on generalization and maintenance, and reporting ES separately for experiments with treatment integrity	1. ES for intervention were PND = 80% (range 29–100%, $N=22$ studies), for maintenance were PND = 83% (35–100%, $N=18$ studies), and for generalization were PND = 74% (range 22–100%, $N=7$ studies) 2. Intervention ESs were large to moderate for functional skills, social communication skills, and behavioral functioning (PND = 89%, 77%, and 76% respectively) 3. VM and VSM were both moderately equally effective (PNDs = 88% and 77%) 4. Studies with treatment fidelity data were as effective as studies that did not (Intervention PND = 85%)	"video-modeling and VSM meet the criteria for designation as an evidence-based practice" (p. 281)
Wang et al. (2011)	1. $N=13$ papers on peer or VM (1995–2007) 2. $N=0$ RCTs 3. $N=43$ participants (aged 4–15 years, mean = 7 years) 4. Used a standard measure of study quality	1. Using hierarchical linear modeling, they showed that the mean ES was 1.27 (range 0.65–2.31) which was significantly different from 0 2. There was little difference between peer or VM	"peer-mediated and video-modeling are both effective in improving the social behavior of children with autism" (p. 566)
Mason et al. (2012)	1. $N=42$ small N experiments (1989–2010) 2. $N=0$ RCTs 3. $N=126$ participants, 84% with ASD 16% with developmental disability 79% were children and adolescents and 21% were adults 4. Did not measure study quality	1. Overall IRD = 0.82 (0.81, 0.83) "high magnitude of change" 2. ESs were larger for elementary-aged children than other age groups and larger for those with ADS (IRD = 0.83) than those with developmental disability (IRD = 0.68) 3. For those with ASD, ESs were larger when intervention included reinforcement (IRD = 0.88) and smaller for treatment packages (IRD = 0.71) than VM alone (IRD = 0.81) 4. For individuals with developmental disabilities, VM alone was minimally effective (IRD = 0.40) and was smaller than VM as part of a treatment package (IRD = 0.76)	"V[ideo]M[odeling] O[nly] is highly effective for participants with autism spectrum disorders … and moderately effective for participants with developmental disabilities" (p. 2012)

Mason, Davis et al. (2013)	1. $N = 56$ small N studies with 233 ESs 2. $N = 0$ RCTs 3. $N = 177$ participants with ASD or ID aged 2–72 years 4. Did not include a measure of study quality, but only include experiments	1. Overall IRD = 0.81 (0.80, 0.82) 2. Adult as model has a larger ES (IRD = 0.87 [0.86, 0.88]) than peer models (IRD = 0.70 [0.68, 0.73]) 3. IRD was larger for VM with reinforcement (IRD = 0.88 [0.78, 0.82]) than VM in a package (IRD = 0.74 [0.71, 0.76])	1. "[VM has] large effects with moderate to large effects for nearly all of the included studies which is consistent with Bellini and Akullian's (2007) previous meta-analysis" (p. 120)
Mason, Davis et al. (2013)	1. $N = 14$ high-quality small N experiments. 2. $N = 0$ RCTs 3. $N = 54$ participants of whom 32% were aged over 18 years and all of whom had either ASD (46%) or developmental disabilities (32%) 4. Quality assessed using a checklist and low-quality studies were excluded	1. Mean IRD for point-of-view (POV) VM was 0.78 (0.76, 0.80) 2. ES varied according to the type of POV modeling used. Viewing the entire model first ("priming") and viewing the model step by step ("prompting") were both associated with large IRDs (0.79 and 0.81, respectively) 3. Inclusion of prompts and inclusion of instructions was associated with larger ESs (IRDs = 0.81, and 0.81 respectively)	1. "results indicated a large omnibus effect size" (p. 9) 2. Procedural variations affected ES, specifically addition of priming, prompting, and instructions resulted in larger IRDs

et al., 2013), and point-of-view (POV) VM (Mason, Davis, Boles, & Goodwyn, 2013). (POV VM is a form of VM where the camera is held at the person's eyeline to show what they see from their own perspective when performing the procedure.) These meta-analyses reported the evaluation of VM for a wide range of target behaviors. For example, Bellini and Akullian (2007) reported the application of VM to social communication skills, such as play and social initiations; functional skills, such as purchasing; and behavioral functioning, such as on/off task behavior. Table 2.2 shows that all five meta-analyses concluded that VM resulted in moderate to large ESs. Further, this was true over a range of participant characteristics and target behaviors. Interestingly, the range of ESs was quite large depending upon the way in which experimenters implemented VM. For example, the addition of prompts, reinforcement, etc., may increase ESs (Mason, Ganz et al., 2013). Thus, VM is an EBP.

Staff and parent training

Table 2.3 summarizes three rather varied meta-analyses of staff and parent training including meta-analyses of staff training (Van Oorsouw, Embregts, Bosman, & Jahoda, 2009); a specific staff training package, named "active support" (Hamelin & Sturmey, 2011); and a review of RCTs of a parent training package, *Stepping Stones Triple P* (Tellegen & Sanders, 2013). The reader is also referred to Table 2.1 for a summary of Strauss, Mancini, the SPC Group, and Fava (2013) on the effects of parent training on EIBI and autism. The first and last meta-analyses found good evidence for the effectiveness of staff and parent training on some aspects of both client/child and staff behavior, whereas the meta-analysis of active support found only limited evidence of its effects on both staff and client behavior. Further, Van Oorsouw et al. (2009) reported disaggregations, revealing that ESs varied considerably in method of staff training and type of skills taught. Additionally, Tellegen and Saunders (2013) reported that ESs depended upon the type of parent and child outcomes measured. Thus, although the two large meta-analyses show that staff and parent training is an EBP, the outcomes are highly varied, probably reflecting the way in which training was conducted, the outcome measured, and other contextual variables. Thus, specific forms of staff/parent training for specific problems may not be an EBP (or may even be harmful).

Two meta-analyses of EIBI have also addressed supervisor and parent training and found benefits on child outcomes. Reichow and Wolery (2009) found that supervisor competence correlated strongly with IQ ($r = .750$) and AB ($r = .982$). Strauss et al. (2013) found that the level of parent training correlated positively with AB ($r = .768$) and IQ ($r = .739$). Thus, these two meta-analyses both found that supervisor and parent training can improve child outcomes.

Self-management

Lee, Simpson, and Shogren (2007) conducted a meta-analysis of 11 small N experiments published from 1992 to 2001 with 34 participants with autism (mean age approximately 9 years, range 3–17 years) which generated 78 ESs. The mean

Table 2.3 A Summary of Three Meta-Analyses of Caregiver Training

Reference	Study characteristics	Main findings	Conclusions
Van Oorsouw et al. (2009)	1. $N = 55$ small N studies of staff training 2. $N = 0$ RCTs 3. $N =$ approximately 518 staff 4. Did include minimal inclusion criteria (e.g., at least two baseline and two intervention data points)	1. Studies that trained staff to change client behavior had smaller PNDs (74%, SD = 35%) than those training staff to do nonclient-related duties (PND = 87%, SD = 25%) 2. For staff training interventions to change client behavior, PNDs were 51%, 68%, and 87% ($p < .0001$) and for training other staff skills were 93.9%, 72.9%, and 86.7% ($p < .0001$) for in-service, coaching on the job, and both strategies combined, respectively 3. For staff training to change client behavior, PNDs were larger for packages (PND = 93%) than interventions with individual training methods (PND = 67%)	1. Combined in-service and on the job coaching was the most effective 2. Staff training packages using more than one method were more effective than those using one method
Hamelin and Sturmey (2011)	1. $N = 2$ studies with three experiments evaluating the active support staff training package 2. $N = 0$ RCTs 3. Three multiple baseline designs 4. Reviewed candidate articles using a checklist	1. PND for staff assistance ranged from 28% to 66% ("ineffective") during treatment and from 30% to 50% at follow-up ("ineffective") 2. PND for client engagement ranged from 17–54% (ineffective) to 0–50% ("ineffective")	Active support is a "promising" but not an "effective" treatment
Tellegen and Sanders (2013)	1. $N = 12$ group studies 2. $N = 9$ RCTs 3. $N = 659$ families with children with a variety of developmental disabilities (ASD, Down syndrome, and developmental disability); age range 1–19 years 4. Quality assessed using several measures of and analyses of the effects of potential bias	1. The authors reported Cohen's d's for each of the five program levels and for multiple parents and child variables, most of which indicated medium to large d's 2. Values of $d = 0.537$, 0.725, 0.523, 0.264, 0.421, 0.523, and 0.093 for child problems, parenting style, parenting satisfaction/efficacy, parental adjustment, parental relationship, child observations, and parent observations, respectively	"The overall evidence base supported the effectiveness of S[tepping] S[tones] T[riple] P as an intervention for improving child and parent outcomes in families of children with disabilities" (p. 1556)

PND was 82% (range 0–100%, SD = 31%). The PND was not affected by treatment procedural variables, target behaviors, or participant characteristics, although the small sample size may have mitigated against the possibility of detecting such differences. PNDs were 85% (SD = 10%, 7 experiments) and 75% (SD = 23%, 5 experiments) for generalization and maintenance, respectively. The authors concluded that self-management was "effective" for children and adolescents with autism.

Peer tutoring

Two meta-analyses of peer tutoring, conducted some 20 years apart, both concluded that peer tutoring had benefits to individuals with disabilities. Cook, Scruggs, Mastropieri, and Casto (1985) conducted a meta-analysis of 19 articles which generated 74 ESs, 49 for tutors and 25 for tutees. This section will only discuss data from tutees as few tutors had cognitive disabilities, whereas 18% of tutees had and 20% had learning disabilities. The mean d for tutees was 0.58 and 0.48 for all studies and good quality studies, respectively. When disaggregated by academic outcomes, d's were 0.49 for reading ($N = 13$ studies) and 0.85 ($N = 5$ studies) for math. ESs remained large when peer tutoring was used as a substitute for regular teaching ($d = 0.73$, 17 studies). Further, ESs were robust across dependent variables including academic ($d = 0.65$, 17 studies), objective standardized measures ($d = 0.45$, 12 studies), objective unstandardized ($d = 0.89$, 7 studies), and questionnaire ratings ($d = 0.47$, 6 studies) and were larger for criterion-referenced outcomes ($d = 1.00$, 6 studies) than norm-referenced studies ($d = 0.45$, 11 studies). The authors concluded that "handicapped … tutees achieve gains on academic dependent measures as a result of participation in a tutoring program. Generally, tutees achieved greater gains than tutors" (p. 488).

Stenhoff and Lignugaris/Kraft (2007) conducted a meta-analysis of six group designs and 14 small *N* experiments in which data were available both on tutors and tutees with cognitive disabilities. They conducted a meta-analysis of 20 articles with 89 participants. Tutors and tutees were aged 10–21 years. Most tutors and over 90% of tutees had learning disabilities or ID. The weighted d for group studies was 0.46 (CI = 0.41–0.71, "medium") and for small *N* experiments was 74% (range 50–98%, "effective"), and most outcomes were measures of correct academic responses. The authors concluded that "Peer tutoring … is supported as an evidence-based practice … there is strong support for peer-tutor training prior to the commencement of peer-tutoring … single-subject studies support monitoring peer tutors during peer tutoring as an evidence-based practice" (p. 24). Thus, both meta-analyses concurred on the benefits of peer tutoring to tutees, primarily on academic outcomes.

Reading

Browder and Xin (1998) conducted a literature search of research teaching sight word reading published between 1980 and 1997 which identified 48 studies with 269 participants. Most (63%) participants were elementary school students, 20% were secondary school students, and 17% were adults, and most (177) had moderate/severe ID. They conducted a meta-analysis of 32 small *N* experiments with baseline data which yielded 52 ESs. The median PND was 91% (range 63–100%) which was somewhat larger for participants with mild ID (PND = 95%; range 81–100%) than those with moderate/severe ID (PND = 89%, range 63–100%). PND did not differ by age groups but differed by type of intervention. ESs were larger for repeating words after error correction (PND = 93%, range 63–100%) than not repeating (PND = 88%, range 72–100%). The authors concluded that sight word instruction was highly effective, but they expressed caution because this research focused on response acquisition; there was also a lack of research on generalization and application of sight word reading to real-world settings.

Psychotherapy-related skills

As part of a systematic review, Prout and Nowak-Drabik (2003) conducted a meta-analysis of nine group studies of interventions for assertiveness, behavioral weight loss interventions, social skills, and vocational skills related broadly to mental health and psychotherapy. (It is unclear what the dependent variables were in this subset of studies, but they likely included measures of skill gain.) The number of participants was unclear. The mean Cohen's *d* was 1.01 (range 0.06–1.85, SD = 0.68). The authors concluded that these studies were moderately effective.

National Institute for Clinical Excellence [NICE] (2012) reviewed psychosocial treatments for adults with ASD including behavioral therapies for communication, FC, behavioral therapies for behavior management, CBT, including antivictimization programs, anger management, and CBT for OCD, leisure programs, social learning interventions, supported employment, and programs to support families and caregivers. The searches only included RCTs and group designs with at least 10 participants per arm with less than 50% attrition and excluded small *N* experiments. Due to the small quantity and poor quality of research, they extended the inclusion criteria to permit studies with a mean age of 15 or over and studies of people with ID and without autism. The authors only conducted meta-analyses. They reported only two low-quality RCTs evaluating antivictimization programs in adults with ID which found significant effects. NICE recommended that for adults with ASD without or with mild ID who are at risk for victimization, practitioners should consider antivictimization interventions based on teaching decision-making and problem-solving skills.

Purchasing, money, and mathematical skills

Xin, Grasso, Dipipi-Hoy, and Jitendra (2005) conducted a meta-analysis of 28 small *N* experiments teaching purchasing skills published between 1978 and 2000. There were 115 participants aged 6–74 years most of whom had moderate/severe (43%) or severe (18%) ID. There were few differences between teaching strategies such as modeling/verbal instruction versus fading, time delay, and system of most to least prompts. There was, however, a larger ES for simplifying money skills, for example, by using a money number line or matching money to a preprinted card (PND = 95%) than the next dollar strategy (PND = 85%). Generalization and maintenance data were moderately good with PNDs of 86% (range 0–100%) and 100% (range

67–100%) with studies that programmed generalization producing larger PNDs (95%) than those that did not (PND = 83%). The authors concluded that teaching purchasing skills is moderately effective with reasonable evidence of generalization and maintenance from 1 week to 5 months.

Browder, Spooner, Ahlgrim-Delzell, Harris, and Wakeman (2008) conducted a meta-analysis of teaching math skills to students with significant cognitive disabilities. They found 62 articles with 68 studies of which 54 were small *N* experiments and 14 were group designs. There were 493 participants most of whom had moderate to severe ID and 16 studies included adults. Almost all studies took place in special education classes (57%) or community settings (27%). The authors assessed the quality using a standard checklist and subsequently compared low- and high-quality articles. The mean PND was 92% (range 0–100%, SD = 26%, 54 studies), and the median *d* was 0.79 (mean = 2.18, SD = 2.90, 14 studies). Most high-quality studies taught purchasing and money skills. When broken down into specific teaching methods, there were few differences between teaching strategies—almost all had large ESs with multiple independent replications; however, in vivo instruction and physical guidance had larger ESs than other methods, and massed practice had smaller ESs than other methods. The authors concluded that systematic instruction was an EBP for teaching mathematics to this population and recommended that practitioners should teach skills in vivo and in the context of purchasing.

Exercise

Exercise has been used to improve a variety of academic and behavioral outcomes for individuals with disabilities. Sowa and Meulenbroek (2012) conducted a meta-analysis of 16 studies—presumably group designs—published between 1991 and 2011. There were 133 children with ASD with a mean age of 14 years (range 4–41 years). The most common interventions were swimming and jogging. The meta-analysis did not evaluate study quality. The ES measure was percentage change from baseline to treatment. The average ES was 38% and was larger for individual (49%) than group interventions (32%). Average ESs were similar for motor skills (40%) and social skills (40%) but smaller for other skills (22%). The authors concluded that "there were robust benefits of physical exercise on motor and social functioning" and that individual interventions had larger effects than group interventions.

Social stories

Social Stories™ (Gray, 2000) is a commercial, proprietary product whose aim is to share accurate information in a personal and reassuring manner which may (or may not) result in behavior change. To date, there have been four meta-analyses (Kokina & Kern, 2010; Reynhout & Carter, 2006; Reynhout & Carter, 2011; Test, Richter, Knight, & Spooner, 2011) which have largely made the same conclusions; therefore, this section will only describe the most recent and most comprehensive meta-analysis in detail. Test et al. (2011) identified 28 published and unpublished studies, which reported from 1995 to 2007, and reviewed them in a descriptive analysis; 18 studies were entered into a meta-analysis which used three measures of ES. (Only PND will be discussed here.) The authors carefully measured the quality of the studies with a checklist of indicators. The median overall PND was 50% (range 0–98%, "ineffective") and highly variable. Maintenance data was available from seven studies (median PND = 50%, range 0–92%) and for generalization data from three studies (median PND = 8%, range 0–76%). Only 9 of 28 (38%) studies were judged to have achieved a socially important behavioral change. Thus, Test et al. concluded that "Social stories may be generally ineffective in producing robust behavior change" (p. 58). Recently, Leaf et al. (2012) compared instruction, modeling, and feedback with social stories to teach social skills to people with autism. They found robust evidence that social stories were robustly inferior to behavioral procedures in both acquisition and generalization of social skills. Given that there are highly effective alternate treatments for many of the target behaviors addressed by social stories, such as self-help, social skills, and challenging behavior, there is little reason to use Social Stories at this time.

Special education placement
Segregated special education remains a very common model of service provision, yet its effectiveness remains unclear (Smith, 1996). This remains controversial over the debate about whether or not mainstreaming is an alternate, more effective service model. Carlberg and Kavale (1980) conducted a meta-analysis of 50 studies comparing the academic, social, and other outcomes of students in special education versus regular classes. The average participant age was 11 years, and their average IQ was 74 (range not reported). The authors included good and poor quality studies and later analyzed some measures of study quality on ES. They found a small ES favoring regular classes ($d = -0.12$, CI $= -0.18$ to -0.06). There was little difference between achievement (-0.15) and social/personality outcomes (-0.11). There were, however, larger differences between student categories with students with higher IQs (75–90, "learning disabled" [LD]) being much more disadvantaged by special education than regular classes (d's $= -0.34$ vs. -0.14), although students with behavioral and emotional disabilities (BD/ED) did better in special education than other students ($d = +0.29$). There was little evidence of quality of study directly affecting outcome, such as blinding; however, there were insufficient studies reported data on teacher assignment and teacher practices, so differences may have been affected by these variables. The authors concluded that "special class placement is an inferior alternative to regular class placement … [but] the problems of LD or BD/ED were apparently more tractable in the special class than children whose primary problem was low IQ" (p. 304). This meta-analysis may be limited by the numerous potential confounds between educational placement and other unknown variables, but it places an onus on those claiming benefits of special education

to show that they do indeed exist. Nevertheless, this meta-analysis provides little data that special education improves AB.

Use of technology at work

Finally, Wehmeyer et al. (2006) conducted a meta-analysis of 13 small *N* experiments teaching the use of technology in the context of employment, such as audio prompting devices, video-assisted training, palmtop and desktop computers, and AAC devices, to teach social skill, task sequencing and transition skills, food preparation skills, etc. There were 42 participants aged 12–37 years (mean IQ = 42). The mean PND was 93% (SD = 0.14). Interestingly, the authors compared ESs in studies that used universal design principles, such as flexible, simple intuitive use, and tolerance for error and appropriate size and space of device, and found that studies that used universal design principles had larger PNDs (97%, SD = 0.08) than those that did not (91%, SD = 0.18). The authors concluded that assistive technology could be effective in contributing to vocational and employment outcomes for youth and adults with disabilities.

Summary

There is good and robust evidence that we can teach many specific AB to people with developmental disabilities. These evidence-based interventions are almost completely behavioral methods with little evidence for other forms of intervention. Additionally, the range of skills that can be addressed is very broad. Unlike the target behaviors in the previous section, the social significance of these target behaviors is more limited: Learning to shop or use a palm pilot is less important that broad increases in development and AB. Nevertheless, these specific AB may be quite important to many individuals in certain contexts and may sometimes be crucial in certain very important contexts, such as key skills related to successful adaptation to certain environments, such as social skills at work, and key replacement behaviors during interventions for challenging behavior, such as acquisition of mands during functional communication training.

Meta-analyses of EI, deinstitutionalization, and teaching specific AB reveal that there are many EBP, many of which have medium to large ESs. Most of these EBP are based on or include behavioral interventions. This is not uniformly true. For example, ESs for PECS on adaptive and maladaptive behavior were small. Indeed, there are evidence-based alternatives. If we ask what should we do to teach a non-verbal/minimally verbal child to communicate, then the evidence supports PECS as one evidence-based option to teach simple requesting through pointing, verbal approximations, and words for some. If, however, we wish to improve social behavior, there is little evidence that PECS will help, but interventions such as social skills training or VM may be much more effective. Thus, meta-analyses can assist practitioners and family members to select the most effective methods and avoid ineffective or harmful interventions to increase AB in individuals with developmental disabilities.

References

Bellini, S., & Akullian, J. (2007). A meta-analysis of video modeling and video self-modeling interventions for children and adolescents with autism spectrum disorders. *Exceptional Children, 73*, 264–287.

Bellini, S., Peters, J. K., Benner, L., & Hopf, A. (2007). A meta-analysis of school-based social skills interventions for children with autism spectrum disorders. *Remedial and Special Education, 28*, 153–162.

Browder, D. M., Spooner, F., Ahlgrim-Delzell, L., Harris, A. A., & Wakeman, S. (2008). A Meta-analysis on teaching mathematics to students with significant cognitive disabilities. *Exceptional Children, 74*, 407–432.

Browder, D. M., & Xin, Y. P. (1998). A meta-analysis and review of sight word research and its implications for teaching functional reading to individuals with moderate and severe disabilities. *The Journal of Special Education, 32*, 130–153.

Carlberg, C., & Kavale, K. (1980). The efficacy of special versus regular class placement for exceptional children: A meta-analysis. *Journal of Special Education, 14*, 295–309.

Casto, G., & Mastropieri, M. A. (1986). The efficacy of early intervention programs: A meta-analysis. *Exceptional Children, 52*, 417–424.

Cook, S. B., Scruggs, T. E., Mastropieri, M. A., & Casto, G. C. (1985). Handicapped students as tutors. *The Journal of Special Education, 19*, 483–492.

Eldevik, S., Hastings, R. P., Hughes, C. J., Jahr, E., Eikeseth, S., & Cross, S. (2010). Using participant data to extend the evidence base for intensive behavioral intervention for children with autism. *American Association on Intellectual and Developmental Disabilities, 115*, 381–405.

Flippin, M., Reszka, S., & Watson, L. R. (2010). Effectiveness of the picture exchange communication system (PECS) on communication and speech for children with autism spectrum disorders: A meta-analysis. *American Journal of Speech-Language Pathology, 19*, 178–195.

Ganz, J. B., Davis, J. L., Lund, E. M., Goodwyn, F. D., & Simpson, R. L. (2012). Meta-analysis of PECS with individuals with ASD: Investigation of targeted versus non-targeted outcomes, participant characteristics, and implementation phase. *Research in Developmental Disabilities, 33*, 406–418.

Ganz, J. B., Earles-Vollrath, T. L., Heath, A. K., Parker, R. I., Rispoli, M. J., & Duran, J. B. (2010). A meta-analysis of single case research on aided augmentative and alternative communication systems with individuals with autism spectrum disorders. *Journal of Autism and Developmental Disorders, 42*, 60–74.

Ganz, J. B., Earles-Vollrath, T. L., Mason, R. A., Rispoli, M. J., Heath, A. K., & Parker, R. I. (2011). An aggregate study of single-case research involving aided AAC: Participant characteristics of individuals with autism spectrum disorders. *Research in Autism Spectrum Disorders, 5*, 1500–1509.

Ganz, J. B., Earles-Vollrath, T. L., Mason, R. A., Rispoli, M. J., Heath, A. K., & Parker, R. I. (2012b). A meta-analysis of single case research on aided augmentative communication systems with individuals with autism spectrum disorders. *Journal of Autism and Developmental Disorders, 42*, 60–74.

Gray, C. (2000). *The new social story book: Illustrated edition* (2nd ed.). Arlington, TX: Future Horizons.

Hamelin, J. P., Frijters, J., Griffiths, D., Condillac, R., & Owen, F. (2011). Meta-analysis of deinstitutionalisation of adaptive behaviour outcomes: Research and clinical implications. *Journal of Intellectual & Developmental Disability, 36*, 61–72.

Hamelin, J., & Sturmey, P. (2013). Psychological treatment: What does the evidence tell us? To appear. In E. Tsakanikos & J. McCarthy (Eds.), *Handbook of psychopathology in intellectual disabilities*. New York: Springer.

Hamelin, J. P., & Sturmey, P. (2011). Active support: A systematic review and meta-analysis. *American Journal on Intellectual and Developmental Disabilities, 49,* 166–171.

Hart, S. L., & Banda, D. R. (2010). Picture exchange communication system with individuals with developmental disabilities: A meta-analysis of single subject studies. *Remedial and Special Education, 31,* 476–488.

Horner, R. H., Carr, E. G., Halle, J. U., McGee, G., Odon, S., & Wolery, M. (2005). The use of single-subject research to identify evidence-based practices in special education. *Exceptional Children, 71,* 165–179.

King, R. (2005). Proceeding with compassion while awaiting the evidence: Psychotherapy with individuals with mental retardation. *Mental Retardation, 43,* 448–450.

Kokina, A., & Kern, L. (2010). Social stories interventions for students with autism spectrum disorders: A meta-analysis. *Journal of Autism and Developmental Disabilities, 40,* 812–826.

Kuppens, S., & Onghena, P. (2012). Sequential meta-analysis to determine the sufficiency of cumulative knowledge: The case of early intensive behavioral intervention for children with autism spectrum disorders. *Research in Autism Spectrum Disorders, 6,* 168–176.

Leaf, J. B., Oppenheim-Leaf, M. L., Call, N. A., Sheldon, J. B., Sherman, J. A., Taubman, M., et al. (2012). Comparing the teaching interaction procedure to social stories for people with autism. *Journal of Applied Behavior Analysis, 45,* 281–298.

Lee, S. H., Simpson, R. L., & Shogren, K. A. (2007). Effects and implications of self-management for students with autism: A meta-analysis. *Focus on Autism and Other Developmental Disabilities, 22,* 2–13.

Levy, S., Kim, A.–H., & Olive, M. L. (2006). Interventions for young children with autism a synthesis of the literature. *Focus Autism Other Developmental Disabilities, 21,* 55–62.

Lynch, P. S., Kellow, T. J., & Wilson, V. L. (1997). The impact of deinstitutionalization on the adaptive behavior of adults with mental retardation: A meta-analysis. *Education and Training in Mental Retardation and Developmental Disabilities, 32,* 255–261.

Maffei-Almodovar, L., & Sturmey, P. (2013). Evidence-based practice and crisis intervention. In D. D. Reed, F. D. DiGennaro Reed, & J. K. Luiselli (Eds.), *Handbook of crisis intervention for individuals with developmental disabilities* (pp. 49–70). New York: Springer.

Makrygianni, M. K., & Reed, P. (2010). A meta-analytic review of the effectiveness of behavioural early intervention programs for children with autistic spectrum disorders. *Research in Autism Spectrum Disorders, 4,* 577–593.

Mason, R. A., Davis, H. S., Boles, M. B., & Goodwyn, F. (2013). Efficacy of point-of-view video modeling: A meta-analysis. *Remedial and Special Education.* Advance online publication. doi: 10.1177/0741932513486298.

Mason, R. A., Ganz, J. B., Parker, R. I., Boles, M. B., Davis, H. S., & Rispoli, M. J. (2013). Video-based modeling: Differential effects due to treatment protocol. *Research in Autism Spectrum Disorders, 7,* 120–131.

Mason, R. A., Ganz, J. B., Parker, R. I., Burke, M. B., & Camargo, S. P. (2012). Moderating factors of video-modeling with other as model: A meta-analysis of single-case studies. *Research in Developmental Disabilities, 33,* 1076–1086.

Mastropieri, M. A., & Scruggs, T. E. (1985). Early intervention for socially withdrawn children. *The Journal of Special Education, 19,* 429–441.

National Institute for Clinical Excellence; The British Psychological Society. (2012). *Autism. The NICE guideline on recognition, referral diagnosis and management of adults on the autism spectrum*. Leicester, UK: British Psychological Society and The Royal College of Psychiatrists.

Ospina, M. B., Krebs, S., Clark, B., Karkhaneh, M., Hartling, L., Tjosvold, L., et al. (2008). Behavioural and developmental interventions for autism spectrum disorder: A clinical systematic review. *PLoS ONE, 3*(11), e3755.

Peters-Scheffer, N., Didden, R., Korzilius, H., & Sturmey, P. (2011). A meta-analytic study on the effectiveness of comprehensive ABA-based early intervention programs for children with autism spectrum disorders. *Research in Autism Spectrum Disorders, 5*, 60–69.

Preston, D., & Carter, M. (2009). A review of the efficacy of the picture exchange communication system intervention. *Journal of Autism and Developmental Disorders, 39*, 1471–1480.

Prout, T. H., & Nowak-Drabik, K. M. (2003). Psychotherapy with persons who have mental retardation: An evaluation of effectiveness. *American Journal on Mental Retardation, 108*, 82–93.

Reichow, B. (2011). Overview of meta-analyses on early intensive behavioral intervention for young children with autism spectrum disorders. *J Autism Developmental Disorders, 42*, 512–520.

Reichow, B., & Volkmar, F. (2009). Social skills interventions for individuals with autism: Evaluation for evidence-based practices within a best evidence synthesis framework. *Journal of Autism and Developmental Disorders, 40*, 149–166.

Reichow, B., & Wolery, M. (2009). Comprehensive synthesis of early intensive behavioral interventions for young children with autism based on the UCLA young autism project model. *Journal of Autism and Developmental Disorders, 39*, 23–41.

Reynhout, G., & Carter, M. (2006). Social stories for children with disabilities. *Journal of Autism and Developmental Disabilities, 36*, 445–469.

Reynhout, G., & Carter, M. (2011). Evaluation of the efficacy of social stories using three single subject metrics. *Research in Autism Spectrum Disorders, 5*, 885–900.

Sallows, G. O., & Graupner, T. D. (2005). Intensive behavioral treatment for children with autism four-year outcome and predictors. *American Journal on Mental Retardation, 110*, 417–438.

Schlosser, R. W. (2008). Effects of augmentative and alternative communication intervention on speech production in children with autism. A systematic review. *American Journal of Speech-Language Pathology, 17*, 212–230.

Schlosser, R. W., & Lee, D. L. (2000). Promoting generalization and maintenance in augmentative and alternative communication: A meta-analysis of 20 years of effectiveness research. *Augmentative and Alternative Communication, 16*, 208–226.

Schlosser, R. W., & Raghavendra, P. (2004). Evidence based practice in augmentative and alternative communication. *Augmentative and Alternative Communication, 20*, 1–21.

Schlosser, R. W., & Wendt, O. (2008). Effects of augmentative and alternative communication intervention on speech production in children with autism: A systematic review. *American Journal of Speech-Language Pathology, 17*, 212–230.

Schneider, N., Goldstein, H., & Parker, R. (2008). Social skills interventions for children with autism: A meta-analytic application of percentage of all non-overlapping data (PAND). *Evidence-Based Communication Assessment and Intervention, 2*, 152–162.

Schwartz, J. B., & Nye, C. (2006). Improving communication for children with autism: Does sign language work? *EBP Briefs, 1*, 1–17.

Scruggs, T. E., Mastropieri, M. A., Forness, S. R., & Kavale, K. (1988). Early language intervention: A quantitative synthesis of single-subject research. *The Journal of Special Education, 22*, 259–283.

Scruggs, T. E., Mastropieri, M. A., & McEwen, I. (1988). Early intervention for developmental functioning: A quantitative synthesis of single-subject research. *Journal of the Division for Early Childhood, 12*, 359–367.

Shonkoff, J. P., & Hauser-Cram, P. (1987). Early intervention for disabled infants and their families: A quantitative analysis. *Pediatrics, 80*, 650–658.

Smith, T. (1996). Are other treatments effective? In C. Maurice, G. Green, & S. C. Luce (Eds.), *Behavioral intervention for young children with autism*. Austin, TX: Proed.

Smith, T. (1999). Outcome of early intervention for children with autism. *Clinical Psychology: Science and Practice, 6*, 33–49.

Smith, T., Eisketh, S., Sallows, G. O., & Grauper, T. D. (2009). Efficacy of applied behavior analysis in autism. Letter to the editor. *Journal of Pediatrics, 154*, 151–152.

Sowa, M., & Meulenbroek, R. (2012). Effects of physical exercise on autism spectrum disorders: A meta-analysis. *Research in Autism Spectrum Disorders, 6*, 46–57.

Spreckley, M., & Boyd, R. (2009). Efficacy of applied behavioral intervention in preschool children with autism for improving cognitive, language, and adaptive behavior: A systematic review and meta-analysis. *The Journal of Pediatrics, 154*, 338–344.

Stenhoff, D. M., & Lignugaris/Kraft, B. (2007). A review of the effects of peer tutoring on students with mild disabilities in secondary settings. *Exceptional Children, 74*, 8–30.

Strauss, K., Mancini, F., the SPC Group, & Fava, L. (2013). Parent inclusion in early intensive behavior interventions for young children with ASD; a synthesis of meta-analysis from 2009–2011. *Research in Developmental Disabilities, 34*, 2967–2985.

Sturmey, P. (2012). Treatment of psychopathology in persons with intellectual and other disabilities. *Canadian Journal of Psychiatry, 57*, 593–600.

Tellegen, C. L., & Sanders, M. R. (2013). Stepping stones triple p-positive parenting program for children with disability: A systematic review and meta-analysis. *Research in Developmental Disabilities, 34*, 1556–1571.

Test, D. W., Richter, S., Knight, V., & Spooner, F. (2011). A comprehensive review and meta-analysis of the social stories literature. *Focus on Autism and Other Developmental Disabilities, 26*, 49–62.

Tincani, M., & Devis, K. (2011). Quantitative synthesis and component analysis of single-participant studies on the picture exchange communication system. *Remedial and Special Education, 32*, 458–470.

Van Oorsouw, W. M. W. J., Embregts, P. J. C. M., Bosman, A. M. T., & Jahoda, A. (2009). Training staff serving clients with intellectual disabilities: A meta-analysis of aspects determining effectiveness. *Research in Developmental Disabilities, 30*, 503–511.

Vaughn, S., Kim, A. H., Morris Sloan, C. V., Hughes, M. T., Elbaum, B., & Sridhar, D. (2003). Social skills interventions for young children with disabilities. A synthesis of group design studies. *Remedial and Special Education, 24*, 2–15.

Virues-Ortega, J. (2010). Applied behavioral analytic intervention for autism in early childhood: Meta-analysis. Meta-regression and dose–response meta-analysis of multiple outcomes. *Clinical Psychology Review, 30*, 387–399.

Walker, V. L., & Snell, M. E. (2013). Effects of augmentative and alternative communication on challenging behavior: A meta-analysis. *Augmentative and Alternative Communication, 29*, 117–131.

Wang, P., & Spillane, A. (2009). Evidence-based social skills interventions for children with autism: A meta-analysis. *Education and Training in Developmental Disabilities, 44*, 318–342.

Wang, S. Y., Ciu, Y., & Parrila, R. (2011). Examining the effectiveness of peer-mediated and video-modeling social skills interventions for children with autism spectrum disorders: A meta-analysis in single-case research using HLM. *Research in Autism Spectrum Disorders, 5*, 562–569.

Wang, S. Y., Parilla, R., & Cui, Y. (2013). Meta-analysis of social skills interventions of single case research for individuals with autism spectrum disorders: Results from three-level HLM. *Journal of Autism and Developmental Disorders, 43*, 1701–1716.

Wehmeyer, M. L., Palmer, S. B., Smith, S. J., Parent, W., Davies, D. K., & Stock, S. (2006). Technology use by people with intellectual and developmental disabilities to support employment activities: A single-subject design meta-analysis. *Journal of Vocational Rehabilitation, 24*, 81–86.

White, K. R. (1985). Efficacy of early intervention. *Journal of Special Education, 19*, 401–416.

White, K. R., Buch, D. W., & Castro, G. (1985). Learning from reviews of early intervention efficacy. *The Journal of Special Education, 19*, 417–428.

Xin, Y. P., Grasso, E., Dipipi-Hoy, C. M., & Jitendra, A. (2005). The effects of purchasing skill instruction for individuals with developmental disabilities: A meta-analysis. *Exceptional Children, 71*, 379–400.

3

Maladaptive Behavior

Peter Sturmey

This chapter continues the review of meta-analyses begun in the previous chapter but focuses on treatment of challenging behavior. The chapter breaks down these meta-analyses into three main groups. The first group deals with challenging behavior generally and is itself broken down into three groups of meta-analyses: (a) general meta-analyses of general challenging behavior; (b) meta-analyses of specific maladaptive behavior, such as pica; and (c) meta-analyses of specific interventions. The second section reviews meta-analyses of specific interventions, such as specific behavioral interventions, positive behavior support (PBS), and cognitive behavioral therapy (CBT). The final section reviews meta-analyses that have focused on treatment of challenging behavior in individuals with autism.

General Challenging Behavior

Challenging behavior has received extensive attention as reflected in at least 19 meta-analyses published since 1986. Table 3.1, Table 3.2, and Table 3.3 summarize them. Table 3.1 summarizes the general characteristics of six meta-analyses of treatment of general challenging behavior. The interventions identified are overwhelmingly behavioral and behavior analytic, although the searches were not limited to these intervention methods. All report evidence of treatment effectiveness based on large and, over time, growing samples of participants from anywhere from 20 to nearly 500 studies, almost all of which are small N experiments, with up to nearly 600 participants.

Evidence-Based Practice and Intellectual Disabilities, First Edition.
Edited by Peter Sturmey and Robert Didden.
© 2014 John Wiley & Sons, Ltd. Published 2014 by John Wiley & Sons, Ltd.

Table 3.1 A Summary of General Meta-analyses of Maladaptive Behavior

Reference	Study characteristics	Main findings	Conclusions
Lennox et al. (1988)	1. $N = 162$ studies from 1981 to 1985 2. N RCTs unclear 3. There were 193, 194, and 95 participants exposed to three levels of intrusive treatments. (Ns overlap as some participants experiences more than one level of intrusiveness.) They were aged 2–56 years and had a variety of degrees of ID and other developmental disorders 4. The authors did not report any measure of quality	1. 13/18 behavioral treatments resulted in 50% or more reduction in target behavior; medication was the least effective 2. There were complex interactions between topography and treatment restrictiveness	1. Differential reinforcement and overcorrection were commonly used 2. Functional analysis was underused (in only 36% of studies)
Lundervold and Bourland (1988)	1. $N = 62$ experiments of which 61 were small N experiments on aggression, SIB, and property destruction 2. 0/1 RCTs 3. N participants unclear, but $N > 62$, most (approximately 60%) of whom have severe/profound ID and approximately 20% had ASD and over half aged 11–20 years and 12% aged over 20 years 4. Study quality measured using ratings of experimental design, generalization, and maintenance	1. Using a 3-point rating scale ($0 = <50\%$, $1 = 51–74\%$, $2 = >75\%$ reduction), efficacy was a function of treatment. The mean ESs were 1.8, 1.8, 1.6, 1.2, 1.0, and 0.0 for response interruption + DR, facial screening, DRI, combined antecedent, punishment and consequence package, and DRO based on 13, 5, 14, 5, 6, and 13 evaluations, respectively, meaning that the typical treatment resulted in a 50–75% reduction in the target behavior	1. There was a lack of studies based on functional analysis and reporting generalization and maintenance data 2. Some interventions, such as DRO, may have been implemented suboptimally 3. More research was needed on adults and on aggression

(Continued)

Table 3.1 (Continued)

Reference	Study characteristics	Main findings	Conclusions
Scotti, Evans, Meyer, and Walker (1991)	1. $N = 403$ individual studies including both experiments and nonexperiments (11% of studies) 2. 0 RCTs 3. $N > 403$ participants of whom 9% were preschool, 67% were of school age, and 24% were adults 4. Study quality was measured and reported	1. 20%, 17%, 30%, and 33% of studies had PNDs of <50% ("ineffective"), 50–80% ("questionable"), 80–99% ("fair"), and >99% ("highly effective") 2. There were few differences between 14 different classes of intervention 3. PNDs were somewhat larger for SIB, stereotypy, and inappropriate social behavior than for physical aggression and destructive/disruptive behavior 4. Follow-up was reported in 156 studies of which 46% reported follow-up data of over 6 months. The mean PND at follow-up was approximately 80% 5. There were also interactions between intervention level of intrusiveness, topography, and behavior severity 6. Conducting a functional analysis resulted in larger effects sizes at follow-up on PND, but not PZD	1. "Only 44 of 403 studies reviewed could be judged to be highly effective" (p. 251) 2. There was a lack of attention to generalization, planned programming, maintenance, collateral behaviors, and functional analysis and assessment 3. Professional standards were commonly not adhered to, such as systematic assessment of individual client needs
Didden et al. (1997)	1. $N = 482$ studies (1968–1994) with 1,451 ESs, 34 topographies, and 64 treatments and 116 treatment combinations 2. 0 RCTs 3. Number of participants unclear but probably over 500. The percentage of comparisons by level of ID were profound (46%), severe (28.2%), moderate (14.8%), and mild/borderline (10.5%), and approximately 10% had ASD. The mean age was 16.4 years (SD = 10.8, range 1–66 years) 4. No measure of study quality applied	1. 26.5% of studies had PND >90%; 47.1% fairly effective, PND 70–90%; 23.5% questionable, PND 50–70%; and 2.9% cannot be treated reliably, PND <50% 2. Externally destructive behavior was more difficult to treat than internal maladaptive behavior and socially disruptive behavior 3. Response contingent procedures were more effective than all other treatments 4. Pharmacological treatments were least effective 5. Pretreatment functional analysis was associated with larger ESs	1. The majority of problems can be treated "quite" or "fairly" effective 2. Functional analysis increases ES

Harvey et al. (2009)	1. One hundred and forty-two articles (published 1988–2006) 2. 0 RCTs, 299 small N studies of which 76% were AB designs 3. $N = 316$ participants of whom 40% had ID and 33% had ASD 4. Did not measure study quality or analyze data separately by study quality	1. For single treatments, PNDs were 60%, 79%, and 49% for antecedent, skills replacement, and consequential intervention 2. For combined treatments, PNDs were 57%, 70%, 57%, and 59% for antecedent, skills replacement, consequential intervention, and systems change 3. For combined treatments and systems changes, PNDs were 60%, 59%, and 58% for no systems change, systems change, and single treatment 4. The authors reported ESs using SMD, PZD, and Allison-MT ESs also which produced divergent outcomes	1. "psychological (behavioral) treatments—compared to no treatment or conditions as usual—can clearly reduce even the most severe challenging behaviours" (p. 76) 2. "...there is no intervention used alone or in combination with others that was associated with highly effective results" (p. 76)
Heyvaert and et al. (2012)	1. $N = 285$ studies 2. N RCTs unclear but probably 0 3. $N = 598$ individuals 4. Meta-analysis did measure study quality which had no effect on ESs	1. The level of challenging behavior was 2.96 lower in treatment compared to baseline ($p < .0001$) 2. ESs were larger for antecedent interventions ($z = -2.67$, $p < .0076$) and for informing, educating, and training the environment ($z = -6.25$, $p < .0076$) 3. ESs were somewhat smaller for aggression and destructive behavior compared to other CBs such as SIB and stereotypy 4. Pretreatment functional analysis did not have an effect on ES	"interventions are on average highly effective in reducing C[hallenging] B[ehavior]" (p. 775)

Early meta-analyses published before 2000 focused on three basic questions: Does any treatment work? Are there effective alternatives to punishments? Does research evaluated functional assessment/analysis? All three used simple univariate analyses, such as reporting of mean effect sizes (ESs), disaggregations by topography, demographic variables or treatment types, and cross tabulations of ES, for example, of intervention restrictiveness by topography. Lennox, Miltenberger, Spengler, and Erfanian (1988) made relatively unqualified conclusions that interventions for general challenging behavior were effective, whereas both Lundervold and Bourland (1988) and Scotti and Evans (1991) qualified the same conclusions because of the relatively small number of high-quality studies, such as studies that included data on generalization, maintenance, and follow-up; however, all of these meta-analyses concluded that behavioral interventions produce some reduction in challenging behavior. More recent meta-analyses used large data sets with hundreds of experiments and participants, and some of them have used multivariate analyses, such as hierarchical linear modeling (Heyvaert, Maes, Van den Noortgate, Kuppens, & Onghena 2012). These last three meta-analyses (Didden, Duker, & Korzilius, 1997; Harvey, Boer, Meyer, & Evans, 2009; Heyvaert et al., 2012) indeed concluded the broad effectiveness of a wide range of behavioral approaches to challenging behavior and provided little data for the effectiveness of other treatments or even some evidence that other treatments such as psychopharmacology are significantly less effective (Didden et al., 1997; Heyvaert et al., 2012). The differences in the confidence of the conclusions made in these meta-analyses may in part reflect both the growing database over the last 40 years and the implicit application of different standards of evidence "effectiveness" in different meta-analyses. For example, applying Chambless and Hollon's (1998) relatively modest criteria, it is possible to meet the criteria for effectiveness with only reduction in the target behavior in three or more small *N* experiments with at least nine participants without social validity and other important considerations. If, however, one applied more rigorous standards in addition to basic requirements of a certain number of well-conducted experiments, such as requiring evidence of generalized change, maintenance, social validity, acquisition of replacement behavior, and lifestyle changes, many fewer studies would meet such rigorous criteria and a meta-analysis would be much less likely to make unqualified conclusions about treatment effectiveness.

Table 3.2 summarizes five meta-analyses focused on treatment of challenging behavior in specific populations such as children in early intervention (Scruggs, Mastropieri, Cook, & Escobar, 1986), autism (Campbell, 2003; Ma, 2009), children with ASD aged under 8 years (Horner, Carr, Strain, Todd, & Reed, 2002), and individuals with mild ID (Didden, Korzilius, van Oorsouw, & Sturmey, 2006). Most of these studies largely reflect the growing interest in ASD, especially in preschoolers and young children, and five of them were published on or after 2002. Although the sample sizes were adequate, the sample sizes were markedly smaller than those reported in Table 3.1 due the more focused questions asked. These meta-analyses were consistently positive in concluding the effectiveness of behavioral treatment of problem behavior within these specific populations, and none consistently identified

Table 3.2 Meta-analyses of Treatment of Challenging Behavior for Specific Populations

Reference	Study characteristics	Main findings	Conclusions
Scruggs et al. (1986)	1. $N=16$ small N studies of which 81% used experimental designs 2. 0 RCTs 3. $N=48$ preschoolers of whom 17% had ID or DD and 22% had ASD 4. Study quality was measured	1. The median PND was 79% (range 0–100%), ("moderate" ES) 2. Tangible reinforcement (mean PND=100) was more effective than attention (mean PND=13.5%) ($p<.007$) but not punishment/time-out (PND=75.5%) was more effective than attention ($p>.05$) 3. PND for generalization=44.5% (range=0–72%, $N=6$ participants) and for maintenance=100% ($N=15$ participants)	1. Tangible reinforcement produced the largest ESs
Horner et al. (2002)	1. $N=9$ articles (published 1996–2000) 2. 0 RCTs 3. $N=24$ participants aged <8 years with ASD 4. Used quality measure and only included better designed experiments	1. Mean reduction in problem behavior was 85% (median=93.2%, mode = –100%) 2. 22/37 comparisons had >90% reduction 3. 6/9 studies with 21/37 comparisons (57%) reported maintenance (mean = 12 weeks, up to 1 year) and in all cases remained within 15% of treatment data 4. 2/9 studies reported generalization data	1. "Reduction in behavior problems was impressive" (p. 432) 2. "there is reason for significant optimism" (p. 434) 3. More attention needs to be paid to base interventions on functional analysis

(Continued)

Table 3.2 (*Continued*)

Reference	Study characteristics	Main findings	Conclusions
Campbell (2003)	1. $N = 117$ articles including both experiments and AB designs (1966–1969) 2. 0 RCTs 3. $N = 181$ participants 4. Used and analyzed measure of article quality	1. Mean reduction in problem behavior as 76% (SD = 29%), PND = 84% (SD = 24%) (ZD = 43%) (all significantly different from 0, p's < .001) 2. There were no differences in ESs between treatments based on aversives, positives, combinations, or extinction 3. ESs were larger if there was a preintervention functional assessment for PND only 4. Quality of study affected ESs	"behavioral treatments were found to be significantly effective in reducing problem behavior in individuals with autism … Treatment was equally effective regardless of problem behavior and type of technique used … pretreatment functional assessment … result[ed] … in higher PZD treatment outcome scores" (p. 133)
Didden et al. (2006)	1. $N = 80$ small N experiments and nonexperiments (1980–2005) 2. $N = 0$ RCTs 3. $N = 150$ participants with mild ID; mean age = 14.5 years (range 2–42 years) 4. Measured and analyzed study quality	1. Mean PND and PZDs were 75% (range 0–100%, SD = 30%) and 35% (range 0–100%, DS = 32%) 2. Pretreatment functional analysis resulted in larger PND = 83% versus 62% ($p < .05$), PZDs = 46% versus 30% ($p < .01$) 3. Better quality studies often had larger ESs than AB studies	"challenging behavior was effectively treated using predominantly behavioral intervention methods and, to a lesser extent, with cognitive behavioral packages, such as anger management" (p. 296)
Ma (2009)	1. $N = 163$ articles 2. $N = 0$ RCTs 3. N individuals unclear, but presumably >163 were individuals with autism, the majority of whom also had ID, most of whom were under 12 years but included some adults 4. Coded experimental design, but no other quality measures	1. Mean PEM = 0.87 (SD = 0.25) "highly effective" and 87.5% of ESs were categorized as "highly effective" (PEM > 0.9) 2. Five most effective treatments (PEM > 0.9) were priming, self-control, training, combined reinforcement and punishment, and presenting preferred activities and reinforcers	Five treatments were considered "highly effective"

other effective treatments for challenging behavior, although Didden et al. (2006) found some qualified support for CBT in individuals with mild ID.

Table 3.3 summarizes two meta-analyses that have focused on the effectiveness of specific intervention methods for general challenging behavior including choice making (Shogren, Fagella-Luby, Jik Bae, & Wehmeyer, 2004) and the effects of different forms of functional assessment methodologies on treatment outcome (Herzinger & Campbell, 2007). These two meta-analyses produced somewhat different results. Namely, although choice making alone was effective, the ESs were somewhat more modest than those reported in previous tables, leading Shogren et al. (2004) to conclude that choice making was desirable as a component of behavioral packages, although they could not conclude that choice making alone was an evidence-based practice. Herzinger and Campbell (2007) reported moderate to large ESs for behavioral interventions but found evidence of somewhat larger ESs for those based on experimental functional analyses on one of the three ES measures.

Summary

Over the last 30 years, there have been 13 meta-analyses of general challenging behavior with different groups of authors. They have reviewed quite different samples of papers and used quite different statistical analyses, but all have concluded that behavioral interventions are effective. Due to the lack of experiments, there is little support from this literature for other forms of intervention, other than limited support for CBT (Didden et al., 2006). Additionally, the ESs for reductions on challenging behavior are typically moderate to large. The growing literature has permitted more refined conclusions over time. For example, some forms of behavioral interventions have smaller ESs than others, such as choice making alone (Shogren et al., 2004), and those not based on functional assessments and analyses (Herzinger & Campbell, 2007). Additionally, there is some evidence that those based on functional analyses have larger ESs than those based on behavioral assessments (Herzinger & Campbell). Thus, the basic three questions from over 30 years ago have largely been answered: There are some treatments for challenging behavior that are effective, there are effective alternatives to punishment, and basing interventions on functional assessment and analysis often produces larger ESs than interventions that are not based on functional analysis.

These meta-analyses have some significant limitations. First, they have focused almost exclusively on reductions in challenging behavior but have almost completely ignored the crucial question of acquisition of adaptive behavior to replace the target behavior. Focus on increasing adaptive behavior is a crucial aspect of PBS and current service ideology; thus, we lack some important information from these meta-analyses. Second, when these meta-analyses did report data on maintenance, generalization, and follow-up, the ES were sometimes similar to treatment ESs but sometime more variable; often, there was much less data available reducing the confidence in any conclusions that could be made. Third, these meta-analyses were

Table 3.3 A Summary of Two Meta-analyses of Specific Interventions Methods for General Challenging Behavior

Reference	Study characteristics	Main findings	Conclusions
Shogren et al. (2004)	1. Thirteen articles (published 1994–2002) 2. 0 RCTs 3. N = 30 participants (mean age 11 years, one participant aged 50 years, 23% with ASD, 17% with developmental disabilities, and 33% with mental retardation) 4. Did not include a quality measure	1. Mean PND and PZD were 66% (56 ESs, range 0–100%) and 42% (range 0–100%, 59 scores) ("questionable")	"[This does not suggest] that this is a moderately beneficial treatment, but rather that if all interventions included a choice-making component, the impact of these treatments might be considerably enhanced (although empirical research is necessary to determine if this hypothesis is true)" (p. 233)
Herzinger and Campbell (2007)	1. N = 56 articles, 21 of which used small N experimental designs (1998–2003) 2. N = 0 RCTs 3. N = 81 participants (78% with ID, 84% with ASD, mean age = 13 years, SD = 9.9)	1. ESs were larger for interventions based on functional than nonexperimental behavioral assessments using PZD (63% and 36%, respectively; p < .05), but not percentage reductions over baseline or PND 2. ESs were generally moderate to large for both experimental and nonexperimental methods (e.g., PNDs = 84% and 77%, respectively) 3. ESs were not different when broken down by function	"intervention packages based on the results of F[unctinal] A[nalyses] are more effective than those based on results of B[ehavioral] A[ssessments]" (p. 1439)

often based on a limited sample of the literature. This included both omission of the earlier literature and most meta-analyses not being updated since publication. Earlier studies may be omitted because they are not readily available on current databases. Meta-analyses are often not updated due to lack of resources to do so or because each meta-analysis is an individual project, rather than part of an ongoing organized effort to surveil the literature. Hence, some conclusions may be outdated and inaccurate, and some questions that are currently important are not addressed. Fourth, there are almost no RCTs addressing this question in these meta-analyses. Finally, almost all the studies have compared one treatment package to no treatment baseline. There was little evidence of parametric analyses of treatment components, component analyses of treatment packages, and head-to-head comparisons of treatment packages.

Specific Maladaptive Behavior

This section reviews meta-analyses of specific maladaptive behaviors. This documents the increasing specificity of meta-analyses as evidence has accumulated and can assist practitioners and family members in answering the more specific questions that are likely to need answers to. This section reviews meta-analyses on self-injurious behavior (SIB), pica, disruptive behavior, stereotyped movement disorder, pediatric feeding problems, and noncompliance.

Self-injurious behavior

This section extends an earlier review of meta-analyses of SIB (Sturmey, Maffei-Almodovar, Madzharova, & Cooper, 2012) which identified four meta-analyses of SIB (Christiansen, 2005, 2009; Kahng, Iwata, & Lewin, 2002) including one of skin picking (Lang et al., 2010) and by the addition of a more recent meta-analysis of SIB in individuals with profound ID (Denis, Van den Noortgate, & Maes, 2011). (See Table 3.4.)

The five meta-analyses all concurred that behavioral treatment was effective in treating SIB. This was true for meta-analyses that focused only on individuals with ASD and on individuals with profound ID. This indicates the robustness of these findings. Some concluded that behavioral treatment was effective, and some concluded that it was highly effective, whereas others tempered such conclusions, noting the potential problem of publication bias (Denis et al., 2011; Kahng et al., 2002). The only nonbehavioral treatment in these meta-analyses with data was sensory integration therapy (SIT), and Christiansen's (2009) meta-analysis found that the ESs for sensory treatments were not different from zero, that is, were ineffective. These meta-analyses suffered from some of the limitations noted elsewhere, namely, there was limited data on increasing replacement behavior, generalization, maintenance, and social validity.

Table 3.4 A Table of Meta-analyses of Psychosocial Treatments for Self-Injurious Behavior

Reference	Study characteristics	Main findings	Conclusions
Kahng et al. (2002)	1. $N = 393$ small N experiments (1964–2000) 2. $N = 0$ RCTs 3. $N = 706$ participants (71% with profound ID, 41% aged 19 years or older, 10% with ASD) 4. No measure of study quality but only included experiments	1. Mean ES was 84% reduction over baseline 2. Most behavioral treatment, including antecedent interventions, extinction, punishment, response blocking, and restraint, had at least an 80% reduction in SIB over baseline 3. ESs were smaller for reinforcement alone or combined with response blocking (approximate ESs = 73% in both cases) 4. Follow-up was reported in 14% of cases (range 2 weeks to 7 years) 5. Generalization was reported in 11% of cases mostly across settings (5% of cases) and therapists (4% of cases)	1. "Most treatments have been highly effective in reducing SIB" (p. 212) 2. High reported success rate may reflect publication bias
Christiansen (2005)	1. $N = 20$ studies, including both AB designs and small N experiments (1965–2003) 2. $N = 0$ RCTs 3. $N = 21$ participants with ASD aged up to 21 years 4. No quality measure reported	1. Using ITSACORR analysis mean ES as −2.32 2. The most effective treatment was aversives (ES = −2.83) 3. Interventions with positive and combined interventions had smaller effects (ES = −0.52 and −0.67, respectively) than aversives, but a second ES measure did not find these differences, indicating the ESs were the same magnitude	Concluded that behavioral treatment of SIB was effective in children with autism

Christiansen (2009)	1. $N = 224$ studies, including AB designs and small N experiments 2. $N = 0$ RCTs 3. $N = 343$ participants 4. No measure of study quality used	1. Mean ES was −3.55 ("large") and significantly different from 0 2. Combined aversives and nonaversives were most effective (ES = −4.19) followed by aversives alone (ES = −3.67), communication interventions (ES = −2.91), and nonaversives alone (ES = −0.89) 3. Sensory interventions had no effects	Behavioral interventions were very effective with large ESs
Lang et al. (2010)	1. $N = 16$ studies 2. $N = 0$ RCTs 3. $N = 19$ participants 4. Analyzed certainty of evidence by explicitly comparing AB designs and small N experimental designs	1. Mean PND was large (97%, range 75–100%) 2. Aversive, restraint, antecedent, and reinforcement-based interventions were all effective 3. Nine studies reported follow-up from 2 to 35 months	"none of the reviewed treatments would qualify as 'well established' … the reviewed studies do provide preliminary evidence that behavioral treatments may be effective for skin-picking topographies" (p. 313) due primarily to the small number of participants
Denis et al. (2011)	1. $N = 18$ studies (2000–2008) of nonaversive and nonintrusive treatments only 2. $N = 0$ RCTs 3. $N = 28$ individuals 4. Measured and analyzed study quality	1. SIB was reduced by approximately 2.5 standard deviations over baseline ($p < .001$)	1. "average effect of treatment was very large" (p. 911) 2. "contingent and non-contingent reinforcement are both effective" (p. 919) 3. Publication bias may be present

Pica

Hagopian, Rooker, and Rolider (2011) conducted a meta-analysis to identify interventions that met criteria for empirically supported treatments for pica. As part of that systematic review, they also calculated percentage reduction in pica from baseline to treatment and hence calculated ESs for these studies. They searched PsycINFO, PubMed, and Web of Science for articles published between 1980 and January 2011 that treated pica. Of 746 potentially relevant articles, only 34 contained sufficient information, all of which were small *N* experiments. They then coded them for participant and study characteristics, experimental design, experimental control, and efficacy with 96% reliability. For a treatment to be coded as effective, there had to be at least an 80% reduction in pica over baseline and that had to be present for at least two-thirds of participants when experiments had more than one participant. Twenty-six of thirty-four studies met this criterion. Of the 50 participants, 38% were adults, 36% were children, and 20% were adolescents, and most (31) had severe/profound or unreported (12) degree of ID.

All interventions were behavioral and included antecedent interventions and interventions using reinforcement and punishment and behavioral skills training. The studies were highly effective: 25 of 26 had an 80% or greater reduction, the other study had a 78% reduction, and 21 of 26 studies had a 90% or greater reduction. There was also sufficient data to report efficacy for separate treatments. Interventions based on functional analysis (26 studies) and reinforcement combined with response reduction procedures (response blocking, response effort manipulations, and punishment) (12 studies) met the criteria for *well-established* treatments, whereas treatments using reinforcement alone (6 studies) and response reduction alone (8 studies) only met the criteria for *probably efficacious* studies. Thus, there was strong evidence for behavioral treatment of pica as being highly effective and no evidence of the effectiveness of other treatments for pica.

McAdam, Breidbord, Dahl, and Williams (2012) independently conducted a meta-analysis of an overlapping set of 35 studies with 59 participants and made very similar conclusions. Like Hagopian et al. (2011), they concluded that behavioral treatment of pica was moderately effective (mean percentage nonoverlapping data (PND) = 77%) and produced some behavioral suppression (mean percentage zero data (PZD) = 33%). Further, using Chambless and Hollon (1998) criteria, they concluded that (a) noncontingent reinforcement (NCR) and environmental enrichment were nonrestrictive, well-established treatments; (b) overcorrection was a highly restrictive, well-established treatment; (c) physical restraint and response blocking were highly restrictive with limited evidence for short-term effectiveness; and (d) discrimination training, aversive stimuli, habit reversal, and negative practice all had insufficient evidence for short-term reduction in pica.

The literature on treatment of pica is interesting because it allows conclusions concerning specific behavioral treatments for a particular challenging behavior including nonrestrictive, well-established treatments. Further, neither meta-analysis identified any other treatment(s) that was effective.

Disruptive behavior

Chen and Ma (2007) conducted a meta-analysis of small N experiments and AB nonexperimental designs evaluating treatment of disruptive behavior which reported data on individuals with developmental disabilities. The authors defined disruptive behavior as "An excessive behavior that can interfere with the general activities proceeding at that time" (pp. 380–381). They identified 106 studies with 694 ESs. Although they did not report the numbers of individuals with developmental disabilities directly, 149, 28, 14, and 58 ESs were from participants with developmental or intellectual disabilities, ASD, brain damage, and developmental or intellectual disabilities and ASD, respectively, indicating that there was a substantial proportion of individuals with developmental disabilities in this meta-analysis. Almost all participants were children and adolescents (only 9 ESs were from adults). The authors used three measures of ES: PND, percentage exceeding baseline phase (PEM), and a three-point ad hoc rating of effectiveness.

The overall mean ESs were 64% (SD = 29%) and 84% (SD = 21%) for PND and PEM, respectively. Although the authors reported disaggregations of ES by treatment and target behavior, they are not reported here as the authors did not report them separately for individuals with developmental disabilities. The authors concluded that "intervention strategies were effective in the elimination of disruptive behaviors, especially, the strategies of differential reinforcement, the token economy system, and the multicomponent intervention were highly effective" (p. 389). Since there was a substantial proportion of participants with developmental disabilities in this meta-analysis, these conclusions are also likely to hold for individuals with developmental disabilities.

Stereotyped movement disorder

There have been two meta-analyses of treatment of stereotyped movement disorder. Wehmeyer (1995) identified 33 studies with 45 participants aged 3–53 years (mean ages = 14 and 18 years) for females and males, respectively, with a total of 164 ESs. The mean PND was 81% (SD = 32%), and the mean PZD was 36% (SD = 38%). Surprisingly, although there were no significant differences between PNDs between younger (aged 3–9 years) than older (aged 10–53 years), PZDs were 25% and 46%, respectively, indicating the complete elimination of stereotypy was more likely in older than younger participants, including adults. This meta-analysis was limited in that it did not apply a quality measure to the studies it included. (See Chapter 7 for a more detailed review of this topic.)

Pediatric feeding problems

The meta-analysis of pediatric feeding problems by Sharp, Jaquess, Morton, and Herzinger (2010) included approximately three-quarters of participants with some form of developmental delay. They analyzed data from 48 small N experiments (none were AB designs) published between 1989 and 2010. There were 96 participants of whom 31% had developmental delays, 24% had ASD, and 22% had ID and were aged 10 months–14 years (mean = 4 years).

The mean PND was 88% (SD = 30%, range 0–100%, "effective"), mean non-overlap of all pairs (NAPs) = 0.96 (SD = 0.12, range 0.29–1.00), and d = 2.46 ("large"). They concluded that this review provides further support for the use of behavioral intervention in the treatment of severe feeding disorders. "The identified studies represent a sound body of literature demonstrating significant improvement in mealtime behavior" (p. 359). This meta-analysis reported some data on study quality, including high IOA data and the inclusion of only experiments; however, the meta-analysis did not report data on generalization and maintenance.

Compliance

Lee (2005) conducted a meta-analysis of 28 studies on behavioral momentum ("high-probability request sequence"). There were 68 participants of whom approximately three-quarters had ID and/or ASD and 17% were adults.

The mean PND was 77% (SD = 29%). Intervention PNDs ranged from 59% (no disability) to 90% (behavior disorder) with mean PNDs for severe/profound ID, mild/moderate ID, ID with autism, and autism alone being 74%, 65%, 95%, and 94% respectively. ESs were markedly smaller for adults (PND = 49%) than for younger participants. Procedural variations in the high p sequence resulted in different ESs. ESs were larger when change agents reinforced the high p response (PND = 81%, SD = 28%) than when they did not (PND = 65%, SD = 28%). Also, ESs were larger when prompts were given in less than 5 s (PND = 79%, SD = 28%) and from 5 to 9 s (PND = 90%, SD = 15%) than when prompts were given after 10 s or more (PND = 67%, SD = 37%). The mean PND for generalization was 76% (30% of data series) and for follow-up was 71% (25% of series). The authors conclude that the intervention was effective, but "for the procedure to work well, the high-p sequence had to occasion compliance throughout intervention... [and] positive intervener consequences...for compliance to high-p requests seemed to enhance effectiveness" (p. 150).

Comment

The meta-analyses of interventions for specific forms of challenging behavior were uniformly positive about the effectiveness of behavioral interventions. This reflects the growing body of evidence on behavioral interventions that can answer questions related not only to maladaptive behavior generally, but to specific forms of challenging behavior.

Specific Interventions

Specific behavioral interventions

Function-based noncontingent reinforcement
Carr, Severtson, and Lepper (2009) conducted a meta-analysis of function-based NCR to treat challenging behavior. NCR included several procedural variations of NCR including fixed-time (FT) and variable-time (VT) schedule and packages that included schedule thinning with or without extinction. The authors screened articles fairly carefully to ensure they met a rather strict definition of function-based NCR, for example, articles must have conducted an experimental functional analysis of the target behavior and interventions. The authors identified 24 studies with 49 participants whose challenging behavior was treated by NCR. The participants' mean age was 18 years (range 3–56), 82% of whom were diagnosed with ID and 33% with ASD, most commonly treated for aggression (51%) and SIB (55%). The authors applied Chambless and Hollon (1998) and the APA Division 12 Task Force criteria. Namely, a "well-established treatment" required at least nine studies by at least two groups of researchers, a "probably efficacious" treatment needed three to eight studies, and if there were fewer than three studies, the treatment was "experimental." Based on this, the only treatment that met criteria for "well established" was FT schedule thinning (mean PND = 71%, SD = 38%, 11 studies). The following two treatments met the criteria for "probably efficacious": FT + extinction (EXT) (PND = 67%, SD = 39%, 8 studies) and VT schedule + EXT (3 studies, 7 participants, PND = 81%, SD = 32%). Finally, two treatments met the criteria for "experimental treatments": FT alone (2 studies, 5 participants, PND = 84%, SD = 32%) and FT + schedule thinning (1 study, 2 participants, PND = 93%, SD = 11%). (The authors also reported mean baseline reduction (MBLR) data.) The authors concluded that NCR "has produced robust effects across a variety of response topographies and reinforcement functions" (p. 54).

Augmentative and alternative communication
Chapter 2 contains an extensive discussion of the evidence for the effectiveness of augmentative and alternative communication (AAC) including PECS on acquisition of communication skills. Walker and Snell (2013) also reported a meta-analysis of the effects of AAC on challenging behavior. They meta-analyzed data from 54 small N experiments with 111 participants. Most (70%) participants were aged less than 12 years, although 14% were aged over 18 years and most had diagnoses of ID (75%) and/or ASD (35%). They used NAPs as the ES. The overall NPA was 0.88 (SD = 0.18, range 0.11–1.00, "medium" to "moderate"). Interestingly, NAPs were larger for functional communication training (FCT) (mean = 0.87) than PECS (0.74) and larger for studies using a functional assessment (0.88) than those that did not (0.72), although NAPs did not differ when experimental and descriptive functional assessments were compared (0.90 and 0.85, respectively). NAPs were also larger for younger children than older children and adults and for those with better

communication skills prior to intervention. The authors concluded that AAC was effective in treating challenging behavior, that effects were larger when AAC is based on a FBA, and that FCT was superior to PECS in the communication-based treatment of challenging behavior. The reader is referred back to Chapter 2 for a review of the rather modest effects of PECS on challenging behavior.

Positive behavioral support

Carr et al. (1999) defined the goals of PBS as "to apply behavioral principles in the community in order to reduce problem behavior and build appropriate behavior that result in durable change and a rich lifestyle" (p. 3). This is done by (a) remediating deficient contexts, by providing choice, teaching adaptive behavior, and providing appropriate materials and activities and appropriate routines, and (b) remediating deficient behavioral repertoires through teaching skills and having an environment that support use of these skills. PBS intervention methods include proactive interventions based on functional assessment and analysis that teaches skills in context in typical settings (not institutions or segregated day services), provides a better lifestyle, using nonaversive antecedent and consequential interventions. Interventions such as punishment, including time-out and DRO, are excluded, although the status of extinction as PBS intervention is unclear. Finally, PBS involves consumer participation and evaluation system-wide change, such as school-wide reduction in punishment, such as office discipline procedures.

Table 3.5 summarizes three meta-analyses of PBS. One focused on PBS generally (Carr et al., 1999; Marquis et al., 2000), one on school settings (Goh & Bambara, 2010), and one only on system interventions (Solomon, Klein, Hintze, Cressey, & Peller, 2012). Carr et al.'s early meta-analysis reported ESs for PBS studies on aggression, SIB, tantrums, and property destruction. There was evidence of moderate reductions in challenging behavior in about half of cases, and approximately half of the studies were rated as "effective." There were only moderate quantity of data on generalization and maintenance, very little data on social validity, and lifestyle changes, and few studies addressed systems interventions, such as environmental reorganization.

Nearly 20 years later, Goh and Bambara (2010) also found similar positive outcomes for function-based interventions that use both antecedents and consequences in natural settings, etc., but little research addressing system-wide and lifestyle interventions. Finally, Solomon et al. could only conclude that school-wide interventions were "promising," but not "well established," due to the modest but highly variable ESs, small number of experiments, and almost complete absence of treatment integrity data.

Since the inception some 30 years ago, the PBS movement has documented individual outcomes on challenging and adaptive behavior similar to those reported for its ABA components, such as function-based antecedent and consequential interventions. To date, there is little evidence to support either the PBS-specific

Table 3.5 A Summary of Three Meta-analyses of Positive Behavioral Support

Reference	Study characteristics	Main findings	Conclusions
Carr et al. (1999)	1. $N = 109$ small N experiments (1985–1996) 2. $N = 0$ RCTs 3. $N = 230$ participants mostly aged 5–19, although 72 were adults; most had ID, ASD, or both 4. Quality assurance took place through articles selection that met criteria for small N experiments on PBS	1. Only 41% of articles reported data on skill acquisition with 37, 31, 25, and 22 outcomes involving 0–15, 25–50, 50–75, and 75–100% increase in adaptive behavior over baseline 2. Approximately two-thirds resulted in 80% or greater reduction in challenging behavior over baseline with slightly larger outcomes for reinforcement- than antecedent-based interventions (67% vs. 72% with >80% reduction in target behavior) 3. Few studies reported stimulus and response generalization (approximately 7% of articles for each) 4. Reductions over baseline were 69%, 64%, and 71% for follow-up at 1–5, 6–12, and 13–24 months, respectively 5. There were lifestyle change and social validity data for only 24/230 and 29 participants 6. ESs were somewhat larger for interventions using natural change agents than others (55% vs. 42% reduction in challenging behavior) 7. There was little evidence (only 13 ESs) that environmental reorganization resulted in larger reductions in challenging behavior (65% vs. 51%)	1. "slightly less than half the outcomes demonstrated modest to substantial increases in socially desirable responses" (p. 66) 2. "a 90% or more reduction criterion was established that yielded a success rate of 51.6%" (p. 67) 3. "about half of the outcomes could be categorized as successes" (p. 67)

(Continued)

Table 3.5 *(Continued)*

Reference	Study characteristics	Main findings	Conclusions
Goh and Bambara (2010)	1. Eighty-three small *N* experiments (1997–2008) 2. *N* = 145 school-age participants 70 with ID and/or ASD 3. *N* = 0 RCTs 4. Quality of articles addressed through screening for the presence of experimental design, etc.	1. Median PNDs were 88% (range 0–100%), 80% (range 0–100%), and 90% (range 0–100) for overall, challenging behavior and appropriate behavior 2. Median PNDs were 100% (range 0–100, 28 students) and 94% (range 0–100%, 12 students) for maintenance (1 week to 24 months) and generalization, respectively 3. Most PNDs were moderate and some were large 4. Thirty-nine percent of experiments reported social validity data	"FBA interventions applied in school settings can effectively reduce problem behavior of students and increase their use of appropriate skills, with moderate effect sizes for both … interventions yielded effective maintenance… these overall findings for intervention effects are positive"
Solomon et al. (2012)	1. Twenty studies (1993–2008) including 12 small *N* experimental designs and 8 AB designs, which yielded 21 ESs 2. *N* = 0 RCTs 3. *N* participants not available as studies used classrooms and schools as the "subject" 4. Analyzed ESs for experiments and nonexperiments and found no difference in ES, but no other measure of quality was reported	1. There were moderate positive ESs (r-squared ranged from .27 to .60) 2. ESs were larger in structured settings (CI = 0.44–0.63) than classrooms (CI = 0.18–0.36)	"results were promising: … effect sizes on problem behavior was in the low average range … school-wide PBS is moderately effective in reducing problem behavior in students" (p. 2011)

interventions, such as school-wide and lifestyle interventions, or more global outcomes such as lifestyle changes.

Cognitive behavioral therapy

There have been four meta-analyses of CBT: one related to children with ASD (White, 2004), two related to anger management (Hamelin, Travis, & Sturmey, 2013; Nicoll, Beail, & Saxon, 2013), and one related to anger management only with adults (National Institute for Clinical Excellence [NICE], 2012). White's meta-analysis of CBT was unable to find any good-quality studies and so could not perform a meta-analysis; however, this meta-analysis is 10 years old, and hence, its conclusions may be inaccurate due to exclusion of evidence over the last 10 years.

When it comes to CBT for anger in individuals with ID, researchers do not agree if the glass is half full or half empty! Two independently conducted meta-analyses of substantially overlapping group trials of anger management in adults with ID both agreed that ESs were large but disagreed on the interpretation of this finding. Nicoll et al. (2013) conducted a meta-analysis of nine group studies, including two RCTs, and found a mean standard difference of 0.88 (CI = 0.55–2.03, $N = 168$); two additional meta-analyses of subsets of these nine studies also found ESs with similar magnitude. The authors also rated the quality of the studies using a standard quality checklist and concluded that the quality of studies had improved over time and some were of good quality as they used reliable and valid measures of anger and "a good level of methodological rigor in the studies" (p. 60). Hamelin et al. meta-analyzed eight group-design studies including two RCTs which overlapped considerably with the previous meta-analysis. They reported a between-groups ES of $d = 1.52$ and $d = 0.89$ for other studies (both "large"). In contrast to Nicoll et al., they concluded that "anger management is not an empirically supported treatment in individuals with ID." They did so because of the poor quality of the studies, citing problems such as the failure to report clinical significance, treatment integrity, and the possibility that effects were due to changes in staff behavior before and after the treatment. Finally, NICE (2012) conducted a meta-analysis of three poor-quality quasiexperiments evaluating anger management in adults and reported a statistically significant effect. Thus, at this time, there is disagreement about the status of the evidence for the effectiveness of anger management with individuals with ID.

Summary

This chapter has summarized evidence from multiple meta-analyses of psychosocial treatment of maladaptive behavior in children and adults with developmental disabilities, both general challenging behavior, specific forms of challenging behavior, and specific interventions for challenging behavior. These meta-analyses had several common characteristics. First, almost all of the evidence was related to behavioral and behavior analytic interventions, although some relates to CBT and other psychosocial interventions. Almost all reported relatively large ESs for the effectiveness of behavioral and behavior analytic interventions. Exceptions to that can be found when meta-analyses asked questions focused on specific interventions and specific problems. Although evidence is accumulating for the effectiveness of CBT, most of this evidence comes from RCTs and other group designs, where issues of treatment integrity, generalization, maintenance, and social validity have yet to be addressed effectively. Second, the majority were meta-analyses of small *N* experiments. For some, this limits the confidence one can have in these conclusions, since they are largely not based on RCTs. Finally, almost all—but not quite all—evidence related to children and adolescents, although there was a smaller quantity of evidence related to adults with disabilities. Again, this limits the confidence one can have concerning the application of these conclusions to adults from this literature, although there may be many experiments on effectiveness of psychosocial interventions for adults that have not yet been addressed by meta-analysis.

References

Campbell, J. M. (2003). Efficacy of behavioral interventions for reducing problem behavior in persons with autism: A quantitative synthesis of single-subject research. *Research in Developmental Disabilities, 24,* 120–138.

Carr, E. G., Horner, R. H., Turnbull, A. P., Marquis, J. G., McLaughlin, D. M., McAtee, M. L., et al. (1999). *Positive behavior support for people with developmental disabilities: A research synthesis.* Washington, DC: American Association on Mental Retardation.

Carr, J. E., Severtson, J. M., & Lepper, T. L. (2009). Noncontingent reinforcement is an empirically supported treatment for problem behavior exhibited by individuals with developmental disabilities. *Research in Developmental Disabilities, 30,* 44–57.

Chambless, D. L., & Hollon, S. D. (1998). Defining empirically supported therapies. *Journal of Consulting and Clinical Psychology, 66,* 7–18.

Chen, C. W., & Ma, H. H. (2007). Effects of treatment on disruptive behaviors: A quantitative synthesis of single-subject researches using the PEM approach. *The Behavior Analyst Today, 8,* 380–396.

Christiansen, E. (2005). Effectiveness of behavioral treatment for reduction of self-injury in autism: A meta-analysis (Unpublished Masters thesis). *Dissertation Abstracts International: Section B. Sciences and Engineering, 71*(1-B), 647.

Christiansen, E. (2009). Effectiveness of interventions targeting self-injury in children and adolescents with developmental disabilities: A meta-analysis. *Dissertation Abstracts International: Section B. Sciences and Engineering, 71*(1-B), 647.

Denis, J., Van den Noortgate, W., & Maes, B. (2011). Self-injurious behavior in people with profound intellectual disabilities: A meta-analysis of single-case studies. *Research in Developmental Disabilities, 32,* 911–923.

Didden, R., Duker, P., & Korzilius, H. (1997). Meta-analytic study on treatment effectiveness for problem behaviors with individuals who have mental retardation. *American Journal on Mental Retardation, 101,* 387–399.

Didden, R., Korzilius, H., van Oorsouw, W., & Sturmey, P. (2006). Behavioral treatment of challenging behaviors in individuals with mild mental retardation: Meta-analysis of single-subject research. *American Journal on Mental Retardation, 111*, 290–298.

Goh, A. E., & Bambara, L. M. (2010). Individualized positive behavior support in school settings: A meta-analysis. *Remedial and Special Education, 33*, 271–286.

Hagopian, L. P., Rooker, G. W., & Rolider, N. U. (2011). Identifying empirically supported treatments for pica in individuals with intellectual disabilities. *Research in Developmental Disabilities, 32*, 2114–2120.

Hamelin, J., Travis, R., & Sturmey, P. (2013). Anger management and intellectual disabilities: A systematic review. *Journal of Mental Health Research, 6*, 60–70.

Harvey, S. T., Boer, D., Meyer, L. H., & Evans, I. M. (2009). Updating a meta-analysis of intervention research with challenging behaviour: Treatment validity and standards of practice. *Journal of Intellectual & Developmental Disability, 34*, 67–80.

Herzinger, C. V., & Campbell, J. M. (2007). Comparing functional assessment methodologies: A quantitative synthesis. *Journal of Autism and Developmental Disabilities, 37*, 1430–1445.

Heyvaert, M., Maes, B., Van den Noortgate, W., Kuppens, S., & Onghena, P. (2012). A multi-level meta-analysis of single-case and small-n research on the interventions for reducing challenging behavior in persons with intellectual disabilities. *Research in Developmental Disabilities, 33*, 766–780.

Horner, R. H., Carr, E. G., Strain, P. S., Todd, A. W., & Reed, H. K. (2002). Problem behavior interventions for young children with autism: A research synthesis. *Journal of Autism and Developmental Disorders, 32*, 423–446.

Kahng, S., Iwata, B. A., & Lewin, A. B. (2002). Behavioral treatment of self-injury, 1964 to 2000. *American Journal on Mental Retardation, 107*, 212–221.

Lang, R., Didden, R., Machalicekc, W., Rispoli, M., Sigafoos, J., Lancioni, G., et al. (2010). Behavioral treatment of chronic skin- picking in individuals with developmental disabilities: A systematic review. *Research in Developmental Disabilities, 31*, 304–315.

Lee, D. L. (2005). Increasing compliance: A quantitative synthesis of applied research on high-probability request sentences. *Exceptionality, 13*, 141–154.

Lennox, D. B., Miltenberger, R. G., Spengler, P., & Erfanian, N. (1988). Decelerative treatment practices with persons who have mental retardation: A review of five years of the literature. *American Journal on Mental Retardation, 92*, 492–501.

Lundervold, D., & Bourland, G. (1988). Quantitative analysis of treatment aggression, self-injury, and property destructive. *Behavior Modification, 12*, 590–617.

Ma, H. H. (2009). A meta-analysis using percentage of data points exceeding the median of baseline phase (PEM). *Behavior Modification, 33*, 339–359.

Marquis, J. G., Horner, R. H., Carr, E. G., Turnbull, A. P., Thompson, M., Behrens, G. A., et al. (2000). A meta-analysis of positive behavior support. In R. Gersten, E. P. Schiller, & S. Vaughn (Eds.), *Contemporary special education research: Synthesis of the knowledge base on critical issues* (pp. 137–178). Mahwah, NJ: Erlbaum.

McAdam, D., Breidbord, J., Dahl, A., & Williams, D. E. (2012). Pica. In M. Hersen & P. Sturmey (Eds.), *Handbook of evidence-based practice in clinical psychology: Vol. 1. Children and adolescents* (pp. 323–338). New York: Wiley.

National Institute for Clinical Excellence [NICE]. (2012). *Autism. The NICE guideline on recognition, referral diagnosis and management of adults on the autism spectrum.* The British Psychological Society. Leicester, UK: British Psychological Society and The Royal College of Psychiatrists.

Nicoll, M., Beail, N., & Saxon, D. (2013). Cognitive behavioural treatment for anger in adults with intellectual disabilities: A systematic review and meta-analysis. *Journal of Applied Research in Intellectual Disabilities, 26*, 47–62.

Scotti, J. R., & Evans, I. M. (1991). A meta-analysis of intervention research with problem behavior: Treatment validity and standards of practice. *American Journal on Mental Retardation, 96*, 233–256.

Scotti, J. R., Evans, I. M., Meyer, L. H., & Walker, P. (1991). A meta-analysis of intervention research with problem behavior: Treatment validity and standards of practice. *American Journal on Mental Retardation, 96*, 233–256.

Scruggs, T. E., Mastropieri, M. A., Cook, S. B., & Escobar, C. (1986). Early intervention for children with conduct disorders: A quantitative synthesis of single-subject research. *Behavioral Disorders, 11*, 260–271.

Sharp, W. G., Jaquess, D. L., Morton, J. F., & Herzinger, C. V. (2010). Pediatric feeding disorders: A quantitative synthesis of treatment outcomes. *Clinical Child and Family Psychology Review, 13*, 348–365.

Shogren, K. A., Fagella-Luby, M. N., Jik Bae, S., & Wehmeyer, M. L. (2004). The effect of choice-making as an intervention for problem behavior: A meta-analysis. *Journal of Positive Behavior Interventions, 6*, 228–237.

Solomon, B. G., Klein, S. A., Hintze, J. M., Cressey, J. M., & Peller, S. L. (2012). A meta-analysis of school-wide positive behavior support: An exploratory study using single-case synthesis. *Psychology in the Schools, 49*, 105–121.

Sturmey, P., Maffei-Almodovar, L., Madzharova, M., & Cooper, J. (2012). Self-injurious behavior. In P. Sturmey & M. Hersen (Eds.), *The handbook of evidence-based practice in clinical psychology: Vol. 1. Children and adolescents* (pp. 477–492). Hoboken, NJ: Wiley.

Walker, V. L., & Snell, M. E. (2013). Effects of augmentative and alternative communication on challenging behavior: A meta-analysis. *Augmentative and Alternative Communication, 29*, 117–131.

Wehmeyer, M. L. (1995). Intra-individual factors influencing efficacy of interventions for stereotyped behaviours: A meta-analysis. *Journal of Intellectual Disability Research, 39*, 205–214.

White, A. H. (2004). Cognitive behavioural therapy in children with autistic spectrum disorder. *STEER. Succinct and Timely Evaluated Evidence Reviews, 4*(5). Bazian Ltd. and Wessex Institute for Health Research & Development, University of Southampton. Retrieved October 24, 2013, from http://www.signpoststeer.org/

4

But Is It Worth It?

Peter Sturmey

Intellectual Disabilities Services Are Often Expensive

The costs of intellectual disabilities (ID) services are often very great reflecting the lifelong use of services for many individuals and the use of highly staffed services by some. These high costs are exemplified by Knapp, Romeo, and Beecham's (2009) study which estimated the costs for children and adults with autism in the United Kingdom were £2.7 billion and £25 billion per year, respectively. Mean annual costs for children were a function of age, ID, and residence: Services for older children, those in residential care and those with ID were the most expensive. For example, the annual costs for children with ASD and ID in residential care were £16,185, £405,788, and £62,536 for children aged 0–3, 4–11, and 12–17, respectively. Mean annual costs for children with ASD and ID aged 12–17 living with families and in residential care were £36,474 and £62,536, respectively. There were also similar large effects of residence and ID on costs for adults with ASD. The largest cost for children was education, which accounted for approximately three-quarters of the average cost, and the largest costs for adults were accommodation and lost employment. Other evidence of the high cost of services comes from Jarbrink, Fombonne, and Knapp (2003) who estimated that the weekly cost of children with autism was £689.21 (or £35,832 per year) and the largest costs were parental income loss, education, and early intervention therapy. Other economic analyses of autism have confirmed large costs for childhood (Chasson, Harris, & Nely, 2007; Jacobson & Mulik, 2000; Jacobson, Mulik, & Green, 1998; Jarbrink et al., 2003; Leslie & Martin, 2007; Motiwala, Gupta, & Lilly, 2006; Paps & Dyson, 2004; Peng, Hatlestad, Klug, Kerbeshian, & Burd, 2009; Peters-Scheffer, Didden, Korzilius, & Matson, 2012),

Evidence-Based Practice and Intellectual Disabilities, First Edition.
Edited by Peter Sturmey and Robert Didden.
© 2014 John Wiley & Sons, Ltd. Published 2014 by John Wiley & Sons, Ltd.

adults (Cimera & Cowan, 2009), and lifetime costs (Ganz, 2007). For example, Ganz estimated that individual lifetime costs were $3.2 million and lifetime costs of one cohort were $13–$76 billion. Further, the total costs of autism services continue to increase due to increased numbers of individuals (Bouder, Spielman, & Mandell, 2009; Cimera & Cowen, 2009; Leslie & Martin, 2007; Motiwala et al., 2006; Peng et al., 2009), increased costs per individual (Boulder et al., 2009; Leslie & Martin, 2007), and serving children from a younger age than in the past. Such concerns about increasing service costs often take place in the context of expansion of early intervention services and the potential increased costs to states and individuals for health insurance (Boulder et al.) and, as more children are identified than in the past, in the context of larger cohorts of children with ASD coming through preschool, to school, and then to adult services.

These data have important implications for EBP. Yet, despite its importance, it has been largely ignored, although a recent systematic review identified 10 such studies (Romeo & Molosankwe, 2010). Psychosocial interventions that could reduce the costs of education in children could be very socially significant. For example, early intervention that could avoid or delay special education and the costs of adult services and increase the individual's productivity, such as intensive early behavioral intervention, could be highly efficient, cost-effective services. Likewise, services for adults that reduce the costs of accommodation and staffing and increase employment could also have large economic benefits to individuals, their families, and society. In addition, there are probably large individual differences in costs related to behavior management practices, such as one-on-one staffing and out-of-home and out-of-district placements. Any interventions that can delay or avoid these costs could have considerable economic benefits.

Economic data are also useful to evaluate service efficiency. For example, Cimera and Cowan (2009) found that the costs of serving adults with autism in the U.S. vocational system decreased from 2002 to 2006 without any reduction in the hours worked per person served, suggesting that the agency had become more efficient. On the other hand, some services are highly staffed but ineffective. Such services are damned twice: first for spending too much money and second for failing to achieve client outcomes. (Such arguments, e.g., have been applied as partial rationales for deinstitutionalization but also apply to psychosocial treatments.)

Reluctance to Address Economic Evaluations

As noted in earlier chapters, some professionals are reluctant to embrace the implications of EBP. Economic evaluations of EBPs highlight this issue: Who will deny treatment to a person with ID on economic grounds? The reluctance to directly address the economic aspects of EBP is illustrated by Taylor and Knapp (2013), who wrote that "the fundamental purpose of psychological and other therapies is not to save money to achieve cost-effectiveness; it is to improve the health and well-being of individuals with (in this case) mental health needs, as well as the well-being of significant others, such as family members" (p. 9). These authors appear to explicitly oppose economic considerations of treatment but do so by misstating the rationale for economic analysis of EBP. Contrast their quote with how Knapp and McDaid (2012) described economics of EBP: "The primary concerns of anyone working in a mental health system are alleviation of symptoms, promotion of quality of life, support of family caregivers, and improvement of broad family chances. These should also be the primary concerns of those people with responsibility for the allocation of resources, whether it is deciding how many resources can be made available for part or whole of the system, how they are shared between competing use, or how to improve efficiency and fairness in their use. The common threads running through these concerns are that: (a) resources are scarce relative to the needs of the population; (b) therefore careful choices have to be made about how to utilize them; and (c) the criteria employed in making those choices should be linked in some way to the aim of the system, which is to improve the health and quality of life" (p. 71). Thus, economic analysis does indeed concern itself with client outcomes and quality of life but states the rationale for economic analysis explicitly and rationally.

Everyone can understand reluctance to embrace economic analysis of treatment; after an era of economic hardship, deinstitutionalization, reorganization, privatization, outsourcing, downsizing, rightsizing, contracting services, and contracting out of services, many feel battered by economic evaluations of services which mostly seem aimed to save money, rather than serving clients and their families more effectively. But none of us can avoid this issue: When we see one client, we deny resources to another; when we chose one therapy, we deny access to another kind of therapy; when we see clients in groups, we deny them access to individual treatment.

As we have seen elsewhere, some claim that there is no evidence to guide EBP in ID. This is illustrated again by Taylor and Knapp (2013) when they write that "The difficulty that the field of intellectual disabilities and mental health faces is that the interventions that are available and for which there is an evidence base that they work (in terms of improving health and well-being) cannot point to cost savings for public budgets … There has been little investigation of this area" (p. 9). Both previous and subsequent chapters show that there is considerable evidence available and while it is certainly true that there has been much less economic analysis of EBP in ID, it is not true that there is none as this chapter will show.

Methodologies to Evaluate Costs and Benefits

How do we evaluate the cost and benefits of psychosocial treatments? The economics of EBP uses at least four types of methodologies (Foster & McCombs-Thornton, 2012). *Benefit–cost analysis* calculates whether the economic benefits exceed the cost of treatment. If they do, then this is deemed to be a desirable treatment. This then raises the question as to whether society wishes to pay for the resources and outcomes. For example, society may be willing to invest a lot of money in expensive, effective treatment when the benefits are immediate and large, such as returning people to work and eliminating treatments and other costs, but society may be reluctant to do if the benefits only occur (some or many) years in the future. *Cost-effectiveness analysis* (CEA) estimates the costs of a unit of outcome, such as a one-point reduction on a depression scale, obtaining employment for one person for a year, or percentage reduction in the prevalence of a problem. *Cost–utility analysis* is a form of CEA in which the outcome is some global measure of benefit, such as quality-adjusted life year (QALY) (see the succeeding text). Finally, there are *costs of illness studies* which calculate the costs of treatment and the economic effects of treatment on employment, but do not calculate the costs of pain and suffering.

Economic analysis of treatment benefits can be calculated for different program participants. Economic benefits and costs may accrue to direct program participants, such as a person in a supported employment program. Economic benefits and costs may accrue to funding agents, such as the government funding a supported employment program, who expends money funding the program and potentially gains from increased taxes paid and avoiding even more expensive public programs. Other interested parties may also gain benefits or incur costs. For example, an employer may gain from having a better trained, more productive employee or receive tax credits from the funding program. Similarly, a family member may also benefit or incur costs. Benefits may also accrue to family members who may no longer incur lost income and who may gain income if they too can work, when their family with a disability works in a supported employment program (Cimera, 2000, 2002 Conley, Rusch, McCaughran, & Tines, 1989).

Benefits may not accrue to all interested parties. For example, Conley et al. (1989) reported that a supported employment program in Illinois increased participants' income beyond that which they would have otherwise earned by approximately $710 per year. In contrast, the taxpayer received only approximately $0.75 cents back for every dollar invested. Other apparently paradoxical outcomes are also possible, such as when society benefits from a program, but individuals lose money (Lewis, Johnson, Bruininks, Kallen, & Guillery, 1992).

Economic analyses of health and education programs also raise broader questions including whether the economic benefits from psychosocial treatments are more or less than other uses of the same resources. Perhaps money spent on treating depression would result in bigger savings if spent on roads and bridges. Society can also choose to forgo maximum financial gains in order to pursue social justice goals. For example, one might fund a supported employment program that *costs* the taxpayer money in order to pursue socially valued goals such as community integration of adults with disabilities or achieve better outcomes for groups that have historically been discriminated against (Lewis et al., 1992).

This section showed that there are a range of methodologies to conduct economic analyses of psychosocial treatments for individuals with ID. These economic evaluations raise practical and ethical questions over the choices of treatment and make explicit what the benefits of psychosocial treatments might be to different interested parties. The next section goes on to review the examples of economic evaluations of psychosocial treatments for individual with ID.

Applications

Data on the costs and benefits of psychosocial interventions are scattered but have addressed several interventions. These include toilet training, supported employment, early intensive behavioral intervention for autism, behavior management, and reduction of unnecessary psychotropic medication.

Toilet training

Some skills training programs have the potential to save costs by reducing staffing and other costs, such as those that arise from failure to provide treatment, such as medical costs or costs of other ineffective treatments. Incontinence is a highly expensive and avoidable disability that accrues costs from staff, costs of diapers, and the costs of medical complications, such as preventable urinary tract infections and unnecessary medical evaluations and ineffective medical treatments. Further, personal goals such as achieving continence are usually highly valued: Children and adults who are incontinent are often evaluated negatively because of the appearance of diapers, odor, and personal incompetence often assumed by others. Thus, independent toileting is a skill that is consonant with current service ideology which emphasizes autonomy and competence as valued outcomes.

Hyams, McCoull, Smith, and Tyrer (1992) reported a 10-year follow-up on toilet training with 14 individuals with severe and profound ID in which they randomly assigned 15 children with severe and profound ID to three intensities of toilet training. The first group received regular, individual toilet training which involved prompting at set intervals to use the toilet. In the second group, participants were taught to go to the toilet after a toileting accident occurred. The third group received less intense group training. At follow-up, they were aged 18–29 years old. Group 1 had 67, 1, and 8 episodes of incontinence at pretraining, posttraining, and 10-year follow-up, respectively, for a 99% and 88% reduction in toileting accidents at the end of training and 10-year follow-up, respectively. Group 2 had 117, 23, and 30 incidents of incontinence at pretraining, posttraining, and 10-year follow-up, respectively, for and 80% and 52% reduction at posttraining and 10-year follow-up, respectively. Finally, group 3 had 86, 52, and 41 episodes of incontinence at pretraining, posttraining, and 10-year follow-up, respectively, for a 39% and 52% reduction in incontinence at posttraining and 10-year follow-up. Hyams et al. based their estimations that the costs of toileting were primarily due to the time taken to physically prompt and escort to someone to the bathroom after a toileting accident and that verbal or gestural prompts involved insignificant extra staff time. Thus, they estimated that treatment had saved 2.2 and 2.5 staff hours per person per week in groups 1 and 2, respectively, compared to group 3. They estimated that the initial costs of treatment were recouped after 41 and 47 weeks for groups 1 and 2, respectively. They estimated that the total saving for all three groups over 10 years was 52,000 staff hours.

This paper was limited because it did not systematically assess the costs and savings of toilet training. For example, it did not include the savings from reduction of consumption of diapers and assessment and treatment of medical conditions associated with lifelong incontinence. Also, it did not demonstrate that the potential savings in staff hours actually occurred and did not convert the hours saved into monetary units.

Two factors likely influence the economics of toilet training. Greatest savings will accrue from those methods that are most efficient. There are a number of toilet training procedures which vary considerably in their intensity and effectiveness. For example, Azrin's and Foxx (1971) highly effective *Toilet Training in One Day* procedure results in very rapid acquisition of continence and maintenance data. Smith (1979) concluded that intensive toilet training was more cost-effective than less intense interventions. This procedure also reduces staff treatment costs and allows treatment of the greatest number of participants. Second, savings will be increased by starting as early as possible, thereby maximizing the avoidance of subsequent service costs over many years. Thus, intensive toilet training programs started as early as possible for those individuals most likely to not become continent by routine care are likely to be most economically beneficial and enhance individual independence for the longest period of time.

Other skills training programs that increase adaptive behavior, such as dressing, feeding, and transportation, also have the potential for large savings from reducing the cost of care. To date, data are lacking to support this possibility. Future research should address this possibility.

Supported employment

Supported employment may offer economic benefits to society including reduced government subsidies, increased taxes paid, and reduced costs of ineffective programming, such as sheltered workshops. Supported employment also accrues costs, such as the costs of operating the supported employment program and employer tax credits. Several economic analyses have found relatively consistent support for the economic benefits for supported employment using cost efficiency analyses (Cimera, 2010, 2011, 2012), including adults with autism (Cimera & Burgess, 2011; National Institute for Clinical Excellence [NICE], 2012), benefit–cost accounting (Lewis et al., 1992), and benefit–cost analysis (Hill et al., 1987). The most recent review (Cimera, 2012) updated earlier reviews by including research pub-lished since 2000. Cimera concluded that supported employment is robust in providing economic benefits to the individual with disabilities and the taxpayer. Indeed, Cimera (2012) presented data showing that the wages in sheltered work-shops had declined but in supported employment wages had increased during this decade. This resulted in economic benefits to all concerned.

Not all economic analyses have found such cost–benefit analyses of supported employment (Conley et al., 1989). The outcomes also vary by the U.S. state (Cimera,

2010, 2011). These varied outcomes might reflect the factors such as smaller economic benefits when programs are first set up and have high initial costs and the smallest worker benefits and degree of client disability, since clients with more severe disability may require more training and need greater support than clients with less severe disability (Lewis et al., 1992). It may also reflect the ongoing level of unemployment and availability of work for everyone. Additionally, supported employment programs vary in their efficiency in training employees with disabilities to work independently and to be socially acceptable in the workplace, which may reflect program features. Thus, staff training interventions to reduce job coach assistance (Parsons, Reid, Green, & Browning, 1999), maximize client grains through carefully designed and effective simulation training (Lattimore, Parsons, & Reid, 2006), and involve coworkers in job training (Likins, Salzberg, Stowitschek, Lignugaris/Kraft, & Curl, 1989), eliminating the need for staff prompts by using self-management strategies (Sowers, Verdi, Bourbeau, & Sheehan, 1985) and teaching job interview skills to maximize the likelihood of hiring (Hall, Sheldon-Wildgen, & Sherman, 1980; Kelly, Wildman, & Berler, 1980), may maximize the economic efficiency and client outcomes. Finally, some authors have speculated that sheltered workshops may have *harmful* effects on client behavior, thereby attenuating future client employability (Cimera, 2011). Thus, program quality may also contribute to the economic viability of supported employment. Finally, the economic benefits of supported employment are greatest when it is started as early as possible, such as in the final years of high school, and when the school system immediately refers students to supported employment programs before graduation from high school rather than to sheltered workshops (Cimera, 2012). So, although most economic analyses of supported employment have concluded that such programs are economically beneficial to participants and the taxpayer, this generalization must be tempered, perhaps leading to the conclusion that each supported program should receive its own economic analysis. The greatest point of leverage to maximize the personal and economic benefits of supportive employment is to increase the number of individuals with disabilities obtaining jobs after supportive employment. Since only approximately one-third of individuals who participate in supported employment subsequently obtain employment, any increases in the number of individuals employed would result in large economic benefits to all. Additional economic benefits may also accrue by making supportive employment programs more efficient and effective (Cimera, 2012).

Independent support for the economic benefits of supported employment comes from NICE's (2012) review of interventions for adults with autism. NICE located three studies which were not RCTs and were rated as low-quality nonexperiments due to nonrandomization and imprecision over the reported sample size. All three studies, however, reported large ES including significant retention of jobs for up to 8 years in one study. Thus, although study quality was poor, there was consistent evidence of personal and economic benefits. NICE then conducted an economic model based primarily on intervention costs which took the costs of training job skills, job finding, locating and support for potential employers, reduction in residential costs and other services, etc., into account to calculate the additional QALYs that might accrue from supported employment. Using conservative estimates, there was again robust evidence that supported employment was very likely to be both personally beneficial and highly cost-effective. This study was limited in that the data came from studies of individuals with ASD with IQs over 70. Hence, it cannot be assumed that the costs and benefits of supported employment are the same for individuals with more severe cognitive disabilities.

Early intensive behavioral intervention and autism

If teaching individual skills might reduce costs, what savings and other benefits might be made by teaching sufficient skills such that the individual no longer requires services? This issue is current in the literature on the effectiveness of EIBI and the possibility of recovery from ASD. At least four papers have undertaken such economic analyses: All have concluded that EIBI is highly cost-effective.

Jacobson et al. (1998) reported an early economic evaluation of EIBI. Their model assumed that children with ASD are treated at age 3 years and receive 3 years of EIBI and that 20–50% of children achieve typical functioning, 40% achieve moderate gains, and 10% require continuing intense services. The CBA included data for both childhood services and adult services up to age 55 years. They also provided estimates at differing levels of effectiveness of EIBI from 20% to 50% typical functioning. They calculated that cost savings were approximately $250,000–300,000 per child up to age 22 years and approximately $2.4–$2.8 million during adult years up to age 55 years. Since the majority of saving accrues from children who attain typical rather than partial recovery, the largest savings come from the number of children who attain typical functioning. Similar economic evaluations of EIBI that have been reported from economic analyses of services in Ontario (Motiwala et al., 2006), Texas (Chasson et al., 2007), and the Netherlands (Peters-Scheffer et al., 2012) have reached similar conclusions.

Marcus, Rubin, and Rubin (2000) critiqued Jacobson et al.'s analysis. Marcus et al. (2000) and Chasson et al.'s (2007) commentary on it illustrate some important issues and potential limitations in economic analysis of EIBI. Marcus et al. commented that at the time of publication, the only group study on EIBI was that by Lovaas (1987), which was not a true experiment, and, thus, there was limited evidence at the time to be confident in the rate of recovery. Subsequently, more studies have been published such that Peters-Scheffer et al. (2012) could base their estimates of recovery rates on 16 studies from six meta-analyses based on 292 children, thus leading to greater confidence in the likely outcomes (see also Chapter 2 for a review of this literature). Marcus et al. also commented that Jacobson et al. appeared to imply that EIBI was the most effective or only effective form of EIBI. Chassen et al. commented that this was untrue, but Jacobson et al.'s and other such comparisons only compare two treatment options—EIBI and typical services. Clearly, the door is open for anyone to report economic evaluations of other forms of early interventions, and over time, such alternatives may be reported.

Perhaps the most pertinent critique of any economic analysis of psychological or other treatment is that such analyses make assumptions, which may or may not hold true in the future. For example, the assumption of relatively constant costs of adult services might not hold true if governments defund services to adults and shift services and costs to family members, thereby resulting in overestimation of savings. Similarly, the assumption that the lifespan of adults with ASD is only 55 years might be very conservative, resulting in underestimation of savings.

Behavior management

Data on economics of behavior management comes from direct and indirect sources. Some papers have calculated economic benefits of behavioral treatment directly, whereas other have reported data on avoidance of expensive services, such as residential treatment or returning individuals from costly restrictive placements to community placements.

Hassiotis et al. (2009) conducted an RCT evaluating applied behavior analytic interventions for adults with ID in community settings. The treatment group received lower ratings of behavior problems than the control group. The control group also received higher ratings of some psychiatric problems than the treatment group posttreatment. These outcomes were maintained at 2-year follow-up (Hassiotis et al., 2011). Although treatment costs were more than twice a great in the treatment group than the control group, there was a nonsignificant trend toward lower cost in the treatment group posttreatment and no significant difference between the groups at 2-year follow-up. The costs of treatment were offset by large reductions in use and intensity of community- and hospital-based services in the treatment group. This study demonstrated that standard treatment was expensive, resulted in some client harm, and was thus inefficient. In contrast, behavior analytic intervention results in both reduction in behavior problems and reduced service costs (but no overall reduction in service costs) and was thus a more efficient use of money than regular services. These results are even more socially significant, since a recent cost–benefit analysis of risperidone and haloperidol (which are very common psychotropic treatments of challenging behavior) and placebo for treatment of aggression and improvements in quality of life indicated that pharmacological treatment was more costly than placebo (Romeo, Knapp, Tyrer, Crawford, & Oliver-Africano, 2009). Risperidone resulted in higher rates of aggression, and haloperidol results in lower quality of life than placebo. The increase in costs was mostly due to increases in the costs of formal and informal care in the drug groups.

Reduction of unnecessary psychotropic medication

Psychotropic medications are commonly used with individuals with ID in both institutional and community services and contemporary children's services (Aman, Field, & Bridgman, 1985; Logan et al., 2012; Valldovinos, Schroeder, & Kim, 2003) with perhaps one- to two-thirds of children and youth taking psychotropic medication and often multiple psychotropic medications (Logan et al.). Psychotropic medications are primarily used for behavioral issues such as aggression, self-injury, and tantrums (Aman et al., 1985; Wressell, Tyrer, & Berney, 1990), although they are also used less frequently for bona fide mental health problems, such as depression without the presence of challenging behavior.

Despite their almost ubiquitous use, the evidence base for psychotropic medication is small and weak (La Malfa, Lassi, Bertelli, & Castellani, 2006; Sturmey, 2012), and there is considerable evidence of ineffectiveness and harm including sedation, neurological impairments in learning in adaptive behavior, and other negative side effects. Despite this, services continue to spend millions of dollars on psychotropic medication, and it appears the easy default treatment in many situations, absent the availability of alternatives.

There have been several empirical reports of programs to reduce the dosage and total number of individuals taking psychotropic medication. These programs typically involve systematic review of drug use; integration of psychopharmacology with other elements of individual programming; development and implementation of alternate treatments, including the use of placebo-like alternate medications during tapering (Jancar, 1970); multidisciplinary teams; input from pharmacologists and other consultants; systematic data collection to evaluate effects of drugs in specified target behaviors and psychiatric symptoms and negative side effects; and sometimes targeting of specific groups such as individuals on antipsychotic medication without clear diagnoses of psychotic disorders (Luchins, Dojka, & Hanrahan, 1993). Such programs can result in a reduction in the average dose of psychotropic medication, polypharmacy (James, 1983), and the number of individuals taking medication (Ahmed et al., 2000; Branford, 1996; Briggs, 1989; Ellenor & Frisk, 1977; Fielding, Murphy, Reagan, & Peterson, 1980; Finholt & Emmett, 1990; Glaser & Morreau, 1986; Inoue, 1982; James, 1983; Jancar, 1970; Lepler, Hodas, & Cotter-Mack, 1994; Smith et al., 2002; Wressell et al., 1990) and may have behavioral benefits, such as increased alertness and program participation without increase in behavior problems (Ahmed et al.), although not all studies have found these benefits (Smith et al.). At least one study found no increases in injuries during medication tapering (Glaser & Morreau). Some individuals may experience increase in challenging behavior and psychiatric symptoms, but many can be successfully placed back on psychotropic medications at lower than original doses.

Some papers have reported reductions in costs of psychotropic medication (e.g., Ellenor & Frisk, 1977; Finholt & Emmet, 1990; James, 1983), but none have conducted CBAs or other economic analyses of these programs. Thus, at this time, it is unclear if the additional cost of such programs and the development and implementation of other interventions is economically beneficial to the individual or taxpayer. Further, all but one of the papers were not experiments. The one experiment (Ahmed et al., 2000; Smith et al., 2002), however, was severely compromised because randomization resulted in statistically significant differences between the experimental and control groups at baseline. The control group had fewer men, fewer participants living in institutions, and higher baseline dose of antipsychotics than the experimental group. The differences between the groups were very large: 33% of the experimental group (*N* = 36) had complete elimination and 19% had at least a 50% reduction in psychotropic medications. Participants in the control group had no such reductions. Thus, although it seems that the drug reduction protocol caused the change in behavior, we can be more confident if these results are replicated independently in a true experiment.

What Treatments Are Missing?

The list of missing treatments is long: There are no available economic analyses of CBT (NICE, 2012), counseling, and psychotherapy with people with ID. Many common programs, such as typical special education, TEACCH, and nonbehavioral approaches to early intervention for young children with ASD, are also absent from the list. This absence of data is disturbing as large quantities of money spent on such treatments and services. In some cases, this reflects the absence of outcome data on which to base an economic evaluation.

Summary

Contrary to expectations, there are indeed economic evaluations of psychosocial treatments. Some particularly promising interventions include toilet training, early intensive behavioral intervention for autism, and supported employment. Data to support behavioral interventions for high-cost individuals, such as those in out-of-district placements and enhanced staffing levels, is limited, but the potential for cost savings is large but has yet to be demonstrated robustly. Large savings may accrue from deferment of or repatriation from placement in expensive programs, such as residential care and institutionalization, but again at this point in time, the data are not available to support this possibility. The most striking feature of this literature is its small size: We need more economic evaluations of psychosocial treatments for individuals with ID.

References

Ahmed, Z., Fraser, W., Kerr, M. P., Kiernan, C., Emerson, E., Robertson, J., et al. (2000). Reducing anti-psychotic medication in people with a learning disability. *British Journal of Psychiatry, 176*, 42–46.

Aman, M. G., Field C. J., & Bridgman, G. D. (1985). City-wide survey of drug patterns among non-institutionalized mentally retarded persons. *Applied Research in Mental Retardation, 6*, 159–171.

Azrin, N. H., & Foxx, R. M. (1971). A rapid method for toilet training the institutionalized retarded. *Journal of Applied Behavior Analysis, 4*, 89–99.

Bouder, J. N., Spielman, S., & Mandell, D. S. (2009). Brief report: Quantifying the impact of autism coverage on private insurance premiums. *Journal of Autism and Developmental Disorders, 39,* 953–957.

Branford, D. (1996). Factors associated with the successful or unsuccessful withdrawal of antipsychotic drug therapy prescribed for people with learning disabilities. *Journal of Intellectual Disabilities Research, 40,* 322–329.

Briggs, R. (1989). Monitoring and evaluating psychotropic medication drug use for persons with mental retardation: A follow-up report. *American Journal on Mental Retardation, 93,* 633–639.

Chasson, G. S., Harris, G. E., & Nely, W. J. (2007). Cost comparison of early intensive behavioral intervention and special education for children with autism. *Journal of Child and Family Studies, 16,* 401–413.

Cimera, R. E. (2000). The cost-effectiveness of supported employment programs: A literature review. *Journal of Vocational Rehabilitation, 14,* 51–61.

Cimera, R. E. (2002). The monetary benefits and costs of hiring supported employees: A primer. *Journal of Vocational rehabilitation, 17,* 23–32.

Cimera, R. E. (2010). National cost efficiency of supported employees with intellectual disabilities: 2002–2007. *American Journal on Mental Retardation, 115,* 19–29.

Cimera, R. E. (2011). Supported versus sheltered employment: Cumulative costs, hours saved, and wages earned. *Journal of Vocational Rehabilitation, 35,* 85–92.

Cimera, R. E. (2012). The outcomes achieved by previously placed supported employees with intellectual disabilities: Second verse same as the first? *Journal of Vocational Rehabilitation, 36,* 65–71.

Cimera, R. E., & Burgess, S. (2011). Do adults with autism benefit monetarily from working in their communities. *Journal of Vocational Rehabilitation, 34,* 173–180.

Cimera, R. E., & Cowan, R. J. (2009). The cost of services and employment outcomes achieved with adults with autism in the US. *Autism, 13,* 285–302.

Conley, R. W., Rusch, F. R., McCaughran, W. B., & Tines, J. (1989). Benefits and costs of supported employment: An analysis of the Illinois supported employment project. *Journal of Applied Behavior Analysis, 22,* 441–447.

Ellenor, G. L., & Frisk, P. A. (1977). Pharmacist impact on drug use in an institution for the mentally retarded. *American Journal of Health-System Pharmacy, 34,* 604–608.

Fielding, L. T., Murphy, R. T., Reagan, M. W., & Peterson, T. L. (1980). An assessment program to reduce drug use with the mentally retarded. *Hospital and Community Psychiatry, 31,* 771–773.

Finholt, N. E., & Emmett, C. G. (1990). Impact of interdisciplinary team review on psychotropic drug use with persons who have mental retardation. *Mental Retardation, 28,* 41–46.

Foster, E. M., & McCombs-Thornton, K. (2012). The economics of evidence-based practice in disorders of childhood and adolescence. In P. Sturmey & M. Hersen (Eds.), *Handbook of evidence-based practice in clinical psychology: Vol. 1. Children and adolescents* (pp. 103–128). Hoboken, NJ: Wiley.

Ganz, M. L. (2007). The lifetime cost of the incremental societal costs of autism. *Archives of Pediatric and Adolescent Medicine, 161,* 343–349.

Glaser, B. A., & Morreau, L. E. (1986). Effects of interdisciplinary team review on the use of antipsychotic agents with severely and profoundly mentally retarded. *American Journal on Mental Deficiency, 90,* 371–379.

Hall, C., Sheldon-Wildgen, J., & Sherman, J. A. (1980). Teaching job interview skills to retarded clients. *Journal of Applied Behavior Analysis, 13,* 433–442.

Hassiotis, A., Robotham, D., Canagasabey, A., Marston, L., Thomas, B., & King, M. (2011). Impact of applied behaviour analysis (ABA) on carer burden and community participation in challenging behaviour: Results from a randomised controlled trial. *British Journal of Psychiatry, 198,* 490–491.

Hassiotis, A., Robotham, D., Canagasabey, A., Romeo, R., Langridge, D., Blizard, R., et al. (2009). Randomized, single-blind, controlled trial of a specialist behavior therapy team for challenging behavior in adults with intellectual disabilities. *American Journal of Psychiatry, 166,* 1278–1285.

Hill, M. L., Banks, P. D., Handrick, R. R., Wehman, P. H., Hill, J. W., & Shafer, M. S. (1987). Benefit-cost analysis of supported competitive employment for persons with mental retardation. *Research in Developmental Disabilities, 8,* 71–89.

Hyams, G., McCoull, K., Smith, P. S., & Tyrer, S. P. (1992). Behavioral continence training in mental handicap: A 10-year follow-up study. *Journal of Intellectual Disabilities Research, 36,* 551–558.

Inoue, F. (1982). A clinical pharmacy service to reduce psychotropic medication use in an institution for mentally handicapped persons. *Mental Retardation, 20,* 70–74.

Jacobson, J. W., & Mulik, J. A. (2000). System and cost research issues in treatments for people with autistic disorders. *Journal of Autism and Developmental Disabilities, 30,* 585–593.

Jacobson, J. W., Mulik, J. A., & Green, G. (1998). Cost-benefit analysis estimates for early intensive behavioral intervention for young children with autism – general model and single state case. *Behavioral Interventions, 13,* 201–226.

James, D. H. (1983). Monitoring drugs in hospitals for the mentally handicapped. *British Journal of Psychiatry, 142,* 163–165.

Jancar, J. (1970). Gradual withdrawal of tranquilizers with the help of ascorbic acid. *British Journal of Psychiatry, 17,* 238–239.

Jarbrink, K., Fombonne, E., & Knapp, M. (2003). Measuring the parental, service and cost impacts of children with autistic spectrum disorders: A pilot study. *Journal of Autism and Developmental Disorders, 33,* 395–402.

Kelly, J. A., Wildman, B. G., & Berler, E. S. (1980). Small group behavioral training to improve the job interview skills repertoire of mildly retarded adolescents. *Journal of Applied Behavior Analysis, 13,* 461–471.

Knapp, M., & McDaid, D. (2012). Economics of evidence-based practice and mental health. In P. Sturmey & M. Hersen (Eds.), *Handbook of evidence-based practice in clinical psychology: Vol. 1. Children and adolescents* (pp. 71–94). Hoboken, NJ: Wiley.

Knapp, M., Romeo, R., & Beecham, J. (2009). Economic cost of autism in the UK. *Autism, 13,* 317–336.

La Malfa, G., Lassi, S., Bertelli, M., & Castellani, A. (2006). Reviewing the use of antipsychotic drugs in people with intellectual disability. *Human Psychopharmacology, 21,* 73–89.

Lattimore, L. P., Parsons, M. B., & Reid, D. H. (2006). Enhancing job-site training of supported workers with autism: A reemphasis on simulation. *Journal of Applied Behavior Analysis, 39,* 91–102.

Lepler, S., Hodas, A., & Cotter-Mack, A. (1994). Implementation of an interdisciplinary psychotropic drug review process for community-based facilities. *Mental Retardation, 31,* 307–315.

Leslie, D. L., & Martin, A. (2007). Health care expenditure associated with autism spectrum disorders. *Archives of Pediatric and Adolescent Medicine, 161,* 350–355.

Lewis, D. R., Johnson, D. R., Bruininks, R. H., Kallen, L. A., & Guillery, R. P. (1992). Is supported employment cost-effective in Minnesota. *Journal of Disability Policy Studies, 3,* 67–92.

Likins, M., Salzberg, C. L., Stowitschek, J. L., Lignugaris/Kraft, B., & Curl, R. (1989). Co-worker implemented job training: The use of coincidental training and quality – control checking on the food preparation skills of trainees with mental retardation. *Journal of Applied Behavior Analysis, 22*, 381–393.

Logan, S. L., Nicholas, J. S., Carpenter, L. A., King, L. B., Garrett-Mayer, E., & Charles, J. M. (2012). High prescription drug utilization and associated costs among Medicaid-eligible children with autism spectrum disorders identified by a population-based surveillance network. *Annals of Epidemiology, 22*, 1–8.

Lovaas, O. I. (1987). Behavioral treatment and normal educational and intellectual functioning in young autistic children. *Journal of Consulting and Clinical Psychology, 55*, 3–9.

Luchins, D. J., Dojka, D. M., & Hanrahan, P. (1993) Factors associated with reduction in antipsychotic medication doses in adults with mental retardation. *American Journal on Mental Retardation, 98*, 165–172.

Marcus, L. M., Rubin, J. S., & Rubin, M. A. (2000). Benefit-cost analysis and autism services: A response to Jacobson and Mulick. *Journal of Autism and Developmental Disabilities, 30*, 595–598.

Motiwala, S. S., Gupta, S., & Lilly, M. B. (2006). The cost-effectiveness of expanding intensive behavioural intervention all autistic children in Ontario. *Healthcare Policy, 1*, 135–151.

National Institute for Clinical Excellence [NICE]. (2012). *Autism. The NICE guideline on recognition, referral diagnosis and management of adults on the autism spectrum.* Leicester, UK: British Psychological Society and The Royal College of Psychiatrists.

Paps, I., & Dyson, A. (2004). *The cost and benefit of earlier identification and effective intervention. Final report.* Annesley, Nottingham: Department of Education and Skills.

Parsons, M., Reid, D. H., Green, C. W., & Browning, L. B. (1999). Reducing individualized job coach assistance provided to persons with multiple severe disabilities in supported work. *Research and Practice for Persons with Severe Developmental Disabilities, 24*, 292–297.

Peng, C.-Z., Hatlestad, P., Klug, M. G., Kerbeshian, J., & Burd, L. (2009). Health care costs and utilization rates for children with developmental disorders in North Dakota from 1998-2004: Impact on Medicaid. *Journal of Child Neurology, 24*, 140–147.

Peters-Scheffer, N., Didden, R., Korzilius, H., & Matson, J. L. (2012). Cost comparison of early intensive behavioral intervention treatment as usual for children with autism spectrum disorders in the Netherlands. *Research in Developmental Disabilities, 33*, 1763–1772.

Romeo, R., Knapp, M., Tyrer, P., Crawford, M., & Oliver-Africano, P. (2009). The treatment of challenging behaviour in intellectual disabilities: Cost-effectiveness analysis. *Journal of Intellectual Disabilities Research, 53*, 633–643.

Romeo, R., & Molosankwe, I. (2010). Economic evidence in intellectual disabilities: A review. *Current Opinions in Psychiatry, 23*, 427–431.

Smith, C., Felece, D., Ahmed, Z., Fraser, W. I., Kerr, M., Kiernan, C., et al. (2002). Sedation effects on responsiveness: Evaluating the reduction of antipsychotic medication in people with intellectual disability using a conditional probability approach. *Journal of Intellectual Disability Research, 46*, 464–471.

Smith, P. S. (1979). A comparison of different methods of toilet training the mentally handicapped. *Behaviour, Research and Therapy, 17*, 33–43.

Sowers, J.-A., Verdi, M., Bourbeau, P., & Sheehan, M. (1985). Teaching job independence and flexibility to mentally retarded students through the use of a self-control package. *Journal of Applied Behavior Analysis, 18*, 81–85.

Sturmey, P. (2012). Treatment of psychopathology in persons with intellectual and other disabilities. *Canadian Journal of Psychiatry, 57*, 593–600.

Taylor, J. L., & Knapp, M. (2013). Mental health and emotional problems in people with intellectual disabilities. In J. L. Taylor, W. R. Lindsay, R. P. Hastings, & C. Hatton (Eds.), *Psychological therapies for adults with intellectual disabilities* (pp. 1–14). Chichester, UK: Wiley.

Valldovinos, M. G., Schroeder, S. R., & Kim, G. (2003). Prevalence and correlated of psychotropic medication us among adults with developmental disabilities 1970–2000. *International Review of Research in Mental Retardation, 26,* 175–220.

Wressell, S. E., Tyrer, S. P., & Berney, T. P. (1990). Reduction in anti-psychotic drug dosage in mentally handicapped patients. A hospital study. *British Journal of Psychiatry, 157,* 101–106.

Part II

Specific Disorders and Challenging Behaviors

5

Aggressive Behavior

Olive Healy, Sinéad Lydon, and Clodagh Murray

Introduction

The risk for the development of challenging behavior among individuals with an intellectual disability (ID) is high (Matson & Shoemaker, 2009; Murphy, Healy, & Leader, 2009). Aggressive behavior is often cited as the most prevalent of such problem behaviors seen in this population (Benson & Brooks, 2008) and is one of the behaviors most likely to be identified for intervention (Didden, Duker, & Korzilius, 1997). In general, aggression is more common among individuals with ID than in the general population (De Ruiter, Dekker, Verhulst, & Koot, 2007; Holden & Gitlesen, 2006). To date, many studies have reported the prevalence of aggression and its impact (Harris, 1993; Hill & Bruininks, 1984; Sigafoos, Elkins, Kerr, & Attwood, 1994). Such studies have been paralleled by numerous treatment approaches to aggression. Reviews of particular approaches have identified idiosyncratic strategies that greatly impact the frequency and severity of aggression emitted by persons with ID (Carr et al., 2000), while others have shown mixed or negative results (Whitaker, 2001). The purpose of this chapter is to systematically review interventions to reduce or eliminate aggression in individuals with ID and examine their evidence base as empirically supported treatments in this population. We begin by defining aggression and then describing its prevalence among persons with ID. We examine the factors that may contribute to its development and its impact and implications for both the persons themselves and the wider community. We examine some of the methodological issues that arise in the assessment and treatment of this problem

Evidence-Based Practice and Intellectual Disabilities, First Edition.
Edited by Peter Sturmey and Robert Didden.
© 2014 John Wiley & Sons, Ltd. Published 2014 by John Wiley & Sons, Ltd.

behavior. Then, we systematically review the evidence base for the treatment of aggression in people with ID. Finally, we provide guidelines for the treatment of aggression in this target group.

Definition

The literature on aggression among persons with ID does not present a uniform definition (Tyrer et al., 2006). Indeed, the term often encompasses a myriad of problem behaviors ranging from severe outward manifestations, including violent hitting, kicking, throwing, biting, etc. aimed at another person to milder destructive behaviors directed towards the environment. McClintock, Hall, and Oliver (2003) found diverse definitions of aggression provided by various researchers including "physical aggression" (Bhaumik, Branford, McGrother, & Thorp, 1997), "physical assault upon others" (Jacobson, 1982), "threatens or does physical violence" (Eyman & Call, 1977), "aggression" (Hardan & Sahl, 1997; Quine, 1986), "hitting" (Bott, Farmer, & Rohde, 1997), "aggressive–destructive behavior" (Lundqvist, Andersson, & Viding, 2009), "aggressive behavior disorder" (McLean, Brady, & McLean, 1996), and "explosive or assaultive behavior towards property or other individuals" (Davidson et al., 1994).

For the purpose of this chapter, aggression is defined as either *physical* (towards people or property) or *verbal*, and we use operational definitions provided by De Wein and Miller (2009). The authors defined *physical aggression* as:

> hitting, kicking, spitting, biting, shoving, shouldering, elbowing, or grappling that makes contact with another person or is directed toward another person within striking distance; throwing objects at or near others; forceful contact with objects, causing them to be damaged; contact with materials in a way that has a history of causing damage (punching a wall without producing a hole, for example); and throwing objects away from others (p. 237).

and *verbal aggression* as:

> yelling, screaming, or other loud vocalizations (directed at a person and accompanied by threatening body language), name calling, or threats (p. 237).

The physical impact of such behavior varies from bodily harm, emotional distress, to destroyed property. Assessing the extent of aggression in persons with ID can be difficult given this lack of consistent operational definition. The range of topographies reported across studies can be diverse, and quite often, the severity of the behavior is either not reported or described subjectively. Aggressive behaviors have frequently been categorized into one of the following descriptors: physical or verbal aggression directed towards others, destruction/tantrums/disruptive behavior resulting in property damage, and inappropriate social or sexual behavior (Tenneij &

Koot, 2008). Furthermore, studies often report aggression in persons with ID that is directed towards oneself usually referred to as self-injurious behavior (SIB) or "auto-aggression." In general, SIB is usually not considered a type of aggressive behavior; however, an association between frequent aggressive behavior towards others and autoaggressive behavior has been demonstrated (Tenneij, Didden, Stolker, & Koot, 2009). Research has also included anger as a precursor or activator of physical aggression, and some have argued that it is important to include this emotional state when defining aggression (Taylor, 2002).

Prevalence and Risk Factors

There are numerous prevalence studies of aggression in people with ID. For example, Emerson et al. (2001) found that aggression towards others occurs in up to 42% of people with ID. Furthermore, rates of physical aggression have been reported to vary from 2% to 24% (Borthwick-Duffy, 1994; Bruininks, Olson, Larson, & Lakin, 1994; Crocker et al., 2006; Linaker, 1994; Tyrer et al., 2006) as a function of the population sampled, setting, and operational definition of aggression employed (McClintock et al., 2003). The prevalence of aggression varies among populations that reside in community versus institutional settings with percentages of persons showing aggressive behavior found to be consistently higher in institutional place-ments (Harris 1993; Sigafoos et al., 1994; Tyrer et al., 2006).

Benson and Brooks (2008) argued that the prevalence of specific topographies of aggressive behavior among individuals with ID is greater than 50% with a correspondence between mild ID and less intrusive aggression (e.g., verbal aggres-sion only). Others with more severe ID are more likely to emit multiple forms of aggression, and a smaller percentage is likely to engage in aggression with high fre-quency or severity (Benson & Brooks). The variables analyzed within prevalence studies, however, are not always homogeneous and include the definition and severity of aggressive behaviors, setting, geographical location, assessment instru-ments, and severity of ID (McClintock et al., 2003). As a result, interpretation of the prevalence rates of aggression within this group is complicated, and it can be diffi-cult to make comparisons between studies and to assess the extent of the problem in individuals with ID. Differences in terminology and variables analyzed across studies may somewhat explain the variation in reported rates of aggressive behaviors (Allen, 2000).

A comprehensive review of the correlates of aggressive behavior in persons with ID has been provided by McClintock et al. (2003). Risk factors identified in this meta-analysis included the following: gender (males were significantly more likely to show aggression than females; Davidson et al., 1994; Quine, 1986), severity of ID with lower levels of ID showing an increased risk (Davidson et al., 1994; Hardan & Sahl, 1997; Jacobson, 1982), autism as a comorbid condition increased the likelihood of aggression (Ando & Yoshimura, 1979a, 1979ba, 1979b; Bhaumik et al., 1997; Davidson et al., 1994), and poor receptive and expressive communication abilities were also associated with aggressive behavior (Ando & Yoshimura, 1979a, 1979b; Bott et al., 1997; McLean et al., 1996). Additional correlates of aggressive behavior include age (individuals with ID between the ages of 20 and 35 years have been identified as more aggressive (Tyrer et al., 2006)), a dual diagnosis of ASD and ID (Hill & Furnis, 2006; McClintock et al., 2003), a history of anger and violence (Davidson et al., 1994; Linaker, 1994; Novaco & Taylor, 2004), psychopathology (Hemmings, Gravestock, Pickard, & Bouras, 2006; Linaker, 1994; Moss et al., 2000), depression (Sovner, DesNoyers-Hurley, & LaBrie, 1982), impulse control and conduct problems (Rojahn, Matson, Naglieri, & Mayville, 2004), and frustration (Tyrer et al.). Aggression also co-occurs with other forms of challenging behavior including SIB, repetitive behavior, and destructive and disruptive behavior (Borthwick-Duffy, 1994; Emerson et al., 1988; Harris & Russell, 1989; Sigafoos et al., 1994); however, the extent to which other challenging behavior contributes as a risk factor to developing aggression is as yet unknown.

Factors that need to be considered when examining risk markers include the interaction of many variables that may inhibit clear conclusions. For example, the type of setting is not often reported and may play an important role in deciphering whether this impacts particular risk markers. McClintock et al. (2003) cautioned researchers on the possible overlap of variables and give an example of the interaction between greater severity of ID, poor communication abilities, and comorbid autism. They argued that the extent to which each variable contributes to the risk for presenting with aggressive behavior in this population is difficult to determine. Allen (2000), however, argued that despite such issues complicating interpretation, gender, placement in institutional settings, and greater severity of disability all contribute to greater risk for developing aggression in persons with ID.

Etiology

Green, O'Reilly, Itchon, and Sigafoos (2005) suggested that in developmental disabilities challenging behaviors, including aggression, emerge early during development and persist over time. Aggression in persons with ID may present at its worst during the adolescent years (Allen, 2000). Client-specific factors may include level of neurological impairment concomitant with ID (Allen) and neurophysiological mechanisms including fluctuations in particular neurotransmitters (Hagerman, Bregman, & Tirosh, 1998; Lewis, Siva, & Silva, 1995). Physiological factors, psychiatric conditions, mental health problems, and deficiencies in communication abilities, adaptive behavior, and cognitive skills are additional client-specific factors which may act as precipitating factors in developing aggressive behaviors (Gardner & Moffatt, 1990). The presence of aggression may also be functionally related to setting events as well as discriminative stimuli within the environment, and these may be mediated by people, places, and/or objects. From this behavioral viewpoint, aggression may be considered a learned behavior maintained by external factors such as reinforcement, that is, the aggressive behavior becomes functionally related to the consequences that reliably follow it (Foxx & Meindl, 2007). Brosnan and Healy (2011) suggested that aggression towards others is socially mediated as it occurs within a social context (i.e., someone is the recipient of the aggressive act). In this context, the consequence that follows may result in attaining attention from others in the environment (Thompson, Fisher, Piazza, & Kuhn, 1998), accessing tangible items (DeLeon, Fisher, Herman, & Crosland, 2000), avoiding/escaping demands and situations (Horner, Day, Sprague, O'Brien, & Heathfield, 1991), or achieving a mix of such consequences (Braithwaite & Richdale, 2000).

Recently, the Social Information Processing (SIP) model has been proposed to emphasize the importance of social and cognitive factors in aggressive behavior in persons with ID (van Nieuwenhuijzen, Orobio de Castro, van der Valk, Vermeer, & Matthys, 2006). SIP explains aggressive behavior through cognitive processes that occur between stimulus onset and response. This model suggest that cognitive processing tendencies (e.g., interpreting the behavior of others, anticipating outcomes of aggression, recognition of emotions) are deficient in individuals with ID who emit frequent aggression.

Other researchers have suggested that aggressive behavior may be nonsocially mediated. For example, May (2011) provides a description of biobehavioral research which explains why certain individuals with ID persistently show aggression in the absence of social consequences. According to May (2011):

> complex interactions occur in the immediate and long-term context of stimulus–response-reinforcement associations. Based on biochemical manipulation of reward-related brain nuclei, however, it is plausible that aggression produces intrinsic reinforcement for the organism engaging in the behavior. As such, behaviors that are readily available in the repertoire of the organism can produce their own reinforcement (i.e., nonsocial reinforcement) (p. 2217).

Cowley, Newton, Sturmey, Bouras, and Holt (2005) discuss learning history associated with aggression in ID. They argued that individuals with ID are at risk of exposure to abuse as children and are often exposed to quite limited and restrictive residential or educational environments, which have been correlated with increased risk for aggression.

Impact

Aggression in people with ID can produce significant short- and long-term concerns for family members and caregivers. First, aggressive behavior can result in referral for psychiatric evaluation (Rojahn et al., 2004) which may impact on future placement. Many individuals can no longer live in the family home and reside in special residential placements or inpatient mental health services which often involve high levels of security and/or intrusive pharmacological interventions, seclusion, or sedation (Cowley et al., 2005; Gardner & Moffat, 1990; McGillivray & McCabe, 2004).

Frequency and chronicity of aggression have been shown to be highly correlated; the greater the rates of aggression, the more difficult the topographies are to manage (Harris & Russell, 1989; Lowe & Felce, 1995) which also can put pressure on resources and impact on treatment choice by professional staff. Jacobson and Ackerman (1993) found that pharmacotherapy was employed at a greater rate than behavioral methods, and restrictive behavioral programs were more commonly employed than preventative or positive behavioral approaches. Brosnan and Healy (2011) suggested that in many cases aggression can result in a loss of, or exclusion from, educational time, perpetuating the overall problem. Duncan, Matson, Bamburg, Cherry, and Buckley (1999) demonstrated that challenging behavior including aggression results in a restricted range of social behaviors (Kearney & Healy, 2011). Furthermore, aggression within the home and community environments can generate stress for other family members (Benderix & Sivberg, 2007), is correlated with staff burnout and stress (Edwards & Miltenberger, 1991; Freeman, 1994; Hastings & Brown, 2002), and can affect negative attitude and interactions with service users (Lawson & O'Brien, 1994). Some authors have reported the use of weapons while being aggressive towards others (Emerson et al., 1988; Harris & Russell, 1989; Sigafoos et al., 1994) which compromises the personal safety of the aggressor and others.

Search Strategies

Systematic searches were conducted using the following databases: PsycInfo, Psychology and Behavioral Sciences Collection, Web of Knowledge, Medline, and Scopus. The searches included English-language journal articles only, without restriction of publication year, and inputting the term "aggression" with the following keywords: intellectual disability/mental retardation/developmental disability/ Down syndrome/fragile X syndrome/autism/Asperger/pervasive developmental disorder/cerebral palsy/learning disability/behavioral intervention/self-monitoring/ self-management/skills training/relaxation/functional communication training/ social skills/problem solving/cognitive behavioral therapy/counseling/psycho-therapy. Abstracts of the records returned from these electronic searches were reviewed to identify studies for inclusion in the review (see "Inclusion Criteria"). The reference lists for the included studies were also reviewed to identify additional articles for possible inclusion.

Definitions

Studies reviewed included aggression or aggressive behavior ranging from physical or verbal aggression to destruction/tantrums/disruptive behavior directed towards others or the environment in accordance with the definition provided earlier. The definition of ID was significant impairments in intellectual functioning (IQ below 70) and limited abilities in adaptive behavior that begin prior to the age of 18 years (American Psychiatric Association, 2000). Where multiple participants were included, we extracted the data relevant to the participant(s) diagnosed with an ID only.

Inclusion criteria

Included were studies (a) that published in English within a peer-reviewed journal, (b) that included at least one participant diagnosed with an ID who engaged in a form of aggressive behavior, (c) that reported the use of one or more treatments that targeted reducing or eliminating aggressive behavior according to the definition outlined previously with at least one participant with ID, and (d) that used an experimental design to evaluate the results of their intervention.

Treatment classification

There were a range of treatments to reduce aggression in persons with ID including the following: (a) *behavioral interventions* designed to reduce or eliminate aggressive behavior using applied behavior analysis (ABA) and defined as any procedure that involved antecedent manipulations and changes in (instructional) context, reinforcement-based strategies, mixed treatments, and non-function-based interventions; (b) *skills training interventions* to teach individuals replacement skill(s) to decrease aggression; (c) *cognitive behavioral approaches* were any treatment approach that focused on changing a person's dysfunctional thoughts, beliefs, self-perceptions, and feelings including anger management, problem-solving skills training, and relaxation training to ameliorate cognitive process deficits and emotional control; and (d) *other treatment approaches* which did not fit into one of the other three categories including mindfulness-based strategies, vibroacoustic music, teaching family model (TFM), and aromatherapy.

Criteria for evidence-based treatments

To determine if a treatment approach could be considered an "evidence based," we applied the standards outlined by Chambless and Hollon (1998). A treatment approach was considered to be an "evidence-based intervention" if there were at least three small *N* experiments conducted by independent researchers showing treatment success with at least nine participants with ID. Treatment approaches were considered to be "promising" or "lacking sufficient evidence" if initial research results showed positive outcomes, but the number of studies required to classify them as evidence based was less than three or there were less than nine participants (Chambless & Hollon). A treatment approach was considered "inconclusive" if there were at least three studies by independent researchers showing conflicting evidence regarding outcomes of the treatment. Treatment approaches were considered to be "ineffective" if at least three studies within existing research showed that the intervention was ineffective in treating aggression across at least nine individuals with ID. Finally, where a randomized control trial (RCT) was implemented to determine treatment effectiveness, the criterion for "evidence based" outlined by Chambless and Hollon requires two RCTs by different research groups with supportive outcomes.

Treatment Review

Behavioral interventions

In this section, we examine studies that employed behavioral interventions to decrease or eliminate aggression in ID including studies that used antecedent-based and reinforcement-based strategies and mixed-treatment packages. Each of these approaches used behavioral interventions that were function-based. Function refers to the relationship between a person's aggressive behavior and the resulting change in the external environment. Functional behavioral assessment (FBA) is a technology that allows clinicians to determine the causal factors or function(s) of problem behavior such as aggression. FBA can be divided into three main methods: (a) indirect methods involving the use of interviews, rating scales, checklists, and questionnaires; (b) direct observation or descriptive analysis, incorporating antecedent–behavior–consequence (ABC) analyses or scatterplots; and (c) experimental methods involving direct manipulation of the consequences following the behavior, more commonly known as experimental functional analyses (Neilsen & McEvoy, 2004).

Research has consistently demonstrated that using functional assessment or analysis to identify the function of challenging behaviors is an important component of treatment development. Data collected during functional assessment on response classes, antecedents, maintaining contingencies, and setting events are invaluable in crafting appropriate, effective function-based interventions. Such function-based treatments have been shown to be more effective at reducing challenging behavior than alternative non-function-based treatments (Campbell, 2003; Didden et al., 1997). In addition, research has shown that treatments implemented without regard for the function of the challenging behavior can actually lead to increases in the targeted behavior rather than reductions (Devlin, Healy, Leader, & Hughes, 2011; Sigafoos & Kerr, 1994).

We also include studies that employed non-function-based behavioral interventions. We tabulated results to document aggressive topographies, behavioral function, interventions employed, and results demonstrated to determine the effectiveness of each approach.

Function-based antecedent interventions
Antecedent-based behavioral interventions involve manipulation of various aspects of the environment to alter and enhance the probability that the behavior will reduce

or not occur in the future. Antecedent influences on problem behavior include, task presentation, verbal instruction, transition across environments/activities, specific people, and external stimulation (sounds/lighting). Identifying the functional relationship between behavior and such environmental events is useful to determine whether aggression is maintained, for example, by avoidance of, or escape from, such stimuli or situations.

We identified two studies that examined the use of antecedent manipulations. Both used a reversal design to demonstrate treatment effectiveness. Sample size ranged from one to four participants. Topographies included hair pulling, biting, hitting with the hand or head, pushing, pinching, or throwing objects at others. The studies employed different assessment techniques with Horner et al. (1991) conducting a functional analysis of the effect of different demands on aggressive behaviors and Horner, Day, and Day (1997) utilizing the *Functional Assessment Interview* (O'Neill et al., 1997), an experimental functional analysis and an analysis of neutralizing routines. Both studies identified escape from demands as the function of all participants' aggressive behaviors, and Horner et al. (1997) identified a delay in planned activity as an establishing operation.

Interventions involved antecedent manipulations and changes in instructional context. Horner et al. (1991) examined the effects of interspersed requests into the teaching of more difficult tasks. This approach consisted of interspersing simple, previously mastered commands or tasks which had a high probability of being performed correctly to new and/or difficult commands. The intervention led to marked decreases in aggression and a greater number of attempts to complete difficult tasks for all four participants. Social validity data also indicated that participants were more responsive to instructions which included interspersed requests. Horner et al. (1997) evaluated the efficacy of neutralizing routines for reducing aggressive behavior in an adolescent with a severe ID. Postponement of preferred planned activities was identified as an establishing operation for aggressive behavior. Thus, the neutralizing routine involved a brief period of one-to-one staff contact, rescheduling the cancelled preferred event for another day, and spending time reviewing and discussing photographs of the participant's past activities. These procedures were completed approximately 30–40 min prior to the instructional session. This intervention eliminated the participant's aggression. The authors proposed that the treatment effects can be attributed to the neutralizing routine increasing the value of staff praise and decreasing the value of task escape.

Function-based reinforcement procedures
Two reinforcement-based procedures were implemented: noncontingent reinforcement (NCR) and functional communication training (FCT). NCR involves the delivery of the reinforcing consequence identified as the maintaining contingency for aggression independent of the occurrence of aggression which is typically delivered on a fixed-time (FT) or variable-time (VT) schedule. The success of NCR is attributable to abolishing the establishing operations for aggression. Differential reinforcement (DR) involves the delivery of reinforcement contingent on the

absence of the challenging behavior (DRO), the presence of specified alternative behavior (DRA), the occurrence of behavior incompatible to aggressive behavior (DRI), or low rates of the challenging behavior (DRL). While considered a reinforcement-based procedure, DR is typically combined with extinction such that aggression does not result in reinforcement while the DR procedures are in place. For the purpose of this chapter, studies employing combined DR and extinction were categorized as mixed-treatment packages (see the following section). There were no studies which implemented DR without also placing the aggressive behavior on extinction. FCT involves teaching a communicative phrase that is functionally equivalent and that provides a less effortful alternative to the target behavior which will allow individuals to access the desired reinforcement (Durand & Carr, 1991). Studies which implemented FCT alone, as an intervention for aggression, will be described later under the Skills Training section.

We identified four studies that examined the effects of reinforcement-based treatments on aggressive behavior. Each study used a small *N* experimental design, including multielement (Fisher, O'Connor, Kurtz, DeLeon, & Gotjen, 2000; O'Reilly, Lancioni, King, Lally, & Dhomhnaill, 2000; Van Camp, Lerman, Kelley, Contrucci, & Vorndran, 2000) and reversal designs (Tarbox, Wallace, Tarbox, Landaburu, & Williams, 2004; Van Camp et al., 2000). Sample sizes ranged from one to two participants. Topographies of aggressive behavior were similar to those described in antecedent-based intervention studies but also included kicking, scratching, and head butting. In one study, the topographies of aggression were not described (Fisher, O'Connor et al., 2000).

Each study utilized an experimental functional analysis by systematically manipulating environmental events to test behavioral hypotheses. Two studies also employed preference assessments to identify highly preferred stimuli to compete with the reinforcers maintaining aggression to increase alternative appropriate behaviors. Three of the studies identified aggressive behaviors as being multiply controlled. In Fisher, O'Connor et al. (2000), aggression was maintained by attention, escape from demand, and access to tangibles, while in both participants in Tarbox et al.'s (2004) study, aggressive behavior was maintained by both attention and escape from demands. Van Camp et al. (2000) found that aggression was maintained by both escape from demand and access to tangibles for one participant and solely access to tangibles for the other participant. Finally, O'Reilly et al.'s (2000) experimental functional analysis identified diverted parental attention as the discriminative stimulus for aggressive behaviors and attention as the maintaining variable.

Four studies employed NCR, and one employed NCR and FCT to address the differential functions of attention and escape. NCR, implemented on an FT schedule that was gradually thinned, resulted in greatly reduced rates of aggression which were maintained at a 6-month follow-up (O'Reilly et al., 2000). Another study compared NCR, without extinction, with either low- or high-preference stimuli (Fisher, O'Connor et al., 2000). NCR without extinction reduced aggression only when high-preference stimuli were available noncontingently. Van Camp et al. (2000) compared the effects of FT and VT schedules on aggression: Both led to markedly reduced rates of aggression. Tarbox et al. (2004) found that both FCT and NCR reduced aggression to near-zero levels for both participants; however, while NCR and FCT were similarly effective for one participant, FCT led to significantly more variable rates of aggression than NCR for the other participant. Thus, all four studies demonstrated significant reductions in aggression through the use of function-based reinforcement strategies.

Mixed-treatment packages

Mixed-treatment packages incorporating multiple behavioral interventions have been most commonly reported in the literature addressing the treatment of aggressive behaviors of individuals with ID. We identified 25 such studies. Each study used a small *N* experimental design. Sample sizes ranged from one to four. Reversal designs were the most common (13 studies), six used multiple baseline designs, and a further six used multielement designs. Topographies of aggressive behavior involved physical and verbal aggression including spitting, punching, grabbing, shoving, striking with an object, verbal abuse, and throwing furniture at others.

Experimental functional analyses were used in seven studies (Borrero & Vollmer, 2006; Fisher, Thompson, Hagopian, Bowman, & Krug, 2000; Hanley, Piazza, Fisher, Contrucci, & Maglieri, 1997; O'Reilly, Lancioni, & Taylor, 1999; Ringdahl et al., 2009a; Slifer, Ivancic, Parrish, Page, & Burgio, 1986; Vollmer et al., 1998), with all other studies reporting the use of a modified experimental functional analyses and/ or a functional behavior assessment. Twenty-two identified a clear single function for at least one participant that included escape from demand or instruction, escape from social proximity, contingent attention, contingent wheelchair movement, access to tangibles, and access to walks. The remaining three studies found aggression to be multiply controlled with functions including escape from demands, attention, and access to tangibles. Three studies identified establishing operations for participant's aggression including menstrual discomfort, nonpreferred tasks, presence of peers during free play, and low levels of teacher attention (Carr, Smith, Giacin, Whelan, & Pancari, 2003; Richman et al., 1997).

The types of interventions used to implement mixed-treatment packages included a combination of two or more of the following: NCR, FCT, and DR procedures; extinction; response interruption and redirection; antecedent/environment alterations; and punishment procedures (see Carr, Newsom, & Binkoff, 1980; Deleon, Kahng, Rodriguez-Catter, Sveinsdóttir, & Sadler, 2003; Fisher et al., 1993, ; Kahng et al., 2001; Marcus & Vollmer, 1996; Ringdahl, Christensen, & Boelter, 2009; Vollmer, Ringdahl, Roane, & Marcus, 1997; Wacker et al., 1990).

Studies including behavioral interventions within mixed-treatment packages showed significant efficacy in reducing the rates of aggressive behaviors. Two studies reported complete elimination of all topographies of aggression (Bowman, Fisher, Thompson, & Piazza, 1997; Vollmer et al., 1998), one reported the elimination of all topographies of physical aggression but variable rates of verbal aggression (De Zubicaray & Clair, 1998), six reported near-zero levels of aggression at conclusion, while the remaining 17 studies reported either reductions in aggression or low levels of aggression following intervention. Maintenance of treatment effects was reported in three studies 12 weeks later (Slifer et al., 1986) and at 15–22 months (Carr et al., 2003), while the generalization of treatment effects to other settings was reported in only one study (Slifer et al.). Increases in alternative appropriate behaviors, such as compliance, communication, engagement, and appropriate social interactions, were also reported as treatment outcomes in seven studies.

Conclusions   Based on Chambless and Hollon's (1998) criteria, antecedent manipulations based on functional analyses are *promising* but lack sufficient evidence to be an evidence-based practice. Reinforcement-based strategies designed from functional analyses including NCR and FCT are *promising* interventions but lack sufficient evidence based on limited numbers of participants across studies to be considered an evidence-based practice. Additionally, since there are a wide range of parameters of DR schedules, future research should identify which properties of DR schedules affect treatment outcome.

Mixed behavioral treatment packages are clearly *effective* in eliminating and significantly reducing aggression, and this has been reported by 17 experiments conducted by many independent researchers. Thus, mixed behavioral treatments that are based on the outcomes of a functional analysis may therefore be considered an evidence-based approach to treating aggression in ID.

Non-function-based interventions

Despite the importance of function-based interventions, a number of experiments studies have examined the efficacy of behavioral intervention developed without functional assessment or analysis. We identified 10 such experiments, all of which involved single-subject experimental designs with sample sizes ranging from one to six. With the exception of vomiting on others, all other topographies of aggression were similar to studies described in the previous sections. Experimental designs included multiple baseline designs across participants (Cannella-Malone, Tullis, & Kazee, 2011; Sigafoos & Kerr, 1994) and across behaviors (LeBlanc, Hagopian, & Maglieri, 2000), reversal designs, combined reversal and multiple baseline across behaviors design, and a multielement design. Only two studies administered any form of assessment, and these included a preference assessment and a social validity assessment.

Several different types of non-function-based treatments were described including implementation of one or more of the following: DR procedures, time-out from reinforcement, token economy, response cost, contingent exercise, verbal reprimand, antecedent exercise, contingent ammonia spirits, the provision of leisure activities, choice making, response blocking, and overcorrection. The application of these interventions, or a combination of these interventions, was not based on an assessment of the function of aggression.

The outcomes of these experiments were largely positive. Three reported the elimination of aggressive behaviors (Dyer, Dunlap, & Winterling, 1990; LeBlanc et al., 2000; Niemeyer & Fox, 1990), one reported the reduction of aggression to near-zero levels (Cannella-Malone et al., 2011), while five others reported the reduced rates of aggression following intervention (Blum, Mauk, McComas, & Mace, 1996; Bostow & Bailey, 1969; Doke, Cowlery, & Sumberg, 1983; Luce, Delquadri, & Hall, 1980; Repp & Deitz, 1974). The final study (Sigafoos & Kerr, 1994) reported positive outcomes, in the form of decreased aggression, for two participants but increased aggression in response to the intervention for the third. Blum et al. (1996) failed to show that the combined effects of behavioral intervention and medication were greater than their separate effects. Luce et al. (1980) determined that contingent exercise was more effective in reducing rates of aggression than DRO. Increases in engagement and adaptive behavior were reported as additional treatment outcomes in two of the studies (Blum et al., 1996).

Treatments implemented under this heading employed either a single intervention (e.g., antecedent exercise) or multiple interventions (e.g., punishment and DR). Non-function-based behavioral treatment packages including DR procedures met the standard for an evidence-based intervention. Other interventions implemented without analysis of the function of aggression including antecedent exercise, response blocking, and contingent positive punishment lacked sufficient evidence.

Skills training interventions
Skills training approaches are often employed because of the negative correlation between adaptive behavior and challenging behavior (Emerson et al., 2001) and, based on evidence that increases in certain skills, such as communication, are associated with reductions in challenging behaviors (Hudson & Gavidia-Payne, 2002).

This review identified eight experiments which implemented skills training programs in an attempt to reduce the aggressive behaviors of individuals diagnosed with ID. Sample sizes ranged from one to 10 participants. Eight used small *N* experimental designs, including multielement treatment designs, reversal designs, and multiple baseline designs across participants (Durand, 1993; Durand & Carr, 1991) or across settings (Dougherty, Fowlser, & Paine, 1985). Topographies of aggression were similar to earlier studies except for several topographies of aggressive behavior described by Dougherty et al. (1985) which included rough or harmful bodily contact and verbal aggression. Seven experiments identified behavioral function using an experimental functional analysis, a modified experimental functional analysis, or a functional behavior assessment; one did not assess the function of participants' aggressive behaviors (Dougherty et al.) and one used an antecedent analysis (Bailey, McComas, Benavides, & Lovascz, 2002).

Seven experiments studies involved teaching communication skills, six of which used FCT. Four studies used FCT in its typical form. Bailey et al. (2002) compared the efficacy of FCT involving minimal response effort and FCT involving high response effort for reducing aggression. Durand (1993) assessed the efficacy of FCT using assistive communication devices. Ringdahl, Call, Mews, Boelter, and Christensen (2008) failed to determine the function of the participant's aggressive behaviors which precluded the use of FCT. Instead, communication training was used to teach communicative phrases that would allow the participant to access positive reinforcement, in the form of tangibles or edibles, or negative reinforcement, in the form of escape from particular settings. Two studies implemented skills training interventions for behaviors other than communication. Following a successful peer monitoring intervention, Dougherty et al. (1985) taught two participants with ID to self-monitor and report their own behavior.

Outcomes of skills training interventions were quite variable. The experiments employing FCT significantly decreased aggression. Bailey et al. (2002) found that low response effort FCT was significantly more effective than high response effort FCT. Durand (1993) demonstrated the efficacy of FCT using assistive communication devices for reducing the aggression. Najdowski, Wallace, Ellsworth, MacAleese, and Cleveland (2008) found that FCT eliminated both precursor behaviors and more severe target behaviors. Increases in desirable behaviors such as appropriate communication and positive affect were also reported as positive outcomes of FCT among these studies. Generalization of FCT treatment effects were reported in two studies (Durand & Carr, 1992; Najdowski, et al., 2008), and maintenance of treatment effects 1 year later (Day, Horner, & O'Neill, 1994) and 2 years later (Bailey et al.) was reported in two studies. Other studies, which implemented non-function-based skills training interventions, reported less successful outcomes. Ringdahl and colleagues (2008) found that while non-function-based communication training initially had a positive effect on aggression initially, rates of aggression were highly variable at the conclusion. Dougherty et al. (1985) found that following an effective peer monitoring intervention, a self-monitoring intervention, which was subsequently implemented, maintained near-zero levels of aggression; however, poor maintenance and generalization of these treatment effects were reported.

Conclusions Six studies reported the *effective* use of FCT as a skills training intervention, thus qualifying this intervention as an evidence-based approach to treat aggression. Since there was only one experiment demonstrating the effectiveness of self-monitoring, this approach can be considered promising but *lacks sufficient evidence.*

Cognitive behavioral therapy

Cognitive behavioral therapy (CBT) has become increasingly popular in treating aggression, anger, and sexual offences (Taylor, Novaco, Gillmer, & Thorne, 2002). Many studies are based on Novaco's (1975/1994) approach which involves cognitive restructuring, arousal reduction, and behavioral skills training, and some have included relaxation training (Benson, Johnson Rice, & Miranti, 1986; Rose, 2010). (See Chapter 10 on Offenders for discussion of specific application of CBT to offenders with ID).

We identified five experiments that implemented CBT for anger reduction with one of these specifically mentioning physical aggressive behaviors (Taylor, Novaco,

Gilmer, Robertson, & Thorne, 2005). Three experiments conducted standardized pre- and postintervention measures with wait list control groups and random assignment to intervention/control conditions (Hagliassis, Gulbenkoglu, Di Marco, Young, & Hudson, 2005; Taylor et al., 2002, 2005). One experiment employed a single-subject experimental design (ABA reversal; Burns, Bird, Leach, & Higgins, 2003), and another implemented a components analysis with pre- and posttests across four groups. Behavioral function was not examined nor specified in any of the studies. Three experiments utilized Novaco's (1975) model (Hagliassis et al., 2005; Taylor et al., 2002, 2005). The remaining two utilized anger management training that was not based on Novaco's model. The strategies were similar across studies and the methods described included role-playing, psychoeducation, cognitive restructuring, assertiveness, and behavioral skills training and problem-solving skills training. While all of the studies described some improvements on the measures used, many did not reach statistical significance and maintenance over time was problematic.

Burns et al. (2003) utilized anger management training with three participants with ID, two of whom had a comorbid psychiatric disorder. They demonstrated decreased scores on the *Novaco Anger Scale* (NAS; Novaco, 1991) during the intervention, but scores increased again at follow-up, indicating a problem with maintenance effects.

Hagliassis et al. (2005) conducted an RCT of anger management training with 29 participants, 28 of whom had cerebral palsy. Participants used a variety of modes of communication, and the authors were interested to see if any one mode would be associated with greater responsiveness to treatment. A significant between-group difference in scores on the NAS (Novaco, 1991) was observed at posttest; however, the study reported that there were no significant relationships between changes in anger following treatment and age, gender, and mode of communication across participants.

Taylor et al. (2002) utilized anger management training with 19 male offenders with ID who were detained in a secure setting. They implemented a psychoeducational preparatory phase prior to CBT training. The treatment group demonstrated a significant decrease in mean scores on the *Provocation Inventory* (PI; Novaco, 1994). There were no differences in scores on the *Ward Anger Rating Scale* (WARS; Novaco, 1994)—a staff report measure. The *Clinicians Rating Scale* (CRS; Renwick, Black, Ramm, & Novaco, 1997) was also scored, and a modest improvement was reported.

Taylor et al. (2005) used a similar procedure with 36 detained men with borderline ID (IQ 70–85) who had histories of serious aggression. They reported that the intervention group's anger scores on a number of measures were significantly lower following a cognitive behavioral anger treatment compared with the routine care wait list control group; however, the authors noted that the overall findings provided a weak support for the effectiveness of the intervention because the significant between-group differences in change associated with cognitive behavior treatment were only found for the NAS total and its arousal subscale and for only one provocation category index of the PI.

The studies described earlier reported mixed outcomes from CBT-based anger management and treatments for individuals with ID. All but one (Benson et al., 1986) utilized standardized measures, which are useful for statistical analysis; however, none of the studies incorporated direct measurement of aggressive behavior. Aggression may be considered the expression of anger, though it is possible to feel anger without demonstrating aggression. It may be problematic to infer from scales measuring current anger responses that increases or decreases in aggressive behaviors are more or less likely.

Meta-analyses

A meta-analysis is a specific type of statistical method for integrating results from many individual studies. This type of statistic can be useful for obtaining an overall estimate of whether or not an intervention is effective and, if so, what the size of the benefits are. This is referred to as the "effect size" (Healy & Lydon, 2013). Nicoll, Beail, and Saxon (2013) provided a meta-analysis of the effectiveness of CBT interventions for anger in adults with intellectual disabilities. Although research has shown that anger may activate aggressive behavior, it has also been argued that it may not be present or obvious when aggressive acts occur (Novaco, 1994). Nevertheless, anger may be considered a significant issue among the ID population (Nicoll et al., 2013). Effect sizes were calculated for nine studies that employed standardized measures of anger, to determine anger reduction in adults with an ID using CBT, within community or institutional settings. Six studies were group based and three were individual treatment studies. The meta-analysis revealed a large effect size (Cohen's $d = 0.88$, $N = 168$) for the treatment of anger in adults with ID. Based on their analysis, the authors argue that "an emerging evidence base for cognitive behavioral anger interventions in adults with intellectual disabilities" (p. 60) is evident; however, they also note that findings were restricted by the small study sample sizes and recommend that future studies involve larger sample sizes to strengthen any conclusions about the effectiveness of anger treatment in populations with ID.

Hamelin, Travis, and Sturmey (2013) provided a meta-analysis of anger management interventions for adults with ID and identified eight studies that used multicomponent interventions mainly drawn from CBT frameworks. Intervention components included cognitive restructuring, arousal reduction, relaxation training, problem solving, role-play, and behavioral skills training. Standardized anger measures were used to determine treatment effectiveness in all eight studies. Effect sizes across studies were reported to range from medium to large, highlighting the effectiveness of anger management approaches in persons with ID. However, the authors highlight that all studies used either self-reports or staff reports of behavior change, without actual observation of target behaviors, making interpretation of the results difficult. Furthermore, all studies were not well controlled, lacked treatment integrity, and employed interventions that used multiple components, some of which were drawn from CBT and behavioral interventions. Examination of the actual therapeutic constituents of such interventions is necessary in future research. Hamelin et al. (2013) conclude that anger management, using the techniques outlined earlier, cannot at this time be considered an effective intervention in this population.

Conclusion   Clearly, there is a growth in the popularity in cognitive behavioral approaches in treating anger and aggression in individuals with ID. Some positive outcomes on specific standardized measures (or subscales of such measures) were noted across studies on cognitive behavioral approaches, including CBT and anger management; however, the majority of studies demonstrated either mixed outcomes or no change on a wide range of measures. Based on Chambless and Hollon's (1998) criteria, this approach may be considered *inconclusive* and requires further investigation to determine which core elements affect anger and aggression and whether altering anger as an emotional response directly affects the probability of aggressive acts. A greater focus on experimental evaluation using direct observation of the target behaviors with participants with a range of participants with ID will be required in the future.

Other treatments

Mindfulness
Adkins, Singh, Winton, McKeegan, and Singh (2010) conducted an experiment using a multiple baseline design across three participants with ID and mental illness in which aggression was the target behavior for two participants. The authors employed the "Meditation on the Soles of the Feet" procedure (Singh, Wahler, Adkins, & Myers, 2003) in which individuals learned to divert their attention to the soles of their feet when they experienced difficult emotions or recognized one of their triggers for anger or aggression. The frequency of aggressive behaviors (verbal and physical aggression and property destruction) decreased to zero levels for both participants during the training period. For one participant, a zero level was maintained at follow-up, while the other participant demonstrated a slight increase in aggressive behavior.

Teaching family model
De Wein and Miller (2009) applied *the* TFM, a system that addresses aggression and quality of life for individuals with ID and their families. The authors targeted physical and verbal aggression in two adults with ID by designing a "Quality of Life Plan" (QLP) based on their strengths and weaknesses. Information obtained from the QLP was used to target skills that would help the participants learn alternatives to aggression. Functional assessment was used to determine the functions of aggressive behavior and identify incompatible and competing skills. The least-to-most prompting was implemented to teach novel skills including sharing with others, recovering property appropriately, expanding vocabulary, and identifying and labelling feelings. DRO was incorporated into a motivation system whereby participants earned money that allowed them access to preferred items and activities contingent

on the absence of physical aggression at the end of prespecified time blocks throughout the day as well as at the end of the week.

Physical and verbal aggression significantly decreased for both participants, and staff reported that aggression no longer interfered with daily activities with one participant resuming home visits. Quality of life indicators, such as independent living, employment, relationships, and self-determination, increased following participation in the TFM program. Future research is necessary to determine the degree to which the procedures employed within TFM result in reduction of aggression and increases in quality of life measures in persons with ID.

Vibroacoustic music
We identified one experiment (Lundqvist et al., 2009) that used vibroacoustic music to decrease aggression in 20 participants with developmental disabilities, 10 of whom had a comorbid diagnosis of ASD. Thirteen participants demonstrated a combination of SIB, stereotypic behaviors, and aggressive–destructive behaviors. Two participants demonstrated both stereotypic and aggressive–destructive behaviors. The participants were randomized into two groups in an RCT evaluation. The intervention involved the use of chairs or beds with speakers installed inside them. The speakers played low-frequency sound vibrations so that the participants could hear the music and physically feel the vibrations concurrently. The mean frequency of aggression was highly variable across the intervention period with no observed decrease in aggression following the intervention.

Aromatherapy
One study (Ramandi, Daneshfar, & Shojaei, 2012) utilized aromatherapy as an intervention for aggression in 50 individuals with ID aged between 12 and 16 years. Participants were randomly assigned to aromatherapy, play, combined aromatherapy/play, and a control condition whereby participants did not perform any activities. An aggression questionnaire was administered to teachers pre- and postintervention. Aromatherapy involved participants inhaling vaporized lavender in a room. The play component involved a series of unspecified play activities. Mean aggression rates decreased for the aromatherapy, play, and combination groups but not for the control group. Participants in the experimental groups received significantly lower scores on the anger questionnaire following the intervention period, while no change was observed in the control group; however, there was no significant difference between the three intervention groups, making it difficult to interpret which component(s) of the intervention(s) was responsible for changes in pre- and posttest scores. In addition, participants were not matched on levels of aggression at pretest, and the RCT standard of "blind" assessment was not achieved in this study.

Conclusion At this time, mindfulness, the TFM, vibroacoustic music, and aromatherapy must each be considered *lacking sufficient evidence* due to the limited number of studies investigating their effectiveness in directly altering rates of aggression in ID. Further investigation of each of these approaches will be required to determine their utility, suitability, and effectiveness with this population.

Conclusions

Table 5.1 summarizes the evidence and conclusions for treatment of aggression. The substantial number of studies, demonstrating the effectiveness of behavioral interventions and skills training interventions to reduce aggression replicated by numerous independent researchers, provides strong evidence that this approach is an effective treatment and supports their use in clinical practice. This is especially true for function-based behavioral treatment packages employing NCR, FCT, and DR procedures. Although non-function-based interventions are also an effective treatment for aggression, this approach is no longer considered a standard practice except in some cases whereby the operant function of aggression may not always be evident or multiple behavioral functions may obfuscate interpretation and make implementation difficult or impossible.

Some individual behavioral procedures including NCR and antecedent manipulations, including neutralizing routines and interspersal of requests, are also promising but lack sufficient evidence due to the limited number of studies and small number of participants. FCT for aggression met the standard for an evidence-based approach; however, other skills training interventions including self-monitoring did not meet the standard for an effective treatment and requires further investigation.

The mixed findings on CBT to treat anger and aggression necessitate further investigation and replication. We recommend that future studies employ direct measures and robust definitions of aggression to determine its utility in clinical practice. Other authors (Beail, 2003; Sturmey, 2004, 2006, 2006) have found limited evidence to support CBT for people with ID through systematic review of available literature.

A number of issues arise when analyzing studies treating aggression. Many studies reporting behavior change did not report the severity of aggression. Severity is an important measure because it describes the possible threat to others and can help when one is seeking to replicate procedures across similar individuals to further determine the success of an approach (Healy, Lydon, Holloway, & Dwyer, 2014). Often, detailed descriptions of aggression are not provided, and this information would be useful in determining the contextual fit of interventions (Healy et al., 2013; Tenneij & Koot, 2008). Furthermore, the range of levels of ID is often not reported. It can be difficult to determine if particular interventions will be equally effective and efficient with persons with all degrees of ID. Overall, the most effective approaches to reduce aggression in people with ID based on an evaluation of the evidence include function-based behavioral interventions and skills training approaches. Some have argued that behavioral interventions have yet to be shown to be effective in more naturalistic settings (Taylor, 2002), yet 22 studies reviewed here

Table 5.1   Summary of Evidence for the Treatment of Aggression

---

Behavioral interventions

Function-based antecedent interventions:
- Antecedent manipulations and changes in context
  - Lacking sufficient evidence

Function-based reinforcement procedures:
- NCR alone
  - Lacking sufficient evidence
- Mixed-treatment packages
  - Evidence-based intervention

Non-function-based interventions:
- DR procedures
  - Evidence-based intervention
- Antecedent exercise
  - Lacking sufficient evidence
- Response blocking
  - Lacking sufficient evidence
- Contingent positive punishment
  - Lacking sufficient evidence

Skills training interventions
- FCT
  - Evidence-based intervention
- Self-monitoring
  - Lacking sufficient evidence

Cognitive behavior therapy
- Inconclusive

Other treatments:
- *Mindfulness*
  - Lacking sufficient evidence
- *TFM*
  - Lacking sufficient evidence
- *Vibroacoustic music*
  - Lacking sufficient evidence
- *Aromatherapy*
  - Lacking sufficient evidence

---

took place in settings such as family homes (Day et al., 1994; Feldman, Condillac, Tough, Hunt, & Griffiths, 2002; LeBlanc et al., 2000; LeBlanc, Hagopian, Marhefka, & Wilke, 2001; O'Reilly et al., 2000), group homes (Bailey et al., 2002; Carr et al., 2003; Sigafoos & Kerr, 1994), and day programs (Cannella-Malone et al., 2011; Carr & Durand, 1985; Dougherty et al., 1985; Durand, 1993; Durand & Carr, 1992; Hanley, Iwata, & Thompson, 2001; Horner et al., 1997; Luce et al., 1980; Marcus & Vollmer, 1996; Najdowski et al., 2008; O'Reilly et al., 1999; Phillips & Mudford, 2011; Richman et al., 1997), demonstrating that behavioral interventions for aggression can indeed be implemented effectively in naturalistic settings. Thus, professionals dealing with aggression should become knowledgeable and competent in implementing and disseminating evidence-based approaches in order to make sound and consistent clinical judgments and change client behavior and quality of life. Newsom and Hovanitz (2005) argued that the implementation of evidence-based approaches is part of the ethical requirements of all professionals providing treatment. Increasing scientific knowledge in the field of clinical practice by thoroughly exerting all treatment approaches to rigorous review will ensure greater outcomes in the future for populations who require such intervention.

Guidelines and Recommendations

- Determining the function of problem behavior and its environmental determinants is important for the design of effective interventions to target aggressive behavior. The ethical guidelines followed by Board Certified Behavior Analysts highlight the importance of using functional assessment prior to the development or implementation of treatment plans (Behavior Analyst Certification Board, 2004). The outcomes of functional assessment/analysis provide clinicians with information to design a treatment program that will determine the outcomes of aggressive behavior for the individual, environmental alterations required, and the behavioral deficits needing intensive instruction.
- The use of behavioral interventions to treat aggression in ID has a long history and has been shown to be successful in reducing or eliminating such behavior, including in typical community settings. Employing such interventions to primarily target the causes of aggression is recommended in clinical practice. Behavioral interventions within individualized mixed-treatment packages that are based on the outcomes of a functional analysis should be employed by clinicians to treat aggression in persons with ID.
- The use of positive treatment approaches including FCT and DR is recommended. Such procedures target behavioral deficits and manipulate the consequences that may be present for aggressive behavior. Reinforcing target skills will increase the probability of the acquisition and demonstration of novel and more appropriate replacement behavior.
- Providing clear operational definitions of aggression along with the severity of such behavior is important to ensure measurement of behavior change. The use of direct and objective measures of frequency and severity of aggression will determine responsiveness to intervention. Maintaining accurate and reliable data of the problem will aid clinical practice by ensuring treatment approaches are altered according to the rate and level of behavior change.
- Clinical supervision of measurement, individualization, and analysis in the design and implementation of treatment approaches to aggression in ID is recommended. Such supervision ensures consistency in adherence to treatment protocol and ongoing evaluation of responsiveness to intervention.

References

Adkins, A. D., Singh, A. N., Winton, A. S. W., McKeegan, G. F., & Singh, J. (2010). Using a mindfulness-based procedure in the community: Translating research to practice. *Journal of Child and Family Studies, 19*, 175–183.

Allen, D. (2000). Recent research on physical aggression in persons with intellectual disability: An overview. *Journal of Intellectual & Developmental Disability, 25*, 41–57.

American Psychiatric Association. (2000). *Diagnostic and statistical manual of mental disorders* (4th ed., text revision). Washington, DC: Author.

Ando, H., & Yoshimura, I. (1979a). Comprehension skill levels and prevalence of maladaptive behaviors in autistic and mentally retarded children: A statistical study. *Child Psychiatry and Human Development, 9*, 131–136.

Ando, H., & Yoshimura, I. (1979b). Speech skill levels and prevalence of maladaptive behaviors in autistic and mentally retarded children: A statistical study. *Child Psychiatry and Human Development, 10*, 85–90.

Bailey, J., McComas, J. J., Benavides, C., & Lovascz, C. (2002). Functional assessment in a residential setting: Identifying an effective communicative replacement response for aggressive behavior. *Journal of Developmental and Physical Disabilities, 14*, 353–369.

Beail, N. (2003). What works for people with mental retardation? Critical commentary on cognitive-behavioural and psychodynamic psychotherapy research. *Mental Retardation, 41*, 468–472.

Behavior Analyst Certification Board. (2004, August). *Guidelines for responsible conduct for behavior analysts*. Retrieved from http://www.bacb.com/index.php?page=100129 (accessed on October 17, 2013).

Benderix, Y., & Sivberg, B. (2007). Siblings' experiences of having a brother or sister with autism and mental retardation: A case study of 14 siblings from five families. *Journal of Pediatric Nursing, 22*, 410–418.

Benson, B. A., & Brooks, W. T. (2008). Aggressive challenging behaviour and intellectual disability. *Current Opinion in Psychiatry, 21*, 454–458.

Benson, B. A., Johnson Rice, C. J., & Miranti, S. V. (1986). Effects of anger management training with mentally retarded adults in group treatment. *Journal of Consulting and Clinical Psychology, 54*, 728–729.

Bhaumik, S., Branford, D., McGrother, C., & Thorp, C. (1997). Autistic traits in adults with learning disabilities. *British Journal of Psychiatry, 170*, 502–506.

Blum, N. J., Mauk, J. E., McComas, J. J., & Mace, F. C. (1996). Separate and combined effects of methylphenidate and a behavioral intervention on disruptive behavior in children with mental retardation. *Journal of Applied Behavior Analysis, 29*, 305–319.

Borrero, C. S., & Vollmer, T. R. (2006). Experimental analysis and treatment of multiply controlled problem behavior: A systematic replication and extension. *Journal of Applied Behavior Analysis, 39*, 375–379.

Borthwick-Duffy, S. A. (1994). Prevalence of destructive behaviors: A study of aggression, self-injury, and property destruction. In T. Thompson & D. B. Gray (Eds.), *Destructive behavior in developmental disabilities: Diagnosis and treatment* (pp. 3–23). Thousand Oaks, CA: Sage.

Bostow, D. E., & Bailey, J. B. (1969). Modification of severe disruptive and aggressive behavior using brief timeout and reinforcement procedures. *Journal of Applied Behavior Analysis, 2*, 31–37.

Bott, C., Farmer, R., & Rohde, J. (1997). Behaviour problems associated with lack of speech in people with learning disabilities. *Journal of Intellectual Disability Research, 41*, 3–7.

Bowman, L. G., Fisher, W. W., Thompson, R. H., & Piazza, C. C. (1997). On the relation of mands and the function of destructive behavior. *Journal of Applied Behavior Analysis, 30*, 251–265.

Braithwaite, K., & Richdale, A. L. (2000). Functional communication training to replace challenging behaviors across two behavioral outcomes. *Behavioral Interventions, 15*, 21–36.

Brosnan, J., & Healy, O. (2011). A review of behavioral interventions for the treatment of aggression in individuals with developmental disabilities. *Research in Developmental Disabilities, 32*, 437–446.

Bruininks, R. H., Olson, K. M., Larson, S. A., & Lakin, K. C. (1994). Challenging behaviors among persons with mental retardation in residential settings. In T. Thompson & D. B. Gray (Eds.), *Destructive behavior in developmental disabilities: Diagnosis and treatment* (pp. 24–48). Thousand Oaks, CA: Sage.

Burns, M., Bird, D., Leach, C., & Higgins, K. (2003). Anger management training: The effects of a structured programme on the self-reported anger experience of forensic inpatients with learning disability. *Journal of Psychiatric and Mental Health Nursing, 10*, 569–577.

Campbell, J. M. (2003). Efficacy of behavioral interventions for reducing problem behavior in persons with autism: A quantitative synthesis of single-subject research. *Research in Developmental Disabilities, 24*, 120–138.

Cannella-Malone, H. I., Tullis, C. A., & Kazee, A. R. (2011). Using antecedent exercise to decrease challenging behavior in boys with developmental disabilities and an emotional disorder. *Journal of Positive Behavior Interventions, 13*, 230–239.

Carr, E. G., & Durand, V. M. (1985). Reducing behavior problems through functional communication training. *Journal of Applied Behavior Analysis, 18*, 111–126.

Carr, E. G., Newsom, C. D., & Binkoff, J. A. (1980). Escape as a factor in the aggressive behavior of two retarded children. *Journal of Applied Behavior Analysis, 13*, 101–117.

Carr, E. G., Smith, C. E., Giacin, T. A., Whelan, B. M., & Pancari, J. (2003). Menstrual discomfort as a biological setting event for severe problem behavior: Assessment and intervention. *American Journal on Mental Retardation, 108*, 117–133.

Carr, J. E., Coriaty, S., Wilder, D. A., Gaunt, B. T., Dozier, C. L., Britton, L. N., et al. (2000). A review of 'noncontingent' reinforcement as treatment for the aberrant behavior of individuals with developmental disabilities. *Research in Developmental Disabilities, 21*, 377–391.

Chambless, D. L., & Hollon, S. D. (1998). Defining empirically supported therapies. *Journal of Consulting and Clinical Psychology, 66*, 7–18.

Cowley, A., Newton, J., Sturmey, P., Bouras, N., & Holt, G. (2005). Psychiatric inpatient admissions of adults with intellectual disabilities: Predictive factors. *American Journal on Mental Retardation, 110*, 216–225.

Crocker, A. G., Mercier, C., Lachapelle, Y., Brunet, A., Morin, D., & Roy, M. E. (2006). Prevalence and types of aggressive behaviour among adults with intellectual disabilities. *Journal of Intellectual Disability Research, 50*, 652–661.

Davidson, P. W., Cain, N. N., Sloane-Reeves, J. E., Van Speybroech, A., Segel, J., Gutkin, J., et al. (1994). Characteristics of community-based individuals with mental retardation and aggressive behavioral disorders. *American Journal on Mental Retardation, 98*, 704–716.

Day, H. M., Horner, R. H., & O'Neill, R. E. (1994). Multiple functions of problem behaviors: Assessment and intervention. *Journal of Applied Behavior Analysis, 27*, 279–289.

De Ruiter, K. P., Dekker, M. C., Verhulst, F. C., & Koot, H. M. (2007). Developmental course of psychopathology in youths with and without intellectual disabilities. *Journal of Child Psychology and Psychiatry, 48,* 498–507.

De Wein, M., & Miller, L. K. (2009). The teaching family model: A program description and its effects on the aggressive behaviors and quality of life of two adults with intellectual disabilities. *Journal of Positive Behavior Interventions, 11,* 235–251.

De Zubicaray, G., & Clair, A. (1998). An evaluation of differential reinforcement of other behavior, differential reinforcement of incompatible behavior, and restitution for the management of aggressive behaviors. *Behavioral Interventions, 13,* 157–168.

DeLeon, I. G., Fisher, W. W., Herman, K. M., & Crosland, K. C. (2000). Assessment of a response bias for aggression over functionally equivalent appropriate behavior. *Journal of Applied Behavior Analysis, 33,* 73–77.

DeLeon, I. G., Kahng, S., Rodriguez-Catter, V., Sveinsdóttir, I., & Sadler, C. (2003). Assessment of aberrant behavior maintained by wheelchair movement in a child with developmental disabilities. *Research in Developmental Disabilities, 24,* 381–390.

Devlin, S., Healy, O., Leader, G., & Hughes, B. M. (2011). Comparison of behavioral intervention and sensory-integration therapy in the treatment of challenging behavior. *Journal of Autism and Developmental Disorders, 41,* 1303–1320.

Didden, R., Duker, P. C., & Korzilius, H. (1997). Meta-analytic study on treatment effectiveness for problem behaviors with individuals who have mental retardation. *American Journal on Mental Retardation, 101,* 387–399.

Doke, L., Cowlery, M., & Sumberg, C. (1983). Treating chronic aggression effects and side effects of response-contingent ammonia spirits. *Behavior Modification, 7,* 531–556.

Dougherty, B. S., Fowler, S. A., & Paine, S. C. (1985). The use of peer monitors to reduce negative interaction during recess. *Journal of Applied Behavior Analysis, 18,* 141–153.

Duncan, D., Matson, J. L., Bamburg, J. W., Cherry, K. E., & Buckley, T. (1999). The relationship of self-injurious behavior and aggression to social skills in persons with severe and profound learning disability. *Research in Developmental Disabilities, 20,* 441–448.

Durand, V. (1993). Functional communication training using assistive devices: Effects on challenging behavior and affect. *Augmentative and Alternative Communication, 9,* 168–176.

Durand, V. M., & Carr, E. G. (1991). Functional communication training to reduce challenging behavior: Maintenance and application in new settings. *Journal of Applied Behavior Analysis, 24,* 251–264.

Durand, V. M., & Carr, E. G. (1992). An analysis of maintenance following functional communication training. *Journal of Applied Behavior Analysis, 25,* 777–794.

Dyer, K., Dunlap, G., & Winterling, V. (1990). Effects of choice making on the serious problem behaviors of students with severe handicaps. *Journal of Applied Behavior Analysis, 23,* 515–524.

Edwards, P., & Miltenberger, R. (1991). Burnout among staff members at community residential facilities for persons with mental retardation. *Mental Retardation, 29,* 125–128.

Emerson, E., Cummings, R., Barrett, S., Hughes, H., McCool, C., & Toogood, A. (1988). Who are the people who challenge services? *Mental Handicap, 16,* 16–19.

Emerson, E., Kiernan, C., Alborz, A., Reeves, D., Mason, H., Swarbrick, R., et al. (2001). The prevalence of challenging behaviors: A total population study. *Research in Developmental Disabilities, 22,* 77–93.

Eyman, R. K., & Call, T. (1977). Maladaptive behavior and community placement of mentally retarded persons. *American Journal of Mental Deficiency, 2,* 137–144.

Feldman, M. A., Condillac, R. A., Tough, S., Hunt, S., & Griffiths, D. (2002). Effectiveness of community positive behavioral intervention for persons with developmental disabilities and severe behavior disorders. *Behavior Therapy, 33*, 377–398.

Fisher, W., Piazza, C., Cataldo, M., Harrell, R., Jefferson, G., & Conner, R. (1993). Functional communication training with and without extinction and punishment. *Journal of Applied Behavior Analysis, 26*, 23–36.

Fisher, W. W., O'Connor, J. T., Kurtz, P. F., DeLeon, I. G., & Gotjen, D. L. (2000). The effects of noncontingent delivery of high-and low-preference stimuli on attention-maintained destructive behavior. *Journal of Applied Behavior Analysis, 33*, 79–83.

Fisher, W. W., Thompson, R. H., Hagopian, L. P., Bowman, L. G., & Krug, A. (2000). Facilitating tolerance of delayed reinforcement during functional communication training. *Behavior Modification, 24*, 3–29.Foxx, R. M., & Meindl, J. (2007). The long term successful treatment of the aggressive/destructive behaviors of a preadolescent with autism. *Behavioral Interventions, 22*, 83–97.

Freeman, S. J. (1994). Organizational downsizing as convergence or reorientation: Implications for human resource management. *Human Resource Management, 33*, 213–238.

Gardner, W. I., & Moffatt, C. W. (1990). Aggressive behaviour: Definition, assessment, treatment. *International Review of Psychiatry, 2*, 91–100.

Green, V. A., O'Reilly, M., Itchon, J., & Sigafoos, J. (2005). Persistence of early emerging aberrant behavior in children with developmental disabilities. *Research in Developmental Disabilities, 26*, 47–55.

Hagerman, R. J., Bregman, J. D., & Tirosh, E. (1998). Clonidine. In S. Reiss & M. G. Aman (Eds.), *Psychotropic medications and developmental disabilities. The international consensus handbook.* Columbus, OH: Ohio State University, Nisonger Centre.

Hagliassis, N., Gulbenkoglu, H., Di Marco, M., Young, S., & Hudson, A. (2005). The anger management project: A group intervention for anger in people with physical and multiple disabilities. *Journal of Intellectual and Developmental Disability, 30*, 86–96.

Hamelin, J., Travis, R., & Sturmey, P. (2013). Anger management and intellectual disabilities: A systematic review. *Journal of Mental Health Research in Intellectual Disabilities, 6*, 60–70.

Hanley, G. P., Iwata, B. A., & Thompson, R. H. (2001). Reinforcement schedule thinning following treatment with functional communication training. *Journal of Applied Behavior Analysis, 34*, 17–38.

Hanley, G. P., Piazza, C. C., Fisher, W. W., Contrucci, S. A., & Maglieri, K. A. (1997). Evaluation of client preference for function-based treatment packages. *Journal of Applied Behavior Analysis, 30*, 459–473.

Hardan, A., & Sahl, R. (1997). Psychopathology in children and adolescents with developmental disorders. *Research in Developmental Disabilities, 18*, 369–382.

Harris, P. (1993). The nature and extent of aggressive behaviour amongst people with learning difficulties (mental handicap) in a single health district. *Journal of Intellectual Disability Research, 37*, 221–242.

Harris, P., & Russell, O. (1989). *The prevalence of aggressive behaviour among people with learning difficulties (mental handicap) in a single health district. Interim report.* Bristol, UK: Norah Fry Research Centre, University of Bristol.

Hastings, R. P., & Brown, T. (2002). Coping strategies and the impact of challenging behaviors on special educators' burnout. *Mental Retardation, 40*, 148–156.

Healy, O., & Lydon, S. (2013). Early intensive behavioural intervention in autism spectrum disorders. In M. Fitzgerald (Ed.), *Recent advances in autism spectrum disorders* (pp. 565–597). Rijeka, Croatia: InTech.

Healy, O., Lydon, S., Holloway, J., & Dwyer, M. (2014). Behavioral interventions for aggression in autism spectrum disorder. In V. B. Patel, V. R. Preedy & C. R. Martin (Eds.), *The comprehensive guide to autism* (pp. 461–486). New York: Springer.

Hemmings, C. P., Gravestock, S., Pickard, M., & Bouras, N. (2006). Psychiatric symptoms and problem behaviours in people with intellectual disabilities. *Journal of Intellectual Disability Research, 50,* 269–276.

Hill, B. K., & Bruininks, R. H. (1984). Maladaptive behavior of mentally retarded individuals in residential facilities. *American Journal of Mental Deficiency, 88,* 380–387.

Hill, J., & Furnis, F. (2006). Patterns of emotional and behavioral disturbance with autistic traits in young people with severe intellectual disabilities and challenging behaviors. *Research in Developmental Disabilities, 27,* 517–528.

Holden, B., & Gitlesen, J. P. (2006). A total population study of challenging behavior in the county of Hedmark, Norway: Prevalence and risk factors. *Research in Developmental Disabilities, 27,* 456–465.

Horner, R. H., Day, H. M., & Day, J. R. (1997). Using neutralizing routines to reduce problem behaviors. *Journal of Applied Behavior Analysis, 30,* 601–614.

Horner, R. H., Day, H. M., Sprague, J. R., O'Brien, M., & Heathfield, L. T. (1991). Interspersed requests: A nonaversive procedure for reducing aggression and self-injury during instruction. *Journal of Applied Behavior Analysis, 24,* 265–278.

Hudson, A., & Gavidia-Payne, S. (2002). Behavioural supports for parents of children with an intellectual disability and problem behaviours: An overview of the literature. *Journal of Intellectual and Developmental Disability, 27,* 31–55.

Jacobson, J. W. (1982). Problem behavior and psychiatric impairment within a developmentally disabled population I: Behavior frequency. *Applied Research in Mental Retardation, 3,* 121–139.

Jacobson, J. W., & Ackerman, L. J. (1993). Who is treated using restrictive behavioral procedures? A population perspective. *Research in Developmental Disabilities, 14,* 51–65.

Kahng, S., Abt, K. A., & Schonbachler, H. E. (2001). Assessment and treatment of low-rate high-intensity problem behavior. *Journal of Applied Behavior Analysis, 34,* 225–228.

Kearney, D. S., & Healy, O. (2011). Investigating the relationship between challenging behavior, co-morbid psychopathology and social skills in adults with moderate to severe intellectual disabilities in Ireland. *Research in Developmental Disabilities, 32,* 1556–1563.

Lawson, D. A., & O'Brien, R. M. (1994). Behavioral and self-report measures of burnout in developmental disabilities. *Journal of Organizational Behavior Management, 14,* 37–54.

LeBlanc, L. A., Hagopian, L. P., & Maglieri, K. A. (2000). Use of a token economy to eliminate excessive inappropriate social behavior in an adult with developmental disabilities. *Behavioral Interventions, 15,* 135–143.

LeBlanc, L. A., Hagopian, L. P., Marhefka, J. M., & Wilke, A. E. (2001). Effects of therapist gender and type of attention on assessment and treatment of attention maintained destructive behavior. *Behavioral Interventions, 16,* 39–57.

Lewis, M. H., Siva, J. R., & Silva, S. G. (1995). Cyclicity of aggression and self-injurious behaviour in individuals with mental retardation. *American Journal on Mental Retardation, 99,* 436–444.

Linaker, O. M. (1994). Assaultiveness among institutionalised adults with mental retardation. *British Journal of Psychiatry, 164*, 62–68.

Lowe, K., & Felce, D. (1995). How do carers assess the severity of challenging behaviour? A total population study. *Journal of Intellectual Disability Research, 30*, 117–127.

Luce, S. C., Delquadri, J., & Hall, R. V. (1980). Contingent exercise: A mild but powerful procedure for suppressing inappropriate verbal and aggressive behavior. *Journal of Applied Behavior Analysis, 13*, 583–594.

Lundqvist, L., Andersson, G., & Viding, J. (2009). Effects of vibroacoustic music on challenging behaviors in individuals with autism and developmental disabilities. *Research in Autism Spectrum Disorders, 3*, 390–400.

Marcus, B. A., & Vollmer, T. R. (1996). Combining noncontingent reinforcement and differential reinforcement schedules as treatment for aberrant behavior. *Journal of Applied Behavior Analysis, 29*, 43–51.

Matson, J. L., & Shoemaker, M. (2009). Intellectual disability and its relationship to autism spectrum disorders. *Research in Developmental Disabilities, 30*, 1107–1114.

May, M. E. (2011). Aggression as positive reinforcement in people with intellectual disabilities. *Research in Developmental Disabilities, 32*, 2214–2224.

McClintock, K., Hall, S., & Oliver, C. (2003). Risk markers associated with challenging behaviours in people with developmental disabilities: A meta-analytic study. *Journal of Intellectual Disability Research, 47*, 405–416.

McGillivray, J. A., & McCabe, P. (2004). Pharmacological management of challenging behavior of individuals with intellectual disability. *Research in Developmental Disabilities, 25*, 523–537.

McLean, L. K., Brady, N. C., & McLean, J. E. (1996). Reported communication abilities of individuals with severe mental retardation. *American Journal on Mental Retardation, 100*, 580–591.

Moss, S., Emerson, E., Kiernan, C., Turner, S., Hatton, C., & Alborz, A. (2000). Psychiatric symptoms in adults with learning disability and challenging behaviour. *British Journal of Psychiatry, 177*, 452–456.

Murphy, O., Healy, O., & Leader, G. (2009). Risk factors for challenging behaviour for 157 children with autism spectrum disorder in Ireland. *Research in Autism Spectrum Disorders, 3*, 474–482.

Najdowski, A. C., Wallace, M. D., Ellsworth, C. L., MacAleese, A. N., & Cleveland, J. M. (2008). Functional analyses and treatment of precursor behavior. *Journal of Applied Behavior Analysis, 41*, 97–105.

Neilsen, S. L., & McEvoy, M. A. (2004). Functional behavioral assessment in early education settings. *Journal of Early Intervention, 26*, 115–131.

Newsom, C. D., & Hovanitz, C. A. (2005). The nature and value of empirically validated clinical services. In J. W. Jacobson, J. A. Mulick, & R. M. Fox (Eds.), *Fads: Dubious and improbable treatments for developmental disabilities*. Mahway, NJ: Lawrence Erlbaum.

Nicoll, M., Beail, N., & Saxon, D. (2013). Cognitive behavioural treatment for anger in adults with intellectual disabilities: A systematic review and meta-analysis. *Journal of Applied Research in Intellectual Disabilities, 26*, 47–62.

Niemeyer, A. J., & Fox, J. (1990). Reducing aggressive behavior during car riding through parent-implemented DRO and fading procedures. *Education and Treatment of Children, 13*, 21–35.

Novaco, R. W. (1975). *Anger control: The development and evaluation of an experimental treatment.* Lexington, MA: D.C. Health.

Novaco, R. W. (1991). *The Novaco anger scale (September 1991 Version).* Irvine, CA: University of California, Irvine.

Novaco, R. W. (1994). Anger as a risk factor for violence among the mentally disordered. In J. Monahan & H. J. Steadman (Eds.), *Violence and mental disorder* (pp. 21–59). Chicago: The University of Chicago Press.

Novaco, R. W., & Taylor, J. L. (2004). Assessment of anger and aggression in male offenders with developmental disabilities. *Psychological Assessment, 16,* 42–50.

O'Neill, R. E., Horner, R. H., Albin, R. W., Sprague, J. R., Storey, K., & Newton, J. S. (1997). *Functional assessment and program development for problem behavior.* Pacific Grove, CA: Brooks/Cole.

O'Reilly, M., Lancioni, G., & Taylor, I. (1999). An empirical analysis of two forms of extinction to treat aggression. *Research in Developmental Disabilities, 20,* 315–325.

O'Reilly, M. F., Lancioni, G. E., King, L., Lally, G., & Dhomhnaill, O. N. (2000). Using brief assessments to evaluate aberrant behavior maintained by attention. *Journal of Applied Behavior Analysis, 33,* 109–112.

Phillips, K. J., & Mudford, O. C. (2011). Effects of noncontingent reinforcement and choice of activity on aggressive behavior maintained by attention. *Behavioral Interventions, 26,* 147–160.

Quine, L. (1986). Behaviour problems in severely mentally handicapped children. *Psychological Medicine, 16,* 895–907.

Ramandi, L., Daneshfar, A., & Shojaei, M. (2012). Effects of aromatherapy and play on intellectually disables' [sic] aggression. *Annals of Biological Research, 3,* 5211–5215.

Renwick, S. J., Black, L., Ramm, M., & Novaco, R. W. (1997). Anger treatment with forensic hospital patients. *Legal and Criminological Psychology, 2,* 103–116.

Repp, A. C., & Deitz, S. M. (1974). Reducing aggressive and self-injurious behavior of institutionalized retarded children through reinforcement of other behaviors. *Journal of Applied Behavior Analysis, 7,* 313–325.

Richman, D. M., Berg, W. K., Wacker, D. P., Stephens, T., Rankin, B., & Kilroy, J. (1997). Using pretreatment and posttreatment assessments to enhance and evaluate existing treatment packages. *Journal of Applied Behavior Analysis, 30,* 709–712.

Ringdahl, J. E., Call, N. A., Mews, J. B., Boelter, E. W., & Christensen, T. J. (2008). Assessment and treatment of aggressive behavior without a clear social function. *Research in Developmental Disabilities, 29,* 351–362.

Ringdahl, J. E., Christensen, T. J., & Boelter, E. W. (2009). Further evaluation of idiosyncratic functions for severe problem behavior: Aggression maintained by access to walks. *Behavioral Interventions, 24,* 275–283.

Ringdahl, J. E., Falcomata, T. S., Christensen, T. J., Bass-Ringdahl, S. M., Lentz, A., Dutt, A., et al. (2009). Evaluation of a pre-treatment assessment to select mand topographies for functional communication training. *Research in Developmental Disabilities, 30,* 330–341.

Rojahn, J., Matson, J. L., Naglieri, J. A., & Mayville, E. (2004). Relationships between psychiatric conditions and behavior problems among adults with mental retardation. *American Journal of Mental Retardation, 109,* 21–33.

Rose, J. (2010). Carer reports on the efficacy of cognitive behavioral interventions for anger. *Research in Developmental Disabilities, 31,* 1502–1508.

Sigafoos, J., Elkins, J., Kerr, M., & Attwood, T. (1994). A survey of aggressive behavior among a population of persons with intellectual disability in Queensland. *Journal of Intellectual Disability Research, 94*, 369–388.

Sigafoos, J., & Kerr, M. (1994). Provision of leisure activities for the reduction of challenging behavior. *Behavioral Interventions, 9*, 43–53.

Singh, N., Wahler, R. G., Adkins, A. D., & Myers, R. E. (2003). Soles of the feet: A mindfulness-based self-control intervention for aggression by an individual with mild mental retardation and mental illness. *Research in Developmental Disabilities, 24*, 158–169.

Slifer, K. J., Ivancic, M. T., Parrish, J. M., Page, T. J., & Burgio, L. D. (1986). Assessment and treatment of multiple behavior problems exhibited by a profoundly retarded adolescent. *Journal of Behavior Therapy and Experimental Psychiatry, 17*, 203–213.

Sovner, R., DesNoyers-Hurley, A., & LaBrie, R. A. (1982). Diagnosing depression in the mentally retarded. *Psychiatric Aspects of Mental Retardation Newsletter, 1*, 1–3.

Sturmey, P. (2004). Cognitive therapy with people with intellectual disabilities: A selective review and critique. *Clinical Psychology and Psychotherapy, 11*, 222–232.

Sturmey, P. (2006). On some recent claims for the efficacy of cognitive therapy for people with intellectual disabilities. *Journal of Applied Research in Intellectual Disabilities, 19*, 109–117.

Tarbox, J., Wallace, M. D., Tarbox, R. S., Landaburu, H. J., & Williams, W. L. (2004). Functional analysis and treatment of low-rate problem behavior in individuals with developmental disabilities. *Behavioral Interventions, 19*, 73–90.

Taylor, J. L. (2002). A review of the assessment and treatment of anger and aggression in offenders with intellectual disability. *Journal of Intellectual Disability Research, 46*, 57–73.

Taylor, J. L., Novaco, R. W., Gillmer, B., & Thorne, I. (2002). Cognitive-behavioural treatment of anger intensity among offenders with intellectual disabilities. *Journal of Applied Research in Intellectual Disabilities, 15*, 151–165.

Taylor, J. L., Novaco, R. W., Gillmer, B. T., Robertson, A., & Thorne, I. (2005). Individual cognitive-behavioural anger treatment for people with mild-borderline disabilities and histories of aggression: A controlled trial. *British Journal of Clinical Psychology, 44*, 367–382.

Tenneij, N. H., Didden, R., Stolker, J. J., & Koot, H. M. (2009). Markers for aggression in inpatient treatment facilities for adults with mild to borderline intellectual disability. *Research in Developmental Disabilities, 30*, 1248–1257.

Tenneij, N. H., & Koot, H. M. (2008). Incidence, types and characteristics of aggressive behaviour in treatment facilities for adults with mild intellectual disability and severe challenging behaviour. *Journal of Intellectual Disability Research, 52*, 114–124.

Thompson, R. H., Fisher, W. W., Piazza, C. C., & Kuhn, D. E. (1998). The evaluation and treatment of aggression maintained by attention and automatic reinforcement. *Journal of Applied Behavior Analysis, 31*, 103–115.

Tyrer, F., McGrother, C. W., Thorp, C. F., Donaldson, M., Bhaumik, S., Watson, J. M., et al. (2006). Physical aggression towards others in adults with learning disabilities: Prevalence and associated factors. *Journal of Intellectual Disability Research, 50*, 295–304.

Van Camp, C. M., Lerman, D. C., Kelley, M. E., Contrucci, S. A., & Vorndran, C. M. (2000). Variable-time reinforcement schedules in the treatment of socially maintained problem behavior. *Journal of Applied Behavior Analysis, 33*, 545–557.

Van Nieuwenhuijzen, M., Orobio de Castro, B., van der Valk, I., Vermeer, A., & Matthys, W. (2006). Do social information-processing models explain aggressive behaviour by children with mild intellectual disabilities in residential care? *Journal of Intellectual Disability Research, 50*, 801–812.

Vollmer, T. R., Progar, P. R., Lalli, J. S., Van Camp, C. M., Sierp, B. J., Wright, C. S., et al. (1998). Fixed-time schedules attenuate extinction-induced phenomena in the treatment of severe aberrant behavior. *Journal of Applied Behavior Analysis, 31*, 529–542.

Vollmer, T. R., Ringdahl, J. E., Roane, H. S., & Marcus, B. A. (1997). Negative side effects of noncontingent reinforcement. *Journal of Applied Behavior Analysis, 30*, 161–164.

Wacker, D. P., Steege, M. W., Northup, J., Sasso, G., Berg, W., Reimers, T., et al. (1990). A component analysis of functional communication training across three topographies of severe behavior problems. *Journal of Applied Behavior Analysis, 23*, 417–429.

Whitaker, S. (2001). Anger control for people with learning disabilities: A critical review. *Behavioural and Cognitive Psychotherapy, 29*, 277–293.

6

Self-Injurious Behavior

Jeff Sigafoos, Mark F. O'Reilly, Giulio E. Lancioni,
Russell Lang, and Robert Didden

Introduction

This chapter considers the nature of self-injurious behavior (SIB) and reviews
evidence for treatments to reduce SIB among people with intellectual disabilities
(ID). The chapter is divided into four sections. The first section gives an overview of the definition of SIB and lists the most common forms of SIB among
individuals with ID. Prevalence rates and risk factors for SIB among people with
ID are also summarized here. This section ends by considering the impact and
cost of SIB. This overview shows that SIB is a major problem for a significant
percentage of individuals with ID. The second section outlines the methodology
undertaken to identify treatment studies for review. The search strategy, search
terms, and the inclusion and exclusion criteria are described. Procedures for clas-
sifying and appraising treatment studies are also described. The third section
reviews the evidence base supporting identified treatments. Treatments were
assessed using Chambless and Hollon's (1998) criteria for determining whether
each treatment approach was either (a) effective or (b) ineffective, (c) has
conflicting evidence regarding its effectiveness, or (d) has not yet been sufficiently researched (i.e., insufficient evidence). The chapter's concluding section
provides clinical guidelines for selecting and implementing SIB treatments. These
guidelines are intended to facilitate evidence-based practice in the treatment of
SIB among individuals with ID.

Evidence-Based Practice and Intellectual Disabilities, First Edition.
Edited by Peter Sturmey and Robert Didden.
© 2014 John Wiley & Sons, Ltd. Published 2014 by John Wiley & Sons, Ltd.

The Nature of SIB among Individuals with ID

Definition

Winchel and Stanley (1991) defined SIB as

> the commission of deliberate harm to one's own body. The injury is done to oneself, without the aid of another person, and the injury is severe enough for tissue damage (such as scarring) to result (p. 306).

Smith, Vollmer, and St. Peter Pipkin (2007), however, noted that behaviors having "the capacity to produce tissue damage to the individual's own body" (p. 188) should also be considered as forms of SIB. In line with these definitions and for the purpose of the present chapter, SIB is defined as behavior directed towards oneself that causes—or has the potential to cause—tissue damage. This definition covers the SIB forms most commonly observed among people with ID.

Common forms of SIB

Table 6.1 lists the most commonly and consistently identified SIB forms based on the collective results of numerous studies (Bienstein & Nussbeck, 2009; Emerson et al., 2001; Griffin et al., 1987; Holden & Gitlesen, 2006; Murphy et al., 1993; Oliver, Murphy, & Corbett, 1987; Schroeder, Schroeder, Smith, & Dalldorf, 1978; Sigafoos, Elkins, Kerr, & Attwood, 1994; Van Ingen, Moore, Zaja, & Rojahn, 2010). Head hitting and head banging are perhaps the most common form of SIB, occurring in approximately 40% of all SIB cases. Self-induced vomiting and aerophagia (air swallowing), in contrast, are relatively rare in that they occur in only about 2% of all SIB cases; however, it is also important to note that some relatively rare SIB forms are more common among certain subpopulations. Skin picking, for example, is more

Table 6.1 Common Forms of SIB among Individuals with ID

Hits head with hand/body	*Hits head with/against objects*
Skin picking	Bites self
Head punching/slapping	Pinches/scratches self
Pica (eats inedible objects)	Punching/slapping body
Polydipsia	Bruxism (teeth grinding)
Eye poking	Trichotillomania (pulls out hair)
Pinching self	Cutting self with an object
Poking self in the anus	Poking self in other locations
Self-induced vomiting	Aerophagia (swallow air)
Chewing on lips	Nail removal

common among individuals with Prader–Willi syndrome compared to the more general ID population (Didden, Korzilius, & Curfs, 2007).

Prevalence of SIB

SIB occurs in approximately 10–12% of all people with ID (Bienstein & Nussbeck, 2009; Emerson et al., 2001; Griffin et al., 1987; Holden & Gitlesen, 2006; Murphy et al., 1993; Oliver et al., 1987; Schroeder et al., 1978; Sigafoos et al., 1994; Van Ingen et al., 2010); however, other studies have reported prevalence estimates closer to 3–4% figure (Holden & Gitlesen, 2006; Lowe et al., 2007). These varying prevalence estimates are consistent with evidence showing that SIB varies in relation to certain risk factors.

Risk factors

Placement
SIB is more prevalent among people with ID in institutional versus community settings (Holden & Gitlesen, 2006; Lowe et al., 2007). This could reflect a tendency for people with SIB to be placed in institutions, although Oliver et al. (1987) noted that the prevalence of SIB is more difficult to estimate among community samples.

Genetic syndromes
ID is associated with a large number of genetic syndromes, some of which appear to predispose the individual to SIB (Percy et al., 2007). Lesch–Nyhan and Cornelia de Lange syndromes, for example, are associated with an increased risk of SIB, which often takes a precise, syndrome-specific form (Winchel & Stanley, 1991). There also appears to be an increased prevalence of self-injurious skin picking among individuals with Prader–Willi syndrome (Symons, Butler, Sanders, Feurer, & Thompson, 1999). The presence of such behavioral phenotypes means that evidence-based treatments should be viewed in light of whether or not they have been successfully used with individuals with syndrome-associated SIB.

Comorbid conditions
SIB is more prevalent among individuals with ID who also have autism or psychopathology (e.g., depression, bipolar disorder). When these factors are combined, the prevalence of SIB appears to be higher than for any other clinical group (Matson & LoVullo, 2008). Indeed, SIB may be observed in up to 50% of individuals with severe ID who have comorbid autism (Baghdadli, Pascal, Grisi, & Aussilloux, 2003). The presence of significant vision or hearing impairment or seizure disorders also increases the risk of SIB among individuals with ID (Schroeder et al., 1978; Schroeder, Tessel, Loupe, & Stodgell, 1997). SIB may indicate the presence of illness or pain relating to an undiagnosed medical condition (Gunsett, Mulick, Fernald, & Martin,

1989). As noted by Matson and LoVullo, the presence of comorbid conditions could interact with the operant function of SIB in complex ways, necessitating the need for combinations of specialized treatments.

Age

SIB can begin in infancy but more often emerges between 2 and 3 years of age (Schroeder et al., 1997). Some children with ID develop repetitive behaviors that appear to be precursors to SIB (Murphy, Hall, Oliver, & Kissi-Debra, 1999). It is unclear whether treatment of such precursory acts would prevent SIB. What is known, however, is that improvement through the developmental period is unlikely in the absence of effective treatment. Instead, SIB will often become more frequent and severe throughout childhood and into adolescence (Emerson et al., 2001), before moderating somewhat in adulthood. Overall, these age trends indicate that SIB treatments are likely to be needed to cover the entire lifespan.

Intellectual and adaptive functioning

SIB is more prevalent among individuals with severe, as compared to mild/moderate, ID (Schroeder et al., 1997). There is a similar inverse relation between SIB and the level of adaptive behavior functioning. More precisely, impairments in the areas of self-care (e.g., eating, dressing, washing, toileting), gross motor (e.g., mobility), social skills, and communication functioning (e.g., receptive and expressive speech) have been linked to increased frequency and severity of SIB and other problem behaviors among individuals with ID (Emerson et al., 2001; Matson, Anderson, & Bamburg, 2000; Schroeder et al., 1997); however, individuals with more severe intellectual impairment also tend to have greater adaptive behavior deficits. Given this relation, an important question is whether impairments in any specific area of adaptive behavior functioning, such as the communication or social skills domains, are unique risk factors for SIB. This question has significant clinical implications because some SIB treatments (e.g., functional communication training (FCT)) explicitly focus on ameliorating deficits in a specific area of adaptive behavior functioning.

Negative impact and financial costs of SIB

Treatment of SIB is a major priority because of the associated injury and related health problems. The injury and damage caused by SIB can accumulate over time leading to long-term negative health consequences. In addition to injury and long-term health, SIB is associated with significant psychological costs, such as increased rates of medication use, isolation, restriction of opportunities, and the use of physical or mechanical restraint to prevent SIB (National Institutes of Health, 1989).

Given the high potential for injury and long-term trauma, there can also be a high financial cost associated with SIB. The National Institutes of Health (1989) estimated the annual cost of care for a person with severe SIB at $US100,000 per year. It is likely that the cost of care for individuals with SIB varies with the frequency, severity, and form of SIB. And the costs would likely escalate when there is a need for frequent and repeated hospitalizations and emergency medical care. The direct and indirect costs associated with SIB for any given individual are difficult to estimate, but most probably the overall financial cost of caring for an individual with SIB will be much greater than it is for individuals with ID who do not engage in SIB.

In addition to the financial costs, there can be great social costs associated with SIB. SIB is a major cause of institutionalization among individuals with ID (Winchel & Stanley, 1991). For individuals who remain in the community, SIB can greatly restrict their opportunities for community access and prevent successful employment and community integration. Furthermore, SIB is highly distressing to parents, educators, and caregivers, which can negatively affect the quality of their interactions with the individual. This, in turn, might reduce the overall quality of life for all parties involved (Rojahn, Schroeder, & Hoch, 2008).

Given the injury and costs associated with SIB, there is a need to distinguish effective evidence-based treatments from ineffective and unproven treatments. The next section described procedures that we followed to identify and appraise the evidence base related to SIB treatments for individuals with ID.

Methodology for Identifying Treatment Studies

We conducted a systematic search for, and review of, studies that were focused on the treatment of SIB in children, adolescents, or adults with ID. For the purpose of this review, ID was defined as (a) significantly subaverage intellectual functioning (i.e., IQ of 75 or less) and (b) concurrent deficits in adaptive behavior functioning, both of which must be present in the developmental period prior to age 18 years (American Psychiatric Association, 2000).

Search strategies

To identify treatment studies, we conducted systematic searches in three electronic databases: Education Resources Information Center (ERIC), Medline, and PsycINFO. Publication year was not restricted, but the search was limited to English-language journal articles. In all three databases, the terms *self-injurious behavior* (or *SIB* or *self-mutilation*) and *intellectual disability* (or *developmental disability* or *mental retardation*) were inserted into the *Keywords* field. Abstracts of the records returned from these electronic searches were reviewed to identify studies for inclusion in the review (see Section "Inclusion criteria"). The reference lists for the included studies were also reviewed to identify additional articles for possible inclusion.

Inclusion criteria

To be included in this review, the article had to meet three inclusion criteria. First, the study was published in English and in a peer-reviewed journal to ensure that all studies had been subjected to quality control via peer review. Second, the study reported an evaluation of one or more treatments for SIB. Treatment was defined as implementing one or more therapeutic strategies, behavioral interventions, or teaching procedures in an attempt to reduce the frequency or severity of SIB. Treatments involving the use of psychotropic medications were excluded from this review. While antidepressants, antipsychotics, and mood stabilizers have been used to treat severe behavior problems (Morgan, Campbell, & Jackson, 2003), Deb et al. (2008) noted that methodological problems make it difficult to fully evaluate the efficacy of such medications when used on people with ID. Mayville (2007) provided a comprehensive review on the use of psychotropic medications for individuals with ID. Third, the study included objective data, based on either direct observation or use of standardized rating scales, on the frequency and/or severity of SIB in at least one person with ID.

Treatment classification

Treatments meeting the inclusion criteria were classified into one of four categories or broad approaches. First, treatments based on the principles of *applied behavior analysis* (ABA) were defined as any procedure that involved a two-step approach consisting of (a) the prior use of one or more functional assessment procedures to identify the operant function of SIB and (b) the implementation of one or more functional-based treatments that were directed at reducing SIB. Examples of ABA-based treatments include FCT, noncontingent reinforcement (NCR), and function-based extinction. Second, treatments based on the principles of *behavior modification* were considered similar to ABA-based approaches but defined as involving the manipulation of environmental contingencies (i.e., reinforcement and/or punishment schedules) without a prior functional assessment to identify the variables maintaining SIB. Examples of behavior modification procedures include (a) differential reinforcement schedules, (b) punishment procedures, and (c) contingent use of restraints. It should be noted that within the behavior modification approach, restraints are used therapeutically with the aim of reducing future likelihood of SIB, not to physically prevent SIB. Third, *cognitive behavior therapy* (CBT) was defined as any treatment approach that focused on changing a person's dysfunctional thoughts, beliefs, self-perceptions, and feelings. And fourth, *other treatment approaches* were defined as those that did not fit into one of the other three categories. Examples of other treatment approaches include sensory integrative therapy (SIT), Gentle Teaching, and electroconvulsive therapy (ECT).

Evidence appraisal

Treatments were evaluated in terms of the amount and results of available research evidence using the criteria outlined by Chambless and Hollon (1998). From this evaluation, treatment approaches were classified as either (a) effective, (b) ineffective, (c) inconclusive, or (d) lacking sufficient evidence. A treatment approach was considered to be *effective* if there were at least three studies by independent research teams showing that the treatment was successful in producing clinically significant reductions in the frequency or severity of SIB in at least nine individuals with ID. A treatment was considered *ineffective* if there were at least three studies by independent research teams showing that the treatment was unsuccessful in producing clinically significant reductions in the frequency or severity of SIB in at least nine individuals with ID. A treatment approach was considered *inconclusive* if there were at least three studies by independent research teams showing conflicting evidence regarding the success of the treatment. Finally, a treatment was considered as *lacking sufficient evidence* if there were fewer than three studies evaluating that treatment approach. Table 6.2 provides a summary of the evidence for each identified treatments. A more detailed review of each of these treatments is provided in the next section of this chapter.

Table 6.2 Summary of Evidence Base for SIB Treatments

Treatment	Summary of evidence
ABA	
Functional communication training	Effective
Noncontingent reinforcement	Effective
Function-based extinction	Effective
Behavior modification	
Differential reinforcement schedules	Effective
Punishment	Effective
Contingent restraint/protective equipment	Effective
Cognitive behavior therapy	Lacks sufficient evidence
Auditory integration training	Ineffective
Sensory integrative therapy	Ineffective
Weighted vests	Lacks sufficient evidence
Gentle Teaching	Lacks sufficient evidence
Electroconvulsive therapy	Lacks sufficient evidence
Snoezelen rooms	Lacks sufficient evidence
Transcutaneous electric nerve stimulation	Lacks sufficient evidence
Exercise	Lacks sufficient evidence
Room management	Lacks sufficient evidence

Treatment Review

Applied behavior analysis

There is a large amount of evidence to support the use of ABA-based approaches for the treatment of SIB among individuals with ID (Sigafoos, Arthur, & O'Reilly, 2003). The amount and results of this research exceed the criteria outlined by Chambless and Hollon (1998) for an effective treatment. Indeed, the results of several meta-analytic reviews indicate that ABA-based and related behavior modification procedures are the most effective treatments for SIB and other problem behaviors of individuals with ID (Christiansen, 2009; Didden, Duker, & Korzilius, 1997; Didden, Korzilius, van Oorsouw, & Sturmey, 2006; Harvey, Boer, Meyer, & Evans, 2009; Lang et al., 2010; Scotti, Evans, Meyer, & Walker, 1991). Christiansen, for example, undertook a meta-analysis of 224 studies focused on the treatment of SIB. These 224 studies involved 343 participants with ID, autism spectrum disorder, or other developmental disability syndromes. The results of this meta-analysis showed that behavioral treatments, specifically ABA-based and related behavior modification procedures, "generally have a robust effect on the reduction of self-injury" (p. 139). Given the consistent support for ABA-based procedures from the existing meta-analytic studies, this section outlines some of the distinguishing features of the approach and reviews specific ABA-based treatments.

The distinguishing features of ABA-based treatments are (a) the use of a prior functional assessment protocol to identify the operant function of SIB and (b) the implementation of one or more function-based treatments that are conceptually related to, and derived from, more basic principles of learning theory (Baer, Wolf, & Risley, 1987). This two-stage approach to treatment is consistent with evidence showing that SIB often serves one of more operant functions and that function-based treatments are comparatively more effective than nonfunction-based treatments (Smith et al., 2007).

Functional assessment

There is a large amount of data to support the use of a prior functional assessment as the first step in SIB treatment (Didden, 2007; Smith et al., 2007). Functional assessment in this context refers to the use of one or more procedures (e.g., experimental-functional analysis, descriptive analysis, interviews, and rating scales) to identify the operant function of SIB (Rojahn, Whittaker, Hoch, & González, 2007). Smith et al. described the various types of functional assessment procedures that have been used to identify or assess the operant function of SIB among individuals with ID.

In an experimental-functional analysis, for example, the frequency of SIB is recorded during a number of standardized experimental conditions, each of which is designed to test for the influence of a specific variable (e.g., attention, tangibles, task demands, and sensory stimulation). The experimental conditions are typically alternated until each has been presented 7–10 times within a multielement design

(Kennedy, 2005). The experimental-functional analysis protocol described by Iwata, Dorsey, Slifer, Bauman, and Richman (1982/1994) remains the gold standard for undertaking a functional assessment of SIB.

Data from numerous studies involving the use of functional assessment indicate that SIB is often maintained by either positive (e.g., attention from an adult or access to preferred objects or activities), negative (e.g., escape from, or avoidance of, nonpreferred tasks or objects), or automatic reinforcement in the form of sensory stimulation (Iwata et al., 1994; Rojahn et al., 2007; Smith et al., 2007).

Functional assessment is not a treatment but rather an assessment approach that is used to select function-based treatments. There is a large amount of strong evidence showing that functional assessments, particularly the experimental-functional analysis procedure described by Iwata et al. (1982/1994), are highly effective in identifying the operant function of SIB among individuals with ID. The approach has led to a number of function-based treatments to address SIB related to positive, negative, and automatic reinforcement (Smith et al., 2007). Some of the more widely used function-based treatments include FCT, NCR, and function-based extinction. It is important to note, however, that it is not always possible to identify an operant function of SIB using functional assessment procedures (Vollmer, Marcus, & LeBlanc, 1994). It is also important to note that ABA- or function-based approaches are often combined into multicomponent treatment packages (e.g., functional communication plus extinction).

Functional communication training

FCT aims to reduce SIB by teaching appropriate forms of communication that enable the individual to access the same reinforcers that maintain his/her SIB (Durand, 1990; Sigafoos, O'Reilly, & Lancioni, 2009). In FCT, the operant function of SIB is first identified through a functional assessment. Next, an appropriate and functionally equivalent communication response is selected for instruction. For example, if SIB is maintained by attention, then the person might be taught to recruit attention by raising their hand. Alternatively, if SIB is maintained by escape from task demands, then the person might be taught to request a break from nonpreferred tasks using manual signs or by touching a *BREAK* symbol on a picture-based communication board. Instructional procedures associated with FCT include (a) response prompting to ensure the person emits the new communication form under appropriate conditions (e.g., when adults are present but not attending, when confronted with a task demand), (b) reinforcing the prompted communication response with the same consequence (e.g., attention, escape) that maintain SIB, and (c) fading the use of prompts over time to promote self-initiated use of the appropriate communication response (Carr et al., 1994; Durand, 1990; Sigafoos et al., 2009).

A considerable amount of research supports the use of FCT for the treatment of SIB among individuals with ID and related developmental disabilities (Durand & Merges, 2001; Kahng, Iwata, DeLeon, & Worsdell, 1997; Mancil, 2006; Mirenda, 1997; Robinson & Owens, 1995; Shirley, Iwata, Kahng, Mazaleski, & Lerman, 1997; Wacker et al., 1990; Worsdell, Iwata, Hanley, Thompson, & Kahng, 2000). Based on

Chambless and Hollon's (1998) criteria, FCT exceeds the criteria for an effective treatment; however, there has been some debate regarding the mechanisms responsible for the effectiveness of FCT. Hagopian, Fisher, Sullivan, Acquisto, and LeBlanc (1998), for example, demonstrated that extinction (i.e., ensuring that SIB is no longer reinforced) is crucial to the success of FCT. Smith et al. (2007) noted that the FCT could be conceptualized as a type of differential reinforcement schedule.

Noncontingent reinforcement
NCR aims to reduce SIB by providing access to the same reinforcers that maintain SIB. The procedure involves delivering the same consequences that maintain SIB on a noncontingent or fixed-time basis (Tucker, Sigafoos, & Bushell, 1998). To use NCR, one must first identify the type(s) of reinforcement that maintains SIB. This is done through a prior functional assessment. Next, the same type of reinforcement that was shown to maintain SIB in the functional assessment is delivered to the person on a fixed-time schedule (e.g., every 10, 20, or 30 s) regardless of the person's behavior. For example, if SIB is maintained by attention, then the person might receive attention every 30 s. Alternatively, if SIB is maintained by escape from task demands, then the person would receive a break from the task every 30 s. Or, if SIB is maintained by access to preferred objects, then the person would receive access to a preferred object every 30 s. Over time, the delivery schedule is gradually increased (e.g., from 30 to 60 s and then from 60 s to 1, 2, 3, and 5 min) to promote tolerance for delay of reinforcement.

A large amount of research supports the use of NCR as an SIB treatment for individuals with ID (DeLeon, Anders, Rodriguez-Catter, & Neidert, 2000; Kahng, Iwata, DeLeon, & Wallace, 2000; Tucker et al., 1998; Vollmer, Marcus, & Ringdahl, 1995). NCR is an effective treatment based on Chambless and Hollon's (1998) criteria; however, there has been some debate as to whether or not NCR must include delivery of the exact same type of reinforcement that was shown to maintain SIB in the prior functional assessment. Fischer, Iwata, and Mazaleski (1997), for example, demonstrated that noncontingent delivery of arbitrary reinforcers (i.e., preferred items that were not related to the person's SIB) was also effective in reducing SIB. When arbitrary reinforcers are used, NCR would be considered a behavior modification, rather than ABA-based, procedure. NCR appears to reduce SIB indirectly by ameliorating relative states of deprivation and/or reducing exposure to aversive stimuli (Tucker et al.).

Function-based extinction
Function-based extinction aims to reduce SIB by ensuring that it is no longer followed by reinforcement (Sigafoos et al., 2003). The procedure involves ensuring that the consequences that maintain SIB no longer occur during or immediately following SIB. To use function-based extinction, one must first identify the type(s) of reinforcement that maintains SIB. This is done through a prior functional assessment. Next, the clinician must ensure that the maintaining consequences do not occur after SIB. For example, if SIB is maintained by attention, then the clinician must

ensure that attention is no longer given to the person during or following episodes of SIB. This approach is also known as planned or systematic ignoring. Alternatively, if SIB is maintained by escape from task demands, then the clinician must ensure that the person is not allowed to escape from the task if SIB occurs. This approach is known as escape extinction (Zarcone, Iwata, Vollmer et al., 1993). As another example, if SIB is maintained by automatic reinforcement in the form of sensory stimulation, then the clinician must ensure that sensory stimulation does not follow SIB—an approach known as sensory extinction (Luiselli, 1984, 1988).

Function-based extinction is an effective treatment for SIB among individuals with ID according to Chambless and Hollon's (1998) criteria. Data from numerous studies provide strong evidence to support the use of function-based extinction either alone or in combination with other procedures, such as FCT and NCR (Iwata, Pace, Cowdery, & Miltenberger, 1994; Luiselli, 1984; Pace, Iwata, Cowdery, Adree, & McIntyre, 1993; Roscoe, Iwata, & Goh, 1998; Zarcone, Iwata, Hughes, & Vollmer, 1993; Zarcone, Iwata, Vollmer et al., 1993).

Behavior modification

The behavior modification approach is based primarily on the law of effect, in that reinforcement or punishment contingencies are introduced to strengthen alternative behavior and suppress SIB (Foxx, 1996; Kazdin, 2001). Behavior modification procedures have the same historical and conceptual roots as ABA-based treatments (Baer et al., 1987; Foxx, 1996). In addition to sharing common roots, ABA and behavior modification can be viewed as umbrella terms that refer to a wide range of more specific procedures. Overall, meta-analytic studies have shown that ABA-based and behavior modification procedures are highly effective in the treatment of SIB among individuals with ID (Christiansen, 2009; Didden et al., 1997, 2006; Harvey et al., 2009; Scotti et al., 1991).

While ABA-based and behavior modification approaches share common roots, the two can be distinguished by whether or not the resulting behavioral treatment has been informed by the use of a prior functional assessment. Given that functional assessment emerged as a standardized pretreatment protocol during the 1980s, ABA- or function-based approaches could be seen as a contemporary refinement of the prevailing behavior modification approach of the 1960s and 1970s; however, because it may not always be possible to identify an operant function for SIB (Iwata et al., 1994), behavior modification approaches remain relevant.

Specific behavior modification approaches include differential reinforcement and punishment; however, it is important to note, as is the case with ABA-based treatments, that behavior modification treatments often involve a combination of procedures. The use of restraint and protective equipment, for example, is a third class of treatment procedures that are often used in combination within a general behavior modification approach and will therefore be reviewed in this section.

Differential reinforcement schedules

Differential reinforcement schedules have been widely used and their effectiveness well established, for reducing SIB among individuals with ID (Foxx, 1982). Differential reinforcement schedules aim to reduce SIB either by reinforcing the absence of SIB, which is through differential reinforcement of other behavior (DRO), or by reinforcing an alternative or incompatible behavior, which is through differential reinforcement of alternative behavior (DRA) or differential reinforcement of incompatible behavior (DRI).

With DRO, the clinician reinforces the person for increasing periods of time without SIB. Initially, reinforcement might occur every 10 s provided that no SIB has occurred in the previous 10 s. Later, the time interval is increased to teach the person to inhibit SIB for increasingly longer periods of time. With DRA, reinforcement is provided contingent upon an alternative to SIB, such as playing with toys or using academic materials. With DRI, reinforcement is provided for the occurrence of behaviors that are incompatible with SIB. For example, a person who engaged in self-injurious hand biting might be reinforced for keeping their hands in contact with work materials.

DRO, DRA, and DRI meet the criteria for effective treatments based on Chambless and Hollon's (1998) criteria. Numerous studies from different research teams have demonstrated successful use of differential reinforcement schedules to reduce SIB among individuals with ID. Smith et al. (2007) and Vollmer and Iwata (1992) have reviewed this literature. Vollmer and Iwata noted that differential reinforcement schedules are more likely to be successful when they make use of the same the type of reinforcement that currently maintains the person's problem behavior. That is, function-based differential reinforcement is more effective than the use of preferred, yet arbitrary, items within a differential reinforcement program. The use of functionally related reinforcement within a differential reinforcement program represents a clear example of how behavior modification procedures can be refined by incorporating information about the variables that maintain SIB, information that would be gained from a prior functional assessment.

As with many ABA-based and behavior modification treatments, differential reinforcement schedules are often combined with other procedures. Azrin, Besalel, and Wisotzek (1982), for example, showed that a combination of DRI and response interruption (i.e., momentarily interrupting SIB) was more effective than DRI alone in reducing SIB in two adults with severe ID. Differential reinforcement is also often combined with extinction procedures.

Punishment

As with differential reinforcement schedules, a variety of punishment-based procedures have been developed, and their effectiveness established, for reducing SIB among individuals with ID (Foxx, 1982). Punishment procedures aim to reduce SIB by either removal of reinforcement (i.e., time-out, response cost) or delivery of aversive stimulation (e.g., water mist to the face, electric shock, aromatic ammonia) contingent upon SIB.

Time-out and response cost are similar in that each involves removing the person from reinforcement or removing a source of positive reinforcement contingent upon SIB. Nunes, Murphy, and Ruprecht (1977), for example, showed that the contingent withdrawal of reinforcement following SIB was effective in reducing SIB in two adolescents with severe ID. Sigafoos and Pennell (1995) also showed that contingent removal of tactile stimulation, which was presumably reinforcing, was effective in reducing SIB in a 10-year-old boy with severe ID.

A variety of types of aversive stimulation have been delivered contingent upon SIB to reduce its frequency in people with ID. Altman, Haavik, and Cook (1978), for example, successfully used contingent aromatic ammonia to reduce SIB in two young children with ID. Mayhew and Harris (1979) contingently applied citric acid to the mouth of a 19-year-old man in response to SIB and showed that this procedure reduced SIB and tantrums. Other researchers have used ice to the mouth (Drabman, Ross, Lynd, & Cordua, 1978), forced arm movements (DeCatanzaro & Baldwin, 1978), water mist sprayed in the person's face (Bailey, Pokrzywinski, & Bryant, 1983), facial screening (Singh, 1980), overcorrection (Halpern & Andrasik, 1986), and contingent electric shock (Duker & Seys, 1996).

All of these aforementioned punishment procedures meet the criteria for being effective treatments based on Chambless and Hollon's (1998) criteria. Indeed, the evidence base shows punishment to be one of the more rapid and effective treatments for SIB (Didden et al., 2006); however, when the function of SIB is considered in treatment planning, function-based procedures such as FCT appear to be equally rapid and effective to punishment procedures (Iwata et al., 1994). In the meta-analysis conducted by Christiansen (2009), however, the effect size for behavioral treatments involving the use of aversive punishment procedures, or the combined use of aversive and nonaversive procedures (e.g., punishment plus FCT), was significantly more effective than treatments that only used nonaversive procedures. The seemingly differing conclusions made by Iwata et al. and Christiansen could stem from whether or not the selection of the nonaversive treatment was based on the results of a prior, and conclusive, functional assessment of the person's SIB.

Restraint and protective equipment
Various types of restraint and protective equipment (e.g., holding the person's arms, wrist weights, arm splints, and helmets) have been applied, either contingently or noncontingently, to prevent and suppress SIB. There is sufficient evidence to support the use of restraint as a treatment for SIB among individuals with SIB (Ball, Campbell, & Barkemeyer, 1980; Gaylord-Ross, Weeks, Lipner, & Gaylord-Ross, 1983; Hanley, Piazza, Keeney, Blakeley-Smith, & Worsdell, 1998; Konarski & Johnson, 1989; Parrish, Aguerrevere, Dorsey, & Iwata, 1980; Saloviita, 1988; Singh, Dawson, & Manning, 1981). The use of restraint and protective equipment is often combined with other ABA-based and/or behavior modification procedures, such as differential reinforcement schedules and extinction (Radler, Plesa, Senini, & Reicha, 1985; Rolider & Van Houten, 1985; Yang, 2003). Overall, the evidence is sufficient to

conclude that the combined use of restraint with other ABA-based and behavior modification approaches is a well-established and highly effective treatment for SIB among individuals with ID.

A potential problem is that the use of restraints often restricts movement and therefore may limit the person's ability to participate in educational and daily activities. In addition, some individuals may seek to self-restrain in an effort to escape from or avoid certain activities or situations. In such cases, an important treatment objective is to fade the use of restraint and reduce self-restraint, while maintaining low rates and severity of SIB. Fortunately, behavior modification procedures also have been developed and empirically validated via numerous treatment studies for fading the use of restraints and reducing self-restraint among individuals with ID and SIB (Fisher, Piazza, Bowman, Hanley, & Adelinis, 1997; Foxx & Dufrense, 1984; Oliver, Hall, Hales, Murphy, & Watts, 1998; O'Reilly, Murray, Lancioni, Sigafoos, & Lacey, 2003).

Cognitive behavior therapy

CBT has been used with some success in the treatment of various types of behavioral problems in individuals with ID (Dagnan & Lindsey, 2004). The approach is based on changing dysfunctional thoughts, beliefs, self-perceptions, and feelings that appear to underlie problems of adjustment that affect people's lives (Beck, 1976). Operationally, the person is taught to identify the dysfunctional cognitions and adopt alternative thoughts, beliefs, and feelings to deal with problematic situations. The desired outcome is better psychosocial adjustment by adopting the alternative cognitions.

The use of CBT in the treatment of SIB among individuals with ID has rarely been reported in the literature. Van Minnen, Hoogduin, Peeters, and Smedts (1993) described an approach to SIB treatment that appeared to contain elements of CBT. The approach was applied to two adults with mild ID, one of whom presented with SIB. The results were positive, although the study lacked sufficient experimental control to attribute changes in SIB to the treatment. At the present time, while CBT could hold promise as a treatment for individuals with less severe ID, there is currently insufficient evidence to support its use in clinical practice.

Other treatments

Auditory integration training
Auditory integration training (AIT) involves having an individual wear headphones that present filtered music at predetermined frequencies (Mudford & Cullen, 2005). This exposure is supposed to retrain the auditory system and address issues related to suspected hearing problems (e.g., hyperacuity) that some believe may affect the learning and behavior of individuals with developmental disabilities (Berard, 1993). AIT has been evaluated in at least four studies involving over 500 participants and

conducted by three independent research teams (Bettison, 1996; Edelson et al., 1999; Mudford et al., 2000; Rimland & Edelson, 1994, 1995). The studies focused mainly on individuals with autism. Still, the findings of these studies are relevant to this chapter, because some participants had ID diagnoses and researchers included measures of problem behavior.

In a comprehensive review of these studies, Mudford and Cullen (2005) outlined serious methodological problems for three of the studies (Edelson et al., 1999; Rimland & Edelson, 1994, 1995), which negate the positive results reported by this team. The remaining three studies, from three independent investigators, showed that AIT has no beneficial effect on either adaptive functioning or frequency/ severity of problem behavior (Bettison, 1996; Mudford et al., 2000; Zollweg, Palm, & Vance, 1997). Based on the findings of the Mudford and Cullen review, AIT must be viewed as an ineffective treatment.

Sensory integrative therapy
SIT involves exposing the individual to a range of physical sensations and motor activities that are intended to stimulate various sensory systems (Ayres, 1972; Smith, Mruzek, & Mozingo, 2005). To stimulate the vestibular system, for example, it has been proposed that the person should be engaged in various gross motor activities such as "swinging, rolling, jumping on a trampoline, or riding on scooter boards" (Smith et al., 2005, p. 332). To stimulate the tactile and proprioceptive systems, in contrast, the individual's joints are physically manipulated to move them back and forth (i.e., joint compression), or the person's arms and legs might be softly brushed. Another SIT technique is to provide deep pressure by squeezing the person between mats or pillows. These techniques are often combined into 30–60 min sensory-diet sessions that might also include the use of weighted vests (see "Weighted Vests"), altering room lighting, and oral motor exercises (Smith et al.).

Ayres (1972) argued that problems related to integration of the senses were implicated in the problems experienced by individuals with intellectual and other developmental and physical disabilities. Specifically, according to SIT theory, the learning and behavior problems of such individuals are thought to arise from either oversensitivity or undersensitivity of the senses to environmental stimulation (Smith et al., 2005). Following this logic, activities that aim to integrate the vestibular, tactile, and proprioceptive systems are touted as a viable treatment for a range of problems associated with developmental and physical disabilities, including the treatment of SIB (Bright, Bittick, & Fleeman, 1981; Mason & Iwata, 1990; Reisman, 1993).

Mason and Iwata (1990) is one of the few studies to have evaluated the effects of SIT on SIB using a recognized experimental design. This study involved three children with ID and SIB and introduced SIT according to a multiple-baseline across subjects design (Kennedy, 2005). When SIT was introduced, SIB increased for one child and decreased for the other two; however, further analysis showed that decreases in SIB were due to an increase in therapist attention and not to SIT.

The results of Mason and Iwata (1990) are not supportive of the use of SIT as a treatment of SIB. Mason and Iwata's data are consistent with two meta-analyses, which found that SIT had no therapeutic effect across a range of learning and behavioral problems associated with a range of developmental and physical disabilities (Arendt, MacLean, & Baumeister, 1988; Vargas & Camilli, 1999). Christiansen's (2009) meta-analysis "did not find a strong effect of sensory treatments for reducing SIB" (p. 154). Based on these data, SIT must be viewed as ineffective based on Chambless and Hollon's (1998) criteria. In addition to the lack of empirical support, the theory underpinning SIT is highly questionable (Smith et al., 2005).

Weighted vests
Weighted vests are often used within SIT but have also been applied as an independent stand-alone procedure. A weighted vest is a piece of clothing that the individual wears for varying periods of time during the day (e.g., 5 min to 2 hr/ day). The vest is constructed to include ballast (e.g., sand, beads) up to 10% of the person's body weight. Proponents argue that weighted vests alleviate problems arising from over- or undersensitivity to sensory input (Olson & Moulton, 2004). Stephenson and Carter (2009) provided a systematic review of studies that have used weighted vests in the treatment of individuals with developmental disabilities. Of the five peer-reviewed papers in this review, only one study investigated the effects of wearing a weighted vest on SIB (Carter, 2009). Specifically, Carter's study involved a 4-year-old boy with autism with profound deficits in adaptive behavior functioning suggestive of comorbid severe/profound ID. The boy had a history of SIB consisting of head hitting, head banging, and slapping his hand against objects. The child also had a history of sinus infections, which appeared to exacerbate SIB. The frequency of SIB was observed under four conditions (e.g., attention, play, demand, alone), corresponding to the experimental-functional analysis procedures described by Iwata et al. (1982/1994). These conditions alternated in a multielement design (Kennedy, 2005), and the child progressed through a sequence of phases in which he either did or did not wear the weighted vest and either did or did not show symptoms of sinus infection. The results showed that SIB occurred at roughly equal rates under all four functional analysis conditions but varied in relation to the presence or absence of symptoms of sinus infection. That is, SIB was more frequent when there were visible signs of sinus infection and less frequent when the child did not have symptoms of a sinus infection. SIB did not vary in relation to the use of the weighted vest. That is, SIB was low when there were no signs of a sinus infection whether or not the child was wearing a weighted vest. Similarly, SIB was more frequent when signs of sinus infection were present regardless of whether the child was wearing the weighted vest.

Overall, the results of Carter (2009) are not supportive of the use of weighted vests as a treatment of SIB. In addition to the lack of empirical support, the treatment lacks a convincing rationale for why it would be expected to influence SIB. Still, the presence of only a single study, involving only a single participant, means that there are currently insufficient data to support the use of weighted vests for the treatment of SIB.

Gentle Teaching

Gentle Teaching aims to prevent and reduce problem behavior by enhancing the quality of interactions between parents/teachers/staff and the individuals with disabilities that they care for. The techniques and goals of Gentle Teaching include interacting with the person in ways that aim to (a) teach the person to feel safe, (b) teach the person to feel engaged, (c) teach the person to feel unconditionally loved, and (d) teach the person to feel love towards staff (Cullen & Mudford, 2005). Carers might, for example, smile at the person, approach in a nonthreatening manner, and follow the person's interests in an effort to bond with, or build rapport with, the person. In addition to adopting such interaction styles, Gentle Teaching also incorporates a range of additional—and recognizably behavioral—techniques, such as errorless learning, response prompting, prompt fading, and choice-making procedures (Mudford, 1995); however, Cullen and Mudford noted that descriptions of Gentle Teaching by its proponents are often too vague to determine exactly what is to be done by staff in their attempt to achieve the associated teaching goals. The inclusion of behavioral techniques also complicates the evaluation of Gentle Teaching because it remains difficult to determine whether it, or its associated behavioral techniques alone, might have been responsible for any observed changes in behavior.

Despite the difficulties arising from the lack of objective description of Gentle Teaching procedures and inclusion of additional behavioral techniques, several studies have attempted to evaluate the effects of Gentle Teaching on the frequency and severity of SIB among individuals with ID. Cullen and Mappin (1998), for example, used Gentle Teaching on 13 children with severe to profound ID who engaged in severe behavior problems, including SIB. Similarly, McGee and Gonzalez (1990) implemented Gentle Teaching with 15 individuals with ID and serious problem behaviors. Both of these studies are limited, however, by their lack of experimental controls. Two other independently conducted and experimentally controlled case studies have been reported and reviewed by Cullen and Mudford (2005). Jones, Singh, and Kendall (1991) reported a controlled case study of a 44-year-old man with profound ID and self-injurious head slapping. The study involved an alternating treatments design (Kennedy, 2005) comparing the relative effects of Gentle Teaching versus visual screening on the frequency of SIB. Visual screening was more effective in reducing SIB, although Gentle Teaching also produced some modest reductions in SIB relative to baseline and to a third control condition. The amount of rapport or bonding towards staff exhibited by the man was reported to be similar during both visual screening and Gentle Teaching conditions. This is interesting because improved social bonding is purported to be one of the unique benefits of Gentle Teaching. In contrast, Barrera and Teodoro (1990) found no beneficial effect from Gentle Teaching on SIB in a 33-year-old man with profound ID and SIB.

Overall, the number of experimentally controlled studies that have examined the effects of Gentle Teaching on SIB among individuals with ID is few, as is the total number of participants in these studies. So far, the results of these studies have been mixed with one study finding a modest effect (Jones et al., 1991) and the other finding no effect

(Barrera & Teodoro, 1990). Consequently, Gentle Teaching must be considered as lacking sufficient evidence due to the small number of participants who have so far received this treatment within the context of an experimentally controlled evaluation.

Electroconvulsive therapy (ECT)

ECT involves inducing seizures by passing an electric current across the head of an anesthetized person. ECT is primarily used in the treatment of severe [medication-resistant] depression. For this and related conditions, ECT is considered a well-established treatment, although it is not without potential risks (Medda et al., 2010). Wachtel and colleagues (2009) applied ECT to an 8-year-old boy with autism and ID who had a history of extreme SIB. The boy's SIB included forceful blows to the head, which occurred at an average rate of 109 attempts per hour. Due to his frequent and severe SIB, the boy was considered to be at an extremely high risk for brain damage and consequently wore protective restraints, which further limited his participation in daily activities. Fifteen sessions of ECT resulted in a reduction of SIB from an average of 109 instances an hour to an average of 19 attempts per hour. Treatment gains were maintained over a 5-week period, during which time the child continued to receive ECT.

In addition to the Wachtel study, there are two other reports of successful use of ECT as an SIB treatment for individuals with ID. However, each of these reports also included only a single participant (Bates & Smeltzer, 1982; Fink, 1999). Thus, at the present time, support for the use of ECT in the treatment of SIB among individuals with ID must be considered as lacking sufficient evidence due to the small number of participants who have so far received this treatment.

Snoezelen rooms

A Snoezelen room is a room or space fitted with various types of stimulating materials and adaptive devices, such as switches that activate music when touched, colored lights, and soft mats for the person to roll on. The presence of such materials is intended to evoke exploratory behaviors, which may in turn increase adaptive responses that could compete with SIB. Singh et al. (2004) evaluated the effects of exposure to a Snoezelen room on 15 individuals with severe to profound ID. Aggression and self-injury were observed under three conditions: (a) training on daily living skills, (b) training on vocational skills, and (c) during exposure to the Snoezelen room. SIB and aggression were significantly lower under the Snoezelen condition, suggesting that SIB might be effectively suppressed during times when the individual is exposed to the Snoezelen room. While promising, there is currently an insufficient amount of evidence to establish whether the treatment can be classified as effective.

Transcutaneous electric nerve stimulation (TENS)

Transcutaneous electric nerve stimulation (TENS) involves the administration of a mild electric current to stimulate nerve cells. The stimulation is supplied by a battery-operated unit that might be affixed to the person's back. Two studies, involving a total of three individuals with ID, have experimentally evaluated the effects of TENS on rates of SIB (Fisher et al., 1998; Linn, Rojahn, Helsel, & Dixon, 1988). In both studies, TENS reduced SIB. While promising, due to the small number of studies and participants, there is currently an insufficient amount of evidence to establish whether TENS can be classified as an effective treatment for SIB among individuals with ID.

Exercise
Three studies have evaluated the effects of exercise on rates of SIB among individuals with ID. Lancioni, Smeets, Ceccarani, Capodaglio, and Campanari (1984) evaluated whether having three individuals with severe/multiple disabilities and SIB engage in gross motor activities that required considerable physical effort would reduce SIB. They found that all three individuals showed a reduction in the rate of SIB when this treatment was used. Baumeister and MacLean (1984) showed that implementation of a jogging routine reduced SIB in two adults with ID. Whitaker and Saleem (1994) showed that an exercise program initially increased SIB, but as this treatment continued, SIB decreased. Overall these three studies, while promising, involved a total of only six individuals, and therefore, the amount of replication is not sufficient to classify this as an effective treatment for SIB.

Room management
Our literature search identified one study on the use of room management in the treatment of SIB (Crisp & Sturmey, 1987). Room management refers to the systematic alteration of physical and social aspects of the person's environment (e.g., rearrangement of furniture and reorganization of staffing). The study involved six adults with ID and SIB. The results of this study were mixed in that room management was associated with reduction of SIB for some individuals in the study, but not for others. These mixed findings, combined with lack of replication by other investigators, mean that there is currently insufficient evidence to recommend this treatment.

Clinical Guidelines

Functional assessment

There is considerable evidence to support the value of a prior functional assessment of SIB. Information from a prior functional assessment may enable clinicians to select treatments that are matched to the operant function of the person's SIB.

Function-based treatment

When assessment data indicate that SIB serves one or more operant functions, clinicians should implement ABA-based treatments that address that operant function. If SIB is maintained by attention, for example, then intervention should include procedures to address this function, such as teaching the person a better way to recruit attention.

Use a combination of treatments

ABA-based and behavior modification approaches that combine a number of specific procedures have proven to be consistently effective in the treatment of SIB among individuals with ID. Treatment packages that employ DRA and extinction of SIB are among the most well-studied and well-established procedures for the treatment of SIB. In cases where SIB does not respond to such packages, the addition of a punishment component should be considered. The meta-analysis reported by Didden et al. (1997) found that treatment packages that combined well-established procedures (e.g., extinction plus FCT) had higher effect sizes than single-component treatments (e.g., extinction alone).

Ensuring protocol adherence

The success of any treatment protocol depends on how well it is implemented. This in turn depends on the quality of training provided to the interventionists. Parents, teachers, and direct-care staff must often learn how to correctly implement SIB treatments to ensure generalization and maintenance of treatment gains. Training of such persons on protocol implementation should continue until a high level of treatment fidelity is achieved.

Evaluation

Treatments must be objectively evaluated to determine if they are having the desired effect on SIB. Treatment evaluation requires competence in obtaining objective, reliable, and valid data on the frequency and severity of SIB. Repeated measures of the frequency and severity of SIB in combination with an appropriate single-case experimental design will enable the clinician to evaluate the effects of the treatment program in ways that can demonstrate a functional relation between treatment and positive changes in SIB (Barlow & Hersen, 1984).

When data indicate that the treatment program is not having the desired effects, clinicians require the skills to analyze the nature of any such problems and troubleshoot the program. In some cases, a troubleshooting analysis will reveal technical aspects of the procedures that could be corrected to improve effectiveness. In other cases, however, the intervention may be ineffective for a particular case.

While studies evaluating drug treatments were excluded from this review, practitioners working with individuals with ID and SIB are likely to have individuals on their caseloads receiving various types of medications. Practitioners can contribute to the evaluation of such treatments by collecting data on the frequency and severity of SIB while monitoring drug side effects. To this end, several assessment scales have been developed to assess the effects (including side effects) of psychotropic medications in persons with ID (Aman & Singh, 1994; Matson et al., 1998; Mayville, 2007).

Ethical practice

Understanding the concepts of informed consent, confidentiality, breach of confidence, access to information, and reporting laws and how to apply these concepts in practice are basic competencies required of all clinicians (Sales, DeKraai, Hall, & Duvall, 2008). This is particularly the case when addressing SIB in persons with ID. In terms of consenting to treatments, people with ID are often unable to fully comprehend information, and hence, they cannot often provide informed consent. Iacono and Murray (2003) provided guidelines for obtaining informed consent among individuals with ID.

Clinical expertise

Implementing effective evidence-based treatments for SIB requires a high degree of clinical expertise. The design, implementation, and evaluation of SIB treatments are complicated by the very real potential for serious harm and consequent need for immediate and lasting response suppression (Foxx, 1996, 2003, 2005). Expert competencies are therefore required to assess the risk that severe excess behavior poses to the child and others and to determine when more intrusive treatments are indicated.

Risk assessment

The main purpose of undertaking a risk assessment is to prevent harm (McEvoy & McGuire, 2007). One way to prevent harm is to provide effective treatment; however, treatments are rarely immediately effective in preventing or eliminating SIB. Thus, clinicians must consider the risks that SIB represents to the individual and others in the treatment planning.

A risk assessment is also necessary before undertaking a functional assessment to identify the variables that evoke and maintain SIB. Because some such assessments could provoke SIB (Rojahn et al., 2007), it is important to determine whether the information that can be gained from direct assessment methods outweighs the risk that might arise if SIB occurs during the assessment. Clinicians can minimize or prevent this risk by using briefer versions of analogue assessments or by using more indirect assessment protocols (Matson, Terlonge, & Minshawi, 2008).

In some cases, the risks associated with SIB may warrant the use of more intrusive or restrictive treatments, including protective equipment, physical restraint, or response-contingent aversive stimulation (Repp & Singh, 1990). Many jurisdictions have restricted the use of some such procedures in the treatment of persons with ID (Sherman, 1991); however, the use of such procedures may be justified when the risk is high and when less intrusive treatments have failed (Didden et al., 1997; Duker & Seys, 1996; Foxx, 2005). Obviously, clinicians intending to use intrusive treatments must be prepared to justify this decision with evidence, ensure compliance with legal and ethical guidelines, and develop appropriate safeguards. When these conditions can be met, clinicians must gain the necessary expertise to use the procedures prior to implementation. During treatment implementation, clinicians will have to maintain a high degree of oversight and regularly monitor the effects and side effects of the treatment (Duker & Van den Munckhof, 2007). The intensity of the required oversight can be demanding and must be considered in the decision to accept referrals for the treatment of SIB.

References

Altman, K., Haavik, S., & Cook, J. W. (1978). Punishment of self-injurious behavior in natural settings using contingent aromatic ammonia. *Behaviour, Research and Therapy, 16*, 85–96.

Aman, M. G., & Singh, N. N. (1994). *Aberrant behavior checklist—community*. East Aurora, NY: Slosson Educational Publications.

American Psychiatric Association. (2000). *Diagnostic and statistical manual of mental disorders* (4th ed., text revision). Washington, DC: Author.

Arendt, R. E., MacLean, W. E., & Baumeister, A. A. (1988). Critique of sensory integration therapy and its application in mental retardation. *American Journal on Mental Retardation, 92*, 401–411.

Ayres, A. J. (1972). *Sensory integration and learning disorders*. Los Angeles: Western Psychological Services.

Azrin, N. H., Besalel, V. A., & Wisotzek, I. E. (1982). Treatment of self-injury by a reinforcement plus interruption procedure. *Analysis & Intervention in Developmental Disabilities, 2*, 105–113.

Baer, D. M., Wolf, M. M., & Risley, T. R. (1987). Some still current dimensions of applied behavior analysis. *Journal of Applied Behavior Analysis, 20*, 313–327.

Baghdadli, A., Pascal, C., Grisi, S., & Aussilloux, C. (2003). Risk factors for self-injurious behaviors among 222 children with autistic disorders. *Journal of Intellectual Disability Research, 47*, 622–627.

Bailey, S. L., Pokrzywinski, J., & Bryant, L. E. (1983). Using water mist to reduce self-injurious and stereotypic behavior. *Applied Research in Mental Retardation, 4*, 229–241.

Ball, T. S., Campbell, R., & Barkemeyer, R. (1980). Air splints applied to control self-injurious finger sucking in profoundly retarded individuals. *Journal of Behavior Therapy and Experimental Psychiatry, 11*, 267–271.

Barlow, D. H., & Hersen, M. (1984). *Single case experimental designs: Strategies for studying behavior change* (2nd ed.). New York: Pergamon Press.

Barrera, F. J., & Teodoro, G. M. (1990). Flash bonding or cold fusion? A case analysis of gentle teaching. In A. C. Repp & N. N. Singh (Eds.), *Perspectives on the use of non-aversive and aversive interventions for persons with developmental disabilities* (pp. 199–214). Sycamore, IL: Sycamore.

Bates, W., & Smeltzer, D. (1982). Electro-convulsive treatment of psychotic self-injurious behavior in a patient with severe mental retardation. *American Journal of Psychiatry, 139,* 1355–1356.

Baumeister, A. A., & MacLean, W. E. (1984). Deceleration of self-injurious and stereotypic responding by exercise. *Applied Research in Mental Retardation, 5,* 385–393.

Beck, A. (1976). *Cognitive therapy and the emotional disorders.* New York: International Universities Press.

Berard, G. (1993). *Hearing equals behavior.* New Canaan, CT: Keats.

Bettison, S. (1996). The long-term effects of auditory training on children with autism. *Journal of Autism and Developmental Disorders, 26,* 361–374.

Bienstein, P., & Nussbeck, S. (2009). Reliability and validity of a German version of the questions about behavioral function (QABF) scale for self-injurious behavior in individuals with intellectual disabilities. *Journal of Mental Health Research in Intellectual Disabilities, 2,* 249–260.

Bright, T., Bittick, K., & Fleeman, B. (1981). Reduction of self-injurious behavior using sensory integrative techniques. *American Journal of Occupational Therapy, 35,* 167–172.

Carr, E. G., Levin, L., McConnachie, G., Carlson, J. I., Kemp, D. C., & Smith, C. E. (1994). *Communication-based intervention for problem behavior.* Baltimore: Paul H. Brookes Publishing Co.

Carter, S. L. (2009). Use of treatment analysis following ambiguous functional analysis results. *Behavioral Interventions, 24,* 205–213.

Chambless, D. L., & Hollon, S. D. (1998). Defining empirically supported therapies. *Journal of Consulting and Clinical Psychology, 66,* 7–18.

Christiansen, E. A. (2009). *Effectiveness of interventions targeting self-injury in children and adolescents with developmental disabilities: A meta-analysis.* Unpublished doctoral dissertation, University of Utah, Salt Lake City.

Crisp, A. G., & Sturmey, P. (1987). The modification of stereotyped and self-injurious behaviour by room management. *Behavioural Psychotherapy, 15,* 350–366.

Cullen, C., & Mappin, R. (1998). An examination of the effects of gentle teaching on people with complex learning disabilities and challenging behaviour. *British Journal of Clinical Psychology, 37,* 199–211.

Cullen, C., & Mudford, O. C. (2005). Gentle teaching. In J. W. Jacobson, R. M. Foxx, & J. A. Mulick (Eds.), *Controversial therapies for developmental disabilities: Fad, fashion, and science in professional practice* (pp. 423–432). Mahwah, NJ: Lawrence Erlbaum.

Dagnan, D., & Lindsey, W. R. (2004). Cognitive therapy with people with learning disabilities. In E. Emerson, C. Hatton, T. Thompson, & T. Parmenter (Eds.), *International handbook of applied research in intellectual disabilities* (pp. 517–530). Chichester, UK: Wiley.

Deb, S., Chaplin, R., Sohanpal, S., Unwin, G., Soni, R., & Lenotre, L. (2008). The effectiveness of mood stabilizers and antiepileptic medication for the management of behaviour problems in adults with intellectual disability: A systematic review. *Journal of Intellectual Disability Research, 52,* 107–113.

DeCatanzaro, D. A., & Baldwin, G. (1978). Effective treatment of self-injurious behavior through a forced-arm exercise. *American Journal of Mental Deficiency, 82,* 433–439.

DeLeon, I. G., Anders, B. M., Rodriguez-Catter, V., & Neidert, P. L. (2000). The effects of noncontingent access to single- versus multiple-stimulus sets on self-injurious behavior. *Journal of Applied Behavior Analysis, 33,* 623–626.

Didden, R. (2007). Functional analysis methodology in developmental disabilities. In P. Sturmey (Ed.), *Functional analysis in clinical treatment. Practical resources for the mental health professional (pp. 65–86).* San Diego, CA: Elsevier Academic Press.

Didden, R., Duker, P. C., & Korzilius, H. (1997). Meta-analytic study on the treatment effectiveness for problem behaviors with individuals who have mental retardation. *American Journal on Mental Retardation, 101,* 387–399.

Didden, R., Korzilius, H., & Curfs, L. M. G. (2007). Skin-picking in individuals with Prader-Willi syndrome: Prevalence, functional assessment, and its comorbidity with compulsive and self-injurious behaviours. *Journal of Applied Research in Intellectual Disabilities, 20,* 409–419.

Didden, R., Korzilius, H., van Oorsouw, W., & Sturmey, P. (2006). Behavioral treatment of challenging behaviors in individuals with mild mental retardation: Meta-analysis of single-subject research. *American Journal on Mental Retardation, 111,* 290–298.

Drabman, R. S., Ross, J. M., Lynd, R. S., & Cordua, G. D. (1978). Retarded children as observers, mediators, and generalization programmers using an icing procedure. *Behavior Modification, 2,* 371–385.

Duker, P. C., & Seys, D. M. (1996). Long-term use of electrical aversive treatment with self-injurious behavior. *Research in Developmental Disabilities, 17,* 293–301.

Duker, P. C., & Van den Munckhof, M. (2007). Heart rate and the role of the active receiver during contingent electric shock for severe self-injurious behavior. *Research in Developmental Disabilities, 28,* 43–49.

Durand, V. M. (1990). *Severe behavior problems: A functional communication training approach.* Albany, NY: Guilford Press.

Durand, V. M., & Merges, E. (2001). Functional communication training: A contemporary behavior analytic intervention for problem behavior. *Focus on Autism and Other Developmental Disabilities, 16,* 110–119.

Edelson, S. M., Arin, D., Bauman, M., Lukas, S. E., Rudy, J. H., Sholar, M., et al. (1999). Auditory integration training: A double-blind study of behavioral and electrophysiological effects in people with autism. *Focus on Autism and Other Developmental Disabilities, 14,* 73–81.

Emerson, E., Kiernan, C., Alborz, A., Reeves, D., Mason, H., Swarbrick, R., et al. (2001). The prevalence of challenging behaviors: A total population study. *Research in Developmental Disabilities, 22,* 77–93.

Fink, M. (1999). *Electroshock: Healing mental illness.* London: Oxford University Press.

Fischer, S. M., Iwata, B. A., & Mazaleski, J. L. (1997). Noncontingent delivery of arbitrary reinforcers as treatment for self-injurious behavior. *Journal of Applied Behavior Analysis, 30,* 239–249.

Fisher, W. W., Bowman, L. G., Thompson, R. H., Contrucci, S. A., Burd, L., & Alon, G. (1998). Reductions in self-injury produced by transcutaneous electrical nerve stimulation. *Journal of Applied Behavior Analysis, 31,* 493–496.

Fisher, W. W., Piazza, C. C., Bowman, L. G., Hanley, G. P., & Adelinis, J. D. (1997). Direct and collateral effects of restraints and restraint fading. *Journal of Applied Behavior Analysis, 30,* 105–119.

Foxx, R. M. (1982). *Decreasing behaviors of persons with severe retardation and autism.* Champaign, IL: Research Press.

Foxx, R. M. (1996). Twenty years of applied behavior analysis in treating the most severe problem behavior: Lessons learned. *The Behavior Analyst, 19*, 225–235.

Foxx, R. M. (2003). Treating dangerous behaviors. *Behavioral Interventions, 18*, 1–21.

Foxx, R. M. (2005). Severe aggressive and self-destructive behavior: The myth of the nonaversive treatment of severe behavior. In J. W. Jacobson, R. M. Foxx, & J. A. Mulick (Eds.), *Controversial therapies for developmental disabilities: Fad, fashion, and science in professional practice* (pp. 259–310). Mahwah, NJ: Lawrence Erlbaum.

Foxx, R. M., & Dufrense, D. (1984). "Harry": The use of physical restraint as a reinforcer, timeout from restraint, and fading restraint in treating a self-injurious man. *Analysis and Intervention in Developmental Disabilities, 4*, 1–13.

Gaylord-Ross, R. J., Weeks, M., Lipner, C., & Gaylord-Ross, C. (1983). The differential effectiveness of four treatment procedures in suppressing self-injurious behavior among severely handicapped students. *Education & Training of the Mentally Retarded, 18*, 38–44.

Griffin, J. C., Ricketts, R. W., Williams, D. E., Locke, B. J., Altmeyer, B. K., & Stark, M. T. (1987). A community survey of self-injurious behavior among developmentally disabled children and adolescents. *Hospital and Community Psychiatry, 38*, 959–963.

Gunsett, R. P., Mulick, J. A., Fernald, W. B., & Martin, J. L. (1989). Indications for medical screening prior to behavioral programming for severely and profoundly mentally retarded clients. *Journal of Autism and Developmental Disorders, 19*, 167–172.

Hagopian, L. P., Fisher, W. W., Sullivan, M. T., Acquisto, J., & LeBlanc, L. A. (1998). Effectiveness of functional communication training with and without extinction and punishment: A summary of 21 inpatient cases. *Journal of Applied Behavior Analysis, 31*, 211–235.

Halpern, L. F., & Andrasik, F. (1986). The immediate and long-term effectiveness of overcorrection in treating self-injurious behavior in a mentally retarded adult. *Applied Research in Mental Retardation, 7*, 59–65.

Hanley, G. P., Piazza, C. C., Keeney, K. M., Blakeley-Smith, A. B., & Worsdell, A. S. (1998). Effects of wrist weights on self-injurious and adaptive behavior. *Journal of Applied Behavior Analysis, 31*, 307–310.

Harvey, S. T., Boer, D., Meyer, L. M., & Evans, I. M. (2009). Updating a meta-analysis of intervention research with challenging behaviour: Treatment validity and standards of practice. *Journal of Intellectual and Developmental Disability, 34*, 67–80.

Holden, B., & Gitlesen, J. P. (2006). A total population study of challenging behavior in the county of Hedmark, Norway: Prevalence and risk markers. *Research in Developmental Disabilities, 27*, 456–465.

Iacono, T., & Murray, V. (2003). Issues of informed consent in conducting medical research involving people with intellectual disability. *Journal of Applied Research in Intellectual Disabilities, 16*, 41–51.

Iwata, B., Dorsey, M., Slifer, K., Bauman, K., & Richman, G. (1982/1994). Toward a functional analysis of self-injury. *Journal of Applied Behavior Analysis, 1994, 27*, 197–209. Reprinted from *Analysis and Intervention in Developmental Disabilities, 1982, 2*, 3–20.

Iwata, B., Pace, G., Cowdery, G., & Miltenberger, R. (1994). What makes extinction work: An analysis of procedural form and function. *Journal of Applied Behavior Analysis, 27*, 131–144.

Iwata, B., Pace, G., Dorsey, M., Zarcone, J., Vollmer, T., Smith, R., et al. (1994). The functions of self-injurious behavior: An experimental-epidemiological analysis. *Journal of Applied Behavior Analysis, 27*, 215–240.

Jones, J. L., Singh, N. N., & Kendall, K. A. (1991). Comparative effects of gentle teaching and visual screening on self-injurious behaviour. *Journal of Mental Deficiency Research, 35,* 37–47.

Kahng, S. W., Iwata, B. A., DeLeon, I. G., & Wallace, M. (2000). A comparison of procedures for programming noncontingent reinforcement schedules. *Journal of Applied Behavior Analysis, 33,* 223–231.

Kahng, S. W., Iwata, B. A., DeLeon, I. G., & Worsdell, A. S. (1997). Evaluation of the "control over reinforcement" component in functional communication training. *Journal of Applied Behavior Analysis, 30,* 267–277.

Kazdin, A. E. (2001). *Behavior modification in applied settings* (6th ed.). Belmont, CA: Wadsworth/Thomson Learning.

Kennedy, C. H. (2005). *Single-case designs for educational research.* Boston: Allyn & Bacon.

Konarski, E. A., & Johnson, M. R. (1989). The use of brief restraint plus reinforcement to treat self-injurious behavior. *Behavioral Residential Treatment, 4,* 45–52.

Lancioni, G. E., Smeets, P. M., Ceccarani, P. S., Capodaglio, L., & Campanari, G. (1984). Effects of gross motor activities on the severe self-injurious tantrums of multihandicapped individuals. *Applied Research in Mental Retardation, 5,* 471–482.

Lang, R., Didden, R., Machalicek, W., Rispoli, M., Sigafoos, J., Lancioni, G., et al. (2010). Behavioral treatment of chronic skin-picking in individuals with developmental disabilities: A systematic review. *Research in Developmental Disabilities, 31,* 304–315.

Linn, D. M., Rojahn, J., Helsel, W. J., & Dixon, J. (1988). Acute effects of transcutaneous electric nerve stimulation on self-injurious behavior. *Journal of the Multihandicapped Person, 1,* 105–119.

Lowe, K., Allen, D., Jones, E., Brophy, S., Moore, K., & James, W. (2007). Challenging behaviours: Prevalence and topographies. *Journal of Intellectual Disability Research, 51,* 625–636.

Luiselli, J. K. (1984). Use of sensory extinction in treating self-injurious behavior: A cautionary note. *The Behavior Therapist, 7,* 142–160.

Luiselli, J. K. (1988). Comparative analysis of sensory extinction treatments for self-injury. *Education and Treatment of Children, 11,* 149–156.

Mancil, G. R. (2006). Functional communication training: A review of the literature related to children with autism. *Education and Training in Developmental Disabilities, 41,* 213–224.

Mason, S. A., & Iwata, B. A. (1990). Artifactual effects of sensory-integrative therapy on self-injurious behavior. *Journal of Applied Behavior Analysis, 23,* 361–370.

Matson, J. L., Anderson, S. J., & Bamburg, J. W. (2000). The relationship of social skills to psychopathology for individuals with mild and moderate mental retardation. *British Journal of Developmental Disabilities, 46,* 15–22.

Matson, J. L., & LoVullo, S. V. (2008). A review of behavioral treatments for self-injurious behaviors of persons with autism spectrum disorders. *Behavior Modification, 32,* 61–76.

Matson, J. L., Mayville, E. A., Bielecki, J., Barnes, W. H., Bamburg, J. W., & Baglio, C. S. (1998). Reliability of the Matson evaluation of drug side effects scale (MEDS). *Research in Developmental Disabilities, 19,* 501–506.

Matson, J. L., Terlonge, C., & Minshawi, N. F. (2008). Children with intellectual disabilities. In R. J. Morris & T. R. Kratochwill (Eds.), *The practice of child therapy* (4th ed., pp. 337–361). New York: Lawrence Erlbaum.

Mayhew, G., & Harris, F. C. (1979). Decreasing self-injurious behavior: Punishment with citric acid and reinforcement of alternative behavior. *Behavior Modification, 3,* 322–336.

Mayville, E. A. (2007). Psychotropic medication effects and side effects. In J. L. Matson (Ed.), *Handbook of assessment in persons with intellectual disability* (pp. 227–251). San Diego, CA: Academic Press.

McEvoy, J., & McGuire, B. (2007). Risk assessment. In A. Carr, G. O'Reilly, P. Noonan Walsh, & J. McEvoy (Eds.), *The handbook of intellectual disability and clinical psychology practice* (pp. 920–960). London: Routledge.

McGee, J. J., & Gonzalez, L. (1990). Gentle teaching and the practice of human interdependence: A preliminary group study of 15 persons with severe behavioral disorders and their caregivers. In A. C. Repp & N. N. Singh (Eds.), *Perspectives on the use of non-aversive and aversive interventions for persons with developmental disabilities* (pp. 237–254). Sycamore, IL: Sycamore.

Medda, P., Perugi, G., Zanello, S., Ciuffa, M., Rizzato, S., & Cassano, G. B. (2010). Comparative response to electroconvulsive therapy in medication-resistant bipolar patients with depression and mixed state. *Journal of ECT, 26,* 82–86.

Mirenda, P. (1997). Supporting individuals with challenging behavior through functional communication training and AAC. Research review. *Augmentative and Alternative Communication, 13,* 207–225.

Morgan, S. B., Campbell, J. M., & Jackson, J. N. (2003). Autism and mental retardation. In M. C. Roberts (Ed.), *Handbook of pediatric psychology* (3rd ed., pp. 510–528). New York: Guilford Press.

Mudford, O. C. (1995). Review of the gentle teaching data. *American Journal on Mental Retardation, 99,* 345–355.

Mudford, O. C., Cross, B. A., Breen, S., Cullen, C., Reeves, D., Gould, J., et al. (2000). Auditory integration training for children with autism: No behavioral benefits detected. *American Journal on Mental Retardation, 105,* 118–129.

Mudford, O. C., & Cullen, C. (2005). Auditory integration training: A critical review. In J. W. Jacobson, R. M. Foxx, & J. A. Mulick (Eds.), *Controversial therapies for developmental disabilities: Fad, fashion, and science in professional practice* (pp. 351–362). Mahwah, NJ: Lawrence Erlbaum.

Murphy, G., Hall, S., Oliver, C., & Kissi-Debra, R. (1999). Identification of early self-injurious behaviour in young children with intellectual disability. *Journal of Intellectual Disability Research, 43,* 149–163.

Murphy, G. H., Oliver, C., Corbett, J., Crayton, L., Hales, J., Head, D., et al. (1993). Epidemiology of self-injury, characteristics of people with severe self-injury and initial treatment outcome. In C. Kiernan (Ed.), *Research to practice? Implications of research on challenging behaviour of people with learning disability* (pp. 1–35). Avon, UK: British Institute of Learning Disabilities.

National Institutes of Health. (1989). *Treatment of destructive behaviors in persons with developmental disabilities: Vol. 7(9). Consensus development conference statement.* Bethesda, MD. Author.

Nunes, D. L., Murphy, R. J., & Ruprecht, M. L. (1977). Reducing self-injurious behavior of severely retarded individuals through withdrawal of reinforcement procedures. *Behavior Modification, 1,* 499–516.

Oliver, C., Hall, S., Hales, J., Murphy, G., & Watts, D. (1998). The treatment of severe self-injurious behavior by the systematic fading of restraints: Effects on self-injury, self-restraint, adaptive behavior, and behavioral correlates of affect. *Research in Developmental Disabilities, 19,* 143–165.

Oliver, C., Murphy, G. H., & Corbett, J. A. (1987). Self-injurious behaviour in people with mental handicap: A total population study. *Journal of Mental Deficiency Research, 31*, 147–162.

Olson, L. J., & Moulton, H. J. (2004). Use of weighted vests in pediatric occupational therapy practice. *Physical & Occupational Therapy in Pediatrics, 24*(3), 45–60.

O'Reilly, M., Murray, N., Lancioni, G. E., Sigafoos, J., & Lacey, C. (2003). Functional analysis and intervention to reduce self-injurious and agitated behavior when removing protective equipment for brief time periods. *Behavior Modification, 27*, 538–559.

Pace, G. M., Iwata, B. A., Cowdery, G. E., Adree, P. J., & McIntyre, T. (1993). Stimulus (instructional) fading during extinction of self-injurious escape behavior. *Journal of Applied Behavior Analysis, 26*, 205–212.

Parrish, J. M., Aguerrevere, L., Dorsey, M. F., & Iwata, B. A. (1980). The effects of protective equipment on self-injurious behavior. *The Behavior Therapist, 3*, 28–29.

Percy, M., Cheetham, T., Gitta, M., Morrison, B., Machalek, K., Bega, S., et al. (2007). Other syndromes and disorders associated with intellectual and developmental disabilities. In I. Brown & M. Percy (Eds.), *A comprehensive guide to intellectual and developmental disabilities* (pp. 229–267). Baltimore: Paul H. Brookes Publishing Co.

Radler, G. A., Plesa, C., Senini, K., & Reicha, J. (1985). Treatment of self-injurious behaviour in a severely handicapped adolescent: A case study. *Australia & New Zealand Journal of Developmental Disabilities, 11*, 107–112.

Reisman, J. (1993). Using a sensory integrative approach to treat self-injurious behavior in an adult with profound mental retardation. *American Journal of Occupational Therapy, 47*, 403–411.

Repp, A. C., & Singh, N. N. (Eds.). (1990). *Perspectives on the use of nonaversive and aversive interventions for persons with developmental disabilities* (pp. 59–72). Pacific Grover, CA: Brookes/Cole.

Rimland, B., & Edelson, S. M. (1994). The effects of auditory integration training. *American Journal of Speech-Language Pathology, 3*(2), 16–24.

Rimland, B., & Edelson, S. M. (1995). Brief report: A pilot study of auditory integration training in autism. *Journal of Autism and Developmental Disorders, 25*, 61–70.

Robinson, L. A., & Owens, R. E. (1995). Functional augmentative communication and positive behavior change. *Augmentative and Alternative Communication, 11*, 207–211.

Rojahn, J., Schroeder, S. R., & Hoch, T. A. (2008). *Self-injurious behavior in intellectual disability*. Oxford, UK: Elsevier.

Rojahn, J., Whittaker, K., Hoch, T. A., & González, M. L. (2007). Assessment of self-injurious and aggressive behavior. In J. L. Matson (Ed.), *Handbook of assessment in persons with intellectual disability* (pp. 281–319). San Diego, CA: Academic Press.

Rolider, A., & Van Houten, R. (1985). Movement suppression time-out for undesirable behavior in psychotic and severe developmentally delayed children. *Journal of Applied Behavior Analysis, 18*, 275–288.

Roscoe, E. M., Iwata, B. A., & Goh, H. L. (1998). A comparison of noncontingent reinforcement and sensory extinction as treatments for self-injurious behavior. *Journal of Applied Behavior Analysis, 31*, 635–646.

Sales, B. D., DeKraai, M. B., Hall, S. R., & Duvall, J. C. (2008). Child therapy and the law. In R. J. Morris & T. R. Kratochwill (Eds.), *The practice of child therapy* (4th ed., pp. 519–542). New York: Lawrence Erlbaum.

Saloviita, T. (1988). Elimination of self-injurious behaviour by brief physical restraint and DRA. *Scandinavian Journal of Behaviour Therapy, 17*, 55–63.

Schroeder, S. R., Schroeder, C. S., Smith, B., & Dalldorf, J. (1978). Prevalence of self-injurious behaviors in a large state facility for the retarded: A three-year follow-up study. *Journal of Autism and Childhood Schizophrenia, 8*, 261–269.

Schroeder, S. R., Tessel, R. E., Loupe, P. S., & Stodgell, C. J. (1997). Severe behavior problems among people with developmental disabilities. In W. E. MacLean Jr. (Ed.), *Ellis' handbook of mental deficiency, psychological theory and research* (3rd ed., pp. 439–464). Mahwah, NJ: Lawrence Erlbaum.

Scotti, J. R., Evans, I. M., Meyer, L. H., & Walker, P. (1991). A meta-analysis of intervention research with problem behavior: Treatment integrity and standards of practice. *American Journal on Mental Retardation, 96*, 233–256.

Sherman, R. A. (1991). Aversives, fundamental rights and the courts. *The Behavior Analyst, 14*, 197–206.

Shirley, M. J., Iwata, B. A., Kahng, S. W., Mazaleski, J. L., & Lerman, D. C. (1997). Does functional communication training compete with ongoing contingencies of reinforcement? An analysis during response acquisition and maintenance. *Journal of Applied Behavior Analysis, 30*, 93–104.

Sigafoos, J., Arthur, M., & O'Reilly, M. (2003). *Challenging behavior and developmental disability*. Baltimore: Paul H. Brookes Publishing Co.

Sigafoos, J., Elkins, J., Kerr, M., & Attwood, T. (1994). A survey of aggressive behaviour among a population of persons with intellectual disability in Queensland. *Journal of Intellectual Disability Research, 38*, 369–381.

Sigafoos, J., O'Reilly, M. F., & Lancioni, G. E. (2009). Functional communication training and choice-making interventions for the treatment of problem behavior in individuals with autism spectrum disorders. In P. Mirenda & T. Iacono (Eds.), *Autism spectrum disorders and AAC* (pp. 333–353). Baltimore: Paul H. Brookes Publishing Co.

Sigafoos, J., & Pennell, D. (1995). Noncontingent application versus contingent removal of tactile stimulation: Effects on self-injury in a young boy with multiple disabilities. *Behaviour Change, 12*, 139–143.

Singh, N. N. (1980). The effects of facial screening on infant self-injury. *Journal of Behavior Therapy and Experimental Psychiatry, 11*, 131–134.

Singh, N. N., Dawson, M. J., & Manning, P. J. (1981). The effects of physical restraint on self-injurious behaviour. *Journal of Mental Deficiency Research, 25*, 207–216.

Singh, N. N., Lancioni, G. E., Winton, A. S. W., Molina, E. J., Sage, M., Brown, S., & et al. (2004). Effects of Snoezelen room, activities of daily living skills training, and vocational skills training on aggression and self-injury by adults with mental retardation and mental illness. *Research in Developmental Disabilities, 25*, 285–293.

Smith, R. T., Vollmer, T. R., & St. Peter Pipkin, C. (2007). Functional approaches to assessment and treatment of problem behavior in persons with autism and related disabilities. In P. Sturmey & A. Fitzer (Eds.), *Autism spectrum disorders: Applied behavior analysis, evidence, and practice* (pp. 187–234). Austin, TX: Pro-Ed.

Smith, T., Mruzek, D. W., & Mozingo, D. (2005). Sensory integrative therapy. In J. W. Jacobson, R. M. Foxx, & J. A. Mulick (Eds.), *Controversial therapies for developmental disabilities: Fad, fashion, and science in professional practice* (pp. 331–350). Mahwah, NJ: Lawrence Erlbaum.

Stephenson, J., & Carter, M. (2009). The use of weighted vests with children with autism spectrum disorders and other disabilities. *Journal of Autism and Developmental Disorders, 39*, 105–114.

Symons, F. J., Butler, M. G., Sanders, M. D., Feurer, I. D., & Thompson, T. (1999). Self-injurious behavior and Prader-Willi Syndrome: Behavioral forms and body locations. *American Journal on Mental Retardation, 104,* 260–269.

Tucker, M., Sigafoos, J., & Bushell, H. (1998). Use of noncontingent reinforcement in the treatment of challenging behavior: A review and clinical guide. *Behavior Modification, 22,* 529–547.

Van Ingen, D. J., Moore, L. L., Zaja, R. H., & Rojahn, J. (2010). The behavior problems inventory (BPI-01) in community-based adults with intellectual disabilities: Reliability and concurrent validity vis-à-vis the inventory for client and agency planning (ICAP). *Research in Developmental Disabilities, 31,* 97–107.

Van Minnen, A., Hoogduin, C. A., Peeters, L. A., & Smedts, H. T. (1993). An outreach treatment approach for mildly retarded adults with psychiatric disorders. *British Journal of Developmental Disabilities, 39,* 126–133.

Vargas, S., & Camilli, G. (1999). A meta-analysis of research on sensory integration treatment. *American Journal of Occupational Therapy, 53,* 189–198.

Vollmer, T. R., & Iwata, B. A. (1992). Differential reinforcement as treatment for behavior disorders: Procedural and functional variations. *Research in Developmental Disabilities, 13,* 393–417.

Vollmer, T. R., Marcus, B. A., & LeBlanc, L. (1994). Treatment of self-injury and hand mouthing following inconclusive functional analysis. *Journal of Applied Behavior Analysis, 27,* 331–344.

Vollmer, T. R., Marcus, B. A., & Ringdahl, J. E. (1995). Noncontingent escape as treatment for self-injurious behavior maintained by negative reinforcement. *Journal of Applied Behavior Analysis, 28,* 15–26.

Wachtel, L. E., Contrucci-Kuhn, S. A., Griffin, M., Thompson, A., Dhossche, D. M., & Reti, I. M. (2009). ECT for self-injury in an autistic boy. *European Child and Adolescent Psychiatry, 18,* 458–463.

Wacker, D. P., Steege, M. W., Northup, J., Sasso, G., Berg, W., Reimers, T., et al. (1990). A component analysis of functional communication training across three topographies of severe behavior problems. *Journal of Applied Behavior Analysis, 23,* 417–429.

Whitaker, S., & Saleem, A. (1994). The effect of non-contingent exercise on purposeless wandering and self-injury on a man with profound learning difficulty. *Behavioural and Cognitive Psychotherapy, 22,* 99–102.

Winchel, R. M., & Stanley, M. (1991). Self-injurious behavior: A review of the behavior and biology of self-mutilation. *American Journal of Psychiatry, 148,* 306–317.

Worsdell, A. S., Iwata, B. A., Hanley, G. P., Thompson, R. H., & Kahng, S. W. (2000). Effects of continuous and intermittent reinforcement for problem behavior during functional communication training. *Journal of Applied Behavior Analysis, 33,* 167–179.

Yang, L. J. (2003). Combination of extinction and protective measures in the treatment of severely self-injurious behavior. *Behavioral Interventions, 18,* 109–121.

Zarcone, J. R., Iwata, B. A., Hughes, C. E., & Vollmer, T. R. (1993). Momentum versus extinction effects in the treatment of self-injurious escape behavior. *Journal of Applied Behavior Analysis, 26,* 135–136.

Zarcone, J. R., Iwata, B. A., Vollmer, T. R., Jagtiani, S., Smith, R. G., & Mazaleski, J. L. (1993). Extinction of self-injurious escape behavior with and without instructional fading. *Journal of Applied Behavior Analysis, 26,* 353–360.

Zollweg, W., Palm, D., & Vance, V. (1997). The efficacy of auditory integration training: A double blind study. *American Journal of Audiology, 6*(3), 39–47.

7

Stereotypic Behavior

Timothy R. Vollmer, Amanda B. Bosch, Joel E. Ringdahl, and John T. Rapp

Overview

In this chapter, we will introduce the topic of stereotypic behavior by providing a definition, prevalence statistics, and problems in interpreting definitions and prevalence statistics. We will briefly discuss why stereotypic behavior is sometimes a problem, to varying degrees, for individuals with intellectual disabilities (ID). The bulk of the chapter will explore the evidence base for treatments aimed at decreasing stereotypy; however, there are caveats to interpreting treatment efficacy as it relates to stereotypy. For example, a differential reinforcement procedure might only be effective if the reinforcers used can compete effectively with the automatic reinforcement produced by the stereotypic behavior. What works for one individual may not work for other individuals. Nonetheless, generally speaking, the strongest support is for behavioral treatments, so we will further evaluate components of behavioral treatments to suggest a progressive model for intervention.

Definition

The question of what type or form of behavior constitutes stereotypy has been subject to considerable discussion. Dozens of response forms have been called stereotypy. Common examples of stereotypic behavior include but are not limited to body rocking (Newell & Bodfish, 2007), hand flapping or hand waving (Ringdahl et al., 2002), hand mouthing (Vollmer, Marcus, & LeBlanc, 1994), vocalizations or

Evidence-Based Practice and Intellectual Disabilities, First Edition.
Edited by Peter Sturmey and Robert Didden.
© 2014 John Wiley & Sons, Ltd. Published 2014 by John Wiley & Sons, Ltd.

noise making (Miguel, Clark, Tereshko, & Ahearn, 2009), and posturing (Newell & Bodfish), among many others. So many different forms of stereotypy have been reported, that it is difficult to link the behavior by its form. For example, in one study alone, we observed 30 distinct forms of stereotypic behavior displayed by five subjects; one subject himself displayed 11 forms of stereotypy (Rapp, Vollmer, St. Peter, Dozier, & Cotnoir, 2004).

Berkson (1967) differentiated two general categories of stereotypy: repetitive movements (such as rocking) and nonrepetitive movements (such as body posturing). Other researchers have further specified that stereotypy is apparently nonfunctional and is not marked by clear antecedent stimuli (Lewis & Baumeister, 1982). Berkson (1983) later proposed a categorization of stereotypy according to the following criteria: (a) The behavior is voluntary (implying that the behavior is operant as opposed to respondent and ruling out "involuntary" tics), (b) the behavior lacks variability, (c) the behavior persists over time (e.g., for at least several months), (d) the behavior is relatively immutable when faced with environmental changes, and (e) the behavior is out of synchrony with the individual's expected age-related development.

Along with the invariance proposed by Berkson (1983), other authors have proposed that stereotypy contains an element of what is called "periodicity"; however, Rapp and Vollmer (2005) pointed out that both invariance and periodicity might be limited to particular topographies and are almost certainly not a characteristic of all behavior that is called stereotypy. For our purposes, we will consider stereotypy to include repetitive and invariant *operant* behavior that appears to serve no social function (Baumeister, 1978; Rapp & Vollmer, 2005), persists in the absence of social consequences (Lovaas, Newsom, & Hickman, 1987), and is a clinical problem when a significant proportion of an individual's time is allocated to the behavior (Sackett, 1978).

At times, stereotypic behavior and self-injurious behavior (SIB) are categorized or at least conceptualized similarly; however, stereotypic behavior is distinguished from SIB in at least two ways. One, the behavior does not ordinarily produce immediate tissue damage, although sometimes this definitional line is blurry, because, for one example, hand mouthing in the longer-term can produce skin damage. Two, at least by our definition, stereotypic behavior is necessarily automatically reinforced (i.e., not maintained by social reinforcement contingencies) (Ringdahl, 2011). On the other hand, only a percentage of SIB is automatically reinforced. For example, Iwata et al. (1994) reported that automatic reinforcement was the sole function for 25.7% of the SIB exhibited by the 152 individuals in the study. Automatic reinforcement was a maintaining variable in conjunction with a social reinforcer for an additional 7.9% of individuals, bringing the total to 33.6%. SIB that falls into this functional category is sometimes called "stereotypic SIB" (Ringdahl, Vollmer, Marcus, & Roane, 1997). In this chapter, we will at times touch on evaluations of treatments for automatically reinforced SIB as they may relate to stereotypy more generally, but we conceptualized SIB and stereotypy as distinct clinical response forms.

Functions of Stereotypic Behavior

Figure 7.1 shows some functional analysis outcomes from Vollmer et al. (1994) that represent common results when assessing stereotypy or stereotypic SIB. In these cases, the response forms were repetitive head banging/hitting and hand biting (Korey) and repetitive hand mouthing (Rhonda). Note that the proportion of time spent engaging in the behavior is high in all conditions and the behavior persists even in a "no interaction" condition, in which no social reinforcement is delivered following the behavior. Such a functional analysis is commonly used to rule out social reinforcement for stereotypy or stereotypic SIB, as the implications for treatment are very different when the behavior is socially reinforced. Herein, we will emphasize treatments for behavior that is automatically reinforced.

Another functional analysis outcome supporting a conclusion that behavior is automatically reinforced is when the behavior occurs at the highest levels during the

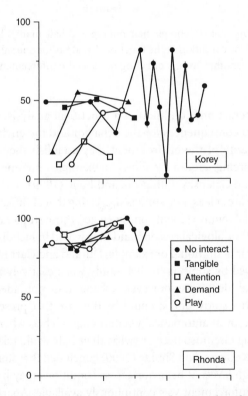

Figure 7.1 Examples of stereotypic behavior during a functional analysis. The percentage of intervals is presented along the *y*-axis, and sessions are presented along the *x*-axis. Korey engaged in repetitive head hitting, head banging, and hand biting, and Rhonda engaged in repetitive hand mouthing. Although these responses produced tissue damage in the long run, they are *functionally* consistent with the topic insofar as the behavior persists in the absence of social reinforcement. Such behavior is maintained by automatic reinforcement. Adapted from Vollmer et al. (1994).

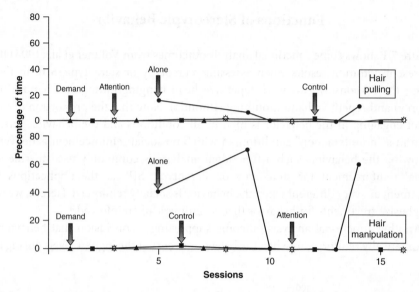

Figure 7.2 Showing that stereotypic hair pulling and hair manipulation occurred almost exclusively in the alone condition of the functional analysis for one subject. Such a functional analysis outcome is another means of ruling out social reinforcement. Adapted from Rapp et al. (1999).

"alone" or "no interaction" condition of a functional analysis. In those conditions, there are no social consequences for the behavior and the environment is relatively austere. The austerity of the environment may establish the stimulus products of behavior as reinforcing. Figure 7.2 shows an example outcome of this pattern from Rapp, Miltenberger, Galensky, Ellingson, and Long (1999).

Although there are at least two studies suggesting that at times stereotypic behavior can enter into social reinforcement contingencies, those studies are not conclusive on the matter for methodological reasons, and they would in fact disqualify the response as stereotypy by our definition. For example, Durand and Carr (1987) concluded that stereotypy displayed by subjects in their study was negatively reinforced by escape from instructional demands; however, escape was not adequately tested as a consequence in that study, and it could be the case that presentation of demands established stereotypy as automatically reinforcing, such as when a person bites their nails in demanding circumstances or twirls their hair while taking a difficult exam. Kennedy, Meyer, Knowles, and Shukla (2000) concluded that stereotypy was multiply controlled, but high levels of behavior across conditions may have indicated merely that automatic reinforcement was continuously available. Apart from these studies, the vast majority of functional analysis research shows that stereotypy is automatically reinforced or what some authors have previously termed "self-stimulatory" (Lovaas et al., 1987). Thus, to remain functionally consistent, throughout the remainder of this paper, we will address treatments for automatically reinforced repetitive behavior.

There are at least five areas of evidence supporting the notion that stereotypy is automatically reinforced operant behavior. First, as previously stated, the behavior persists in the absence of social contingencies in a functional analysis (Piazza, Adelinis, Hanley, Goh, & Delia, 2000; Rapp et al., 1994; Vollmer et al., 1994), such as depicted in Figure 7.1 and Figure 7.2. Second, the provision of alternative sources of reinforcement sometimes has the effect of reducing the frequency of stereotypy (Favell, McGimsey, & Schell, 1982; Horner, 1980; Piazza et al., 2000; Vollmer et al., 1994). This finding is consistent with known principles of operant behavior, such as the matching law (Baum, 1973), which stipulates in part that behavior rate will vary depending on the availability of reinforcement for alternative behavior. Third, the disruption of the contingency between the stereotyped response and the putative sensory products produces an extinction-like effect (Rapp, Dozier, Carr, Patel, & Enloe, 2000; Rincover, 1978; Rincover, Cook, Peoples, & Packard, 1979). Fourth, contingent access to stereotypy can reinforce the occurrence of other behavior (Anderson, Doughty, Doughty, Williams, & Saunders, 2010; Haag & Anderson, 2004; Hanley, Iwata, Thompson, & Lindberg, 2000). Fifth, restricting access to stereotypy results in subsequent increases in the behavior (Forehand & Baumeister, 1973; Lang et al., 2010; Rapp, 2006, 2007; Rapp et al., 2004; Rollings & Baumeister, 1981), which is consistent with known principles of operant behavior, such as establishing operations (Michael, 1982).

Epidemiology

Prevalence studies based on topographical definitions suggest that more than 60% of individuals with ID and as many as 100% of individuals with autism display some form of stereotypy (Bodfish et al., 1995; Campbell et al., 1990). This wide range of estimates is clearly problematic and is reflective of the difficulty in defining the disorder. One difficulty stems from the notion of "repetitiveness." Some behavior occurs in bouts and is only repetitive during bouts. The episodic nature of the behavior is likely to lead some observers to classify the behavior as repetitive and others not to do so. Another difficulty stems from the fact that at some level and under some circumstances, virtually all people engage in repetitive behavior of one kind or another. When do we call it stereotypy and why? For example, Bosch, Vollmer et al. (2010) recently reported in a conference presentation that 100% of typically developing undergraduate students observed while alone engaged in at least some level of repetitive behavior. Thus, it is easy to fall in a trap of splitting hairs when defining stereotypic behavior. Nonetheless, most ID researchers and practitioners generally agree that there is a noticeable quality to repetitive behavior displayed by individuals with ID that leads one to label the behavior as "stereotypic" perhaps relating to the context in which stereotypic behavior tends to occur. You sort of know it when you see it, so to speak, while accepting there very likely will be some grey areas.

On the notion of evidence base

Stereotypic behavior is somewhat unique in its relation to the question of evidence-based treatments. For one reason, there is evidence supporting some treatments, such as punishment procedures, but practitioners may not choose those treatments because the level of intrusiveness does not match the level of behavioral severity. For another reason, there may be evidence supporting some treatments, but those same treatments may be ineffective in individual cases. We will discuss these general issues in the succeeding text.

It may be the case that at times stereotypic behavior is not problematic. The problematic nature of stereotypy is essentially a social validity question (Wolf, 1978): Does the behavior warrant intervention? Also, is the behavior serious enough to warrant intervention if the intervention is somewhat intrusive or labor intensive? For example, a labor-intensive and perhaps intrusive overcorrection procedure may be effective but may not match the level of behavioral severity. Or, a response blocking procedure may be effective, but the level of behavioral severity may not warrant the time allocation spent toward blocking every response. Thus, the utility of any given intervention must be evaluated on an individual basis. At times, stereotypic behavior can be mildly problematic. A parent might report that it is somewhat embarrassing in public or that a child is teased because he rocks back and forth. At other times, the stereotypic behavior can be moderately problematic, such as when a teacher reports that a student is losing valuable instruction time at school because the behavior interferes due to excessive time allocation and resistance to interruption. Finally, the stereotypic behavior can be extremely problematic, such as when the behavior is harmful to the individual (e.g., nearly continuous hand mouthing) or others (e.g., rectal stimulation producing fecal matter on the hands). In the case of mildly problematic, it is unlikely that a family would elect to use punishment even if punishment is shown to be an evidence-based intervention. In the latter case, a family might elect punishment if it effectively suppresses dangerous behavior. The notion of an evidence base, therefore, for the purposes of this chapter, is considered ethically relativistic and contextual. We by no means intend to portray any single procedure as inherently good or bad, only that it has or has not been shown to be effective at least as one *component* of a larger intervention package in the peer-reviewed literature.

Because by our definition stereotypic behavior is not socially reinforced, the efficacy of some reinforcement-based procedures depends on the potency of the reinforcer used in relation to the reinforcer produced by the stereotypic behavior. Thus, a procedure that is effective for one individual may not be effective for another individual. Unfortunately, it is difficult to get a handle on the percentage of cases for which procedures are effective. For one reason, the potency of reinforcers varies from one individual to another. For another reason, editorial practices screen for cases showing a favorable outcome, and/or it is possible that author submission practices screen for cases showing favorable outcomes. Thus, we might know when a procedure is effective in some cases, but we might not know that it is ineffective in other cases. From a clinical perspective, we can safely say that not all procedures reported in the literature consistently work in all cases of stereotypy (Berg et al., in press; Ringdahl et al., 1997). We will stop short of calling any given approach an "evidence-based intervention" and rather stress that some approaches represent evidence-based components of an overall intervention package or model. Thus, one goal for the end of our chapter is to build to an evidence-based *model* for intervention implementation. We will ultimately take a position that a sequential approach to intervention is most appropriate and best supported by the empirical literature.

The Evidence Base for Treatment of Stereotypy

In the following section, we will first describe our method for reviewing the literature. Second, we will discuss specific intervention components by evaluating the evidence base.

Literature reviewed

For over two decades now, Dr. Brian Iwata and his graduate students have carefully selected, reviewed, and keyworded every article published on topics related to SIB (at least to the best of their ability). These articles include studies on stereotypy, self-stimulation, repetitive behavior, and the like. Iwata graciously supplies former members of the lab with updated versions of the electronic files as an outcome of their efforts. As a former member of the lab, the first author of this chapter had access to the most recent version of the files, and the second author utilized the search features using endnote.

Any article keyworded as stereotypy was further reviewed and considered; the second author read each abstract (or title and keywords if the abstract was unavailable) of the 1,007 articles with the keyword stereotypy to determine whether the article presented empirical data on a treatment for stereotypy. Articles on the hyperactivity in ADHD or tics associated with Tourette's syndrome were excluded. Duplicate articles and articles evaluating the reliability and validity of rating scales were also excluded. Of the original 1,007 articles, 426 were sorted into categories based on type of treatment used. If an article presented data on rates of stereotypy (or repetitive behavior or self-stimulation when an independent variable was modified), the article was assigned to one or more group based on the nature of the independent variable(s). For example, an article could be grouped under both differential reinforcement of other behavior (DRO) and timeout if it contained two independent variables (i.e., DRO and timeout).

After the articles were sorted and grouped, each group was examined and read to determine the status of the independent variable as an evidence-based treatment. The group was sorted by date, and the most recent review of the treatment was read (if a review was available). If a review was not available or did not provide sufficient information to determine whether the treatment was evidence-based, articles were read starting with the chronologically most recent until at least one of the criteria set by Chambless and Hollon (1998) is met, that is, at least three small N experiments with a total of at least nine subjects by at least two independent groups. (There were no randomized controlled trials in the data base.)

To find treatments that fell into the category of commonly used, but lacking empirical support, two recent surveys of therapies for autism were reviewed as a beginning point (Green et al., 2006; Hess, Morrier, Heflin, & Ivey, 2008). Any treatment was included for additional review that either of these two studies indicated was used by at least 5% of the subjects surveyed. All medications were excluded from the treatments listed because medications were reviewed using the methods described earlier. Programs such as applied behavior analysis and TEACHH, which consist of multiple treatment components, were excluded. For example, we decided to split applied behavior analysis into categories that included environmental enrichment, extinction, and differential reinforcement. The behavior analysis categories were selected based on the fact that the interventions were described as such. In other words, behavior analysts describe interventions as, for example, "extinction" as opposed to describing it as "applied behavior analysis."

For the remaining list of 35 treatments, an Internet-based search was conducted to determine (a) whether any empirical data existed on each treatment and (b) whether the treatment was recommended to decrease stereotypy by websites or bloggers. The Internet search was conducted in the following manner: A Google Scholar search was conducted for "(name of treatment) treatment for stereotypy." Identical searches were conducted substituting "repetitive behavior," "self-stimulation," or "autism" for stereotypy; "autism" was included because many blogger websites focus on treatments for stereotypy related to autism. Next, a search of the PsycINFO database was conducted using the same search words used for Google Scholar. If no scholarly articles were found as a result of either search, a basic Google web search was conducted for the same terms; the term "stimming" was added because it is a word commonly used by bloggers for stereotypy. If any blogger/autism website cited journal articles, the University of Florida online library was searched for the articles. In addition, the list of "cited by" articles and reference lists within the articles were reviewed to find relevant articles. If a treatment were related to a particular topic, journals specific to that topic would be searched (e.g., nutrition journals for articles pertaining to diet modification and occupational therapy journals for articles pertaining to sensory integration). The web search was terminated when searches yielded the same articles or information. Articles found were reviewed in the same manner described earlier.

Evidence-based approaches

The following were considered to be evidence-based intervention components by virtue of being confirmed by at least three small N experiments with a total of at least nine subjects by at least two independent groups. The intervention components determined to be evidence based include environmental enrichment, extinction, differential reinforcement, punishment, and antecedent exercise.

Environmental enrichment

Studies were considered to be "environmental enrichment" interventions if they involved antecedent provision of presumably or demonstrably reinforcing items. The general notion behind environmental enrichment is that having alternative sources of reinforcement available will reduce the time allocation spent toward engaging in stereotypic behavior. Dozens of published studies have demonstrated the full or partial suppression of stereotypy during environmental enrichment (e.g., Ahearn, Clark, Gardenier, Chung, & Dube, 2003; Athens, Vollmer, Sloman, & St. Peter Pipkin, 2008; Hagopian & Toole, 2009; Rapp, 2004; Rapp et al., 2004; Sidener, Carr, & Firth, 2005), thus qualifying the procedure as an evidence-based approach. Sometimes, enriched environments are given specific names, such as with the so-called "Snoezelen" rooms, but herein, we treat those environments as simply enriched, insofar as the results of research suggest that the same principles of stimulus preference and alternative activity availability apply (e.g., Cuvo, May, & Post, 2001). Given some idiosyncratic outcomes of environment enrichment and given various nuances of the approach, the approach is best considered to be an effective *component* to a larger intervention strategy.

A number of variables influence the efficacy of environmental enrichment (Rapp & Vollmer, 2005). The most obvious factor is the relative potency of the reinforcer or reinforcers used in the intervention. Intuitively, if the items are not more reinforcing or at least at times more reinforcing than the stimulation produced by stereotypy, the intervention would be less effective. For example, Vollmer et al. (1994) showed that for three preschool age children with various developmental disabilities, environmental enrichment was differentially effective if high-preference items were used as opposed to low-preference items as identified in a stimulus preference assessment (Fisher et al., 1992). Figure 7.3 shows an outcome in Vollmer et al.

Another variable discussed by Rapp and Vollmer (2005) is prompting. Where some studies have shown that simple availability of reinforcers decreases stereotypy (e.g., Piazza et al., 2000), other studies have shown that some individuals require prompts to engage with alternative stimuli (Britton, Carr, Landaburu, & Romick, 2002; Singh & Millichamp, 1987). Similarly, idiosyncratic issues arise when some individuals require extraneous reinforcement to at least begin engaging with alternative items (Vollmer et al., 1994) or when additional intervention components such as blocking are required (Lindberg, Iwata, & Kahng, 1999). Presumably, blocking decreases the reinforcement produced by stereotypy and hence limits available reinforcement to those stimuli used in the enriched environment. Combining environmental enrichment with other intervention components will be discussed further when we suggest an evidence-based treatment model at the conclusion of this chapter.

Another variable related to environmental enrichment efficacy is whether the ambient stimuli are "matched" to the stimulation produced by stereotypy. Piazza et al. (2000) and others have concluded that environmental enrichment is more effective if

Te

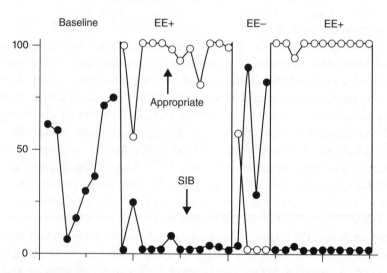

Figure 7.3   Although the target response was SIB (repetitive ear flicking that caused a wound on the ear), it was automatically reinforced SIB (stereotypic SIB) so the example serves. For this subject (Ron) during EE+, a highly preferred stimulus was used. During EE−, a low-preferred stimulus was used. This effect demonstrates the role of and importance of considering stimulus preference in environmental enrichment.

the stimuli are matched (e.g., Higbee, Chang, & Endicott, 2005; Lanovaz & Argumedes, 2009, 2010; Lanovaz, Fletcher, & Rapp, 2009; Lanovaz, Sladeczek, & Rapp, 2011; Rapp, 2007; Simmons, Smith, & Kliethermes, 2003), but conflicting evidence was presented by Ahearn, Clark, DeBar, and Florentino (2005). Piazza et al. showed that a preference assessment could be used to identify matched stimuli that effectively competed with stereotypy, but Ahearn et al. (2007) showed that highly preferred stimuli competed better, even if they were unmatched by stimulus type. A sort of intermediate approach was used by Ringdahl et al. (1997), who used the logic of a stimulus preference assessment to identify the most preferred stimuli but also to gauge levels of stereotypy during exposure to those stimuli. The approach used by Ringdahl et al. will be described in more detail when we propose the evidence-based treatment model at the conclusion of this chapter. Also, some of our preliminary data show that matched stimuli do suppress stereotypy better, and, in fact, we have found that at times highly preferred but unmatched stimuli can *increase* instances of both targeted and untargeted stereotypy (Carroll et al., 2010; Rapp, 2004, 2005).

Extinction
Extinction involves withholding the reinforcing consequence of behavior such that the behavior is no longer reinforced and, hence, the behavior gradually decreases in frequency. When behavior is socially reinforced, extinction procedures can be rather

straightforward because it is possible to identify and manipulate the delivery of rein-forcement: The therapist ensures that the social reinforcement is withheld. When behavior is automatically reinforced, such as is the case with stereotypic behavior, extinction is more difficult to implement as it is more difficult to identify the reinforcer and to manipulate its delivery. In short, because the specific source of reinforcement is often unknown, it can be difficult or impossible to block or withhold that source of reinforcement; however, when termination of reinforcement can be accomplished, there is a sufficient body of evidence to suggest that extinction is at least an evidence-based treatment *component*.

Two lines of research lend support to extinction as an evidence-based component but with some caveats. One is the so-called "sensory extinction" literature and the other is the literature on response blocking. In sensory extinction, the idea is to somehow block the automatic stimulation produced by stereotypy. For example, Rapp et al. (1999) applied gloves to a subject for whom tactile stimulation associated with stereotypic hair manipulation functioned as reinforcement. When the gloves were applied, hair manipulation occurred at near-zero levels. Similar effects have been reported in a variety of related studies across a range of clinical research labo-ratories (Aiken & Salzberg, 1984; Mason & Newsom, 1990; Rincover et al., 1979; also see Rapp & Vollmer, 2005, for a review). One caveat is that some of the proce-dures used may not actually represent extinction per se, but rather effects of alternative stimulation. For example, Mason and Newsom used metal rings on the hands of subjects to reduce hand stereotypy. Although this approach may have pro-duced a withholding of sensory stimulation for hand stereotypy (i.e., extinction), it also fundamentally changed the type of stimulation. Whether or not that procedure technically constitutes extinction is open for debate.

Response blocking is also sometimes associated with extinction procedures and should be considered in the context of extinction insofar as the sensory products of stereotypy are blocked. Numerous studies have shown that response blocking or response redirection has the effect of reducing stereotypy (Ahearn, Clark, MacDonald, & Chung, 2007; Hagopian & Toole, 2009; Rapp, 2006; Rapp et al., 2004; Schumacher & Rapp, 2011; Tarbox, Tarbox, Ghezzi, Wallace, & Yoo, 2007); however, several important caveats should be mentioned. First, it has been shown conclusively that in some circumstances response blocking functions as extinction (Smith, Russo, & Le, 1999), but in other cases, the procedure functions as punish-ment (Lerman & Iwata, 1996). In fact, similar ambiguities have been reported in the use of protective equipment to "block" the sensory consequences of stereotypy. For example, Mazaleski, Iwata, Rodgers, Vollmer, and Zarcone (1994) found that the contingent application of hand mitts reduced hand mouthing in a fashion con-sistent with punishment effects. A second caveat is that several studies have shown that blocking of one stereotypic response produces an increase in other forms of stereotypy (Lerman, Kelley, Vorndran, & Van Camp, 2003; Rapp et al., 2004). A third caveat is that while blocking may suppress stereotypy in the short term, the behavior may rebound to higher levels in the subsequent minutes when blocking stops (Rapp, 2006).

Collectively, the results of sensory extinction approaches, including response blocking and response redirection, suggest that stereotypy can be reduced by extinction-like procedures; however, given possible negative side effects and the possible role of punishment, these approaches should be considered as one component to an overall intervention approach.

Differential reinforcement

Two general types of differential reinforcement procedures were considered in our review: DRO and differential reinforcement of alternative behavior (DRA). The idea behind DRO is to identify potent stimuli to reinforce periods of stereotypy omission. Our review showed overwhelming support for these procedures from dozens of applications across numerous clinical laboratories (e.g., Beare, Severson, & Brandt, 2004; Charlop-Christy & Haymes, 1996; Lanovaz & Argumedes, 2010; Ringdahl et al., 2002; Shabani, Wilder, & Flood, 2001; Taylor, Hoch, & Weissman, 2005; among others). The idea behind DRA is to increase some specific alternative behavior, ideally to functionally replace stereotypy. For example, in our work, we have used DRA to reinforce toy play when enriched environment alone is ineffective (Rapp et al., 2004; Ringdahl et al., 1997; Vollmer et al., 1994). Thus, both DRO and DRA have strong evidence bases.

Like environmental enrichment, the efficacy of DRA depends on the ability to identify reinforcers that can effectively compete with the automatic reinforcers maintaining stereotypy. Although identifying potent reinforcers may seem like a major obstacle, dozens of studies from numerous laboratories have reported success with DRA (Arntzen, Tonnessen, & Brouwer, 2006; Beare et al., 2004; Facon, Beghin, & Riviere, 2007; Kennedy et al., 2000; Nuzzolo-Gomez, Leonard, Ortiz, Rivera, & Greer, 2002; Saunders, Saunders, & Marquis, 1998; among others).

Punishment

Positive punishment involves the response-contingent application of aversive stimulation, such that behavior rates decrease below baseline levels. Negative punishment procedures involve the contingent removal of a stimulus, such as timeout and response cost procedures. This section will focus on positive punishment procedures, and this chapter will address negative punishment procedures later. A wide range of aversive stimuli has been tested as treatment for stereotypy. It is important to reiterate here a point made earlier in the chapter: It is unlikely that some of these aversive stimuli would be used because the stereotypy is not viewed as sufficiently dangerous to require intrusive interventions. In addition, in our present culture, most practitioners defer first to reinforcement-based procedures. Nonetheless, we would be remiss to not mention the types of punishment procedures that have been tested and which have been shown to be effective. We classify punishment procedures as an evidence-based treatment component here, because presumably any number of aversive stimuli *could* be used in treatment, but, again, ethical constraints would limit the list of actual stimuli used in any given clinical setting.

Perhaps the most socially accepted punishment procedure is a verbal reprimand. The reprimand has been shown to be effective in several studies across numerous labs; however, it was often at least initially or sometimes ultimately paired with some other consequence. For example, Charlop, Burgio, Iwata, and Ivancic (1988) showed that stereotypy exhibited by a child with autism could be suppressed by reprimands, timeout, and overcorrection (contingent effort). Reprimands were the least effective, but the general procedure was most effective when all three consequences were alternated. Rapp (2007) and Rapp, Patel, Ghezzi, O'Flaherty, and Titterington (2009) showed that reprimands effectively decreased stereotypy for one subject and two of three subjects, respectively, but one subject required the addition of a response cost procedures (contingent removal of preferred items) in the latter study.

Another procedure that is widely used is blocking (see prior discussion under extinction) or a brief hands-down period for hand stereotypies. For example, Richmond (1983) showed that reprimands were effective, but the procedure was paired with physically guiding the subjects' hands in a downward direction. Vollmer et al. (1994) used a brief (10-s) hands-down procedure for one subject when environmental enrichment and differential reinforcement were not completely effective. Doughty, Anderson, Doughty, Williams, and Saunders (2007) used a 1-s or 10-s hands-down procedure successfully for three subjects.

Extensions of blocking and brief manual restraining procedures include personal and physical restraining, such as using extended holds (personal restraint) or protective equipment (physical restraint). Such procedures were reviewed extensively by Harris (1996) and were found to be both effective and acceptable if combined with fading procedures to eventually eliminate or greatly reduce restraint usage.

Contingent effort is a punishment procedure that involves requiring physical effort contingent on the occurrence of behavior. Perhaps the most widely known and utilized contingent effort procedure is overcorrection. In overcorrection, the subject is typically required to engage in "positive practice" of some response that is deemed to be the correct version of behavior that is now problematic and stereotypic. The prototype studies were presented by Azrin and Foxx (e.g., Azrin, Kaplan, and Foxx, 1973; Foxx & Azrin, 1973). In Azrin et al., for nine individuals with ID, they found large decreases in stereotypy within 0–12 days. Subsequent replications and extensions were reviewed by Miltenberger and Fuqua (1981), who found that virtually all variations of positive practice overcorrection were effective in reducing stereotypy (e.g., Coleman, Whitman, & Johnson, 1979; Epstein, Doke, Sajwaj, Sorrell, & Rimmer, 1974; Harris & Wolchik, 1979; Luiselli, Pemberton, & Helfen, 1978; among many others). The only more recent study we identified was reported by Cole, Montgomery, Wilson, and Milan (2000), who found that relatively short duration positive practice overcorrection (30 s) was as effective as longer duration procedures (2 and 8 min).

The following procedures are mentioned only because of evidence of efficacy; however, it is unlikely that most schools or residential facilities would allow these procedures for student or client rights reasons. Visual screening is a controversial procedure that was widely studied in the 1980s and early 1990s (Barrett, Staub, & Sisson, 1983; Horton, 1987; Jordan, Singh, & Repp, 1989; Singh, Landrum, Ellis, & Donatelli, 1993; Singh & Winton, 1984; among others). Visual screening involves

blocking the person's vision for a brief period (usually less than 1 min) either manually or with a blindfold. The delivery of noxious stimuli is another controversial
procedure that typically involves contingent delivery of bitter or foul tasting substances or odors, such as lemon juice (e.g., Cipani, Brendlinger, McDowell, &
Usher, 1991) or vinegar (e.g., Friman, Cook, & Finney, 1984). Water misting is
another procedure that was initially used as treatment for severe self-injury
(Dorsey, Iwata, Ong, & McSween, 1980) and was extended to the treatment of
stereotypy (e.g., Friman et al., 1984).

When we conclude the chapter, we will present an argument that there is a role for
punishment in treating severe cases of stereotypy, due to its evidence base, but only
when there is an effort to develop inhibitory stimulus control such that punishment
will eventually be reduced or even eliminated (e.g., Rapp et al., 2009) and only after
less intrusive procedures have been attempted.

Antecedent exercise

Antecedent exercise involves some period of physical exertion (i.e., aerobic exercise
including walking, jogging) prior to some subsequent activity. Some of the studies in
this realm have some methodological shortcomings, but collectively there is evidence to support its consideration as one treatment component. Antecedent exercise
has the added value of being important in its own right, so even if the exercise did
not reduce stereotypy, it is presumably good for the individual to receive exercise.
Gabler-Halle, Halle, and Chung (1993) conducted an extensive review of the literature that existed at that time and found support for the procedure. Aerobic exercise
was found to decrease stereotypy when the collective literature was considered (e.g.,
Bachman & Fuqua, 1983; Bachman & Sluyter, 1988; Baumeister & MacLean, 1984;
Kern, Koegel, & Dunlap, 1984; Kern, Koegel, Dyer, Blew, & Fenton, 1982; Watters &
Watters, 1980).

Several additional studies have been published supporting aerobic exercise as
an intervention component (e.g., Morrison, Roscoe, & Atwall, 2011). For example,
Celiberti, Bobo, Kelly, Harris, and Handleman (1997) found that 6 min of jogging
decreased the physical stereotypy of (e.g., hand movements and bouncing) in a
5-year-old boy with autism. Elliot, Dobbin, Rose, and Soper (1994) found that aerobic exercise decreased maladaptive and stereotypic behavior in four of six adults
with ID. Ellis, MacLean, and Gazdag (1989) reported that a regimen of fast walking
and jogging decreased body rocking for an adult male with ID. Others have reported
consistent and similar results (e.g., Morrison et al., 2011; Morrissey, Franzini, &
Karen, 1992; Power, Thibadeau, & Rose, 1992; Prupas & Reid, 2001; Rosenthal-
Malek & Mitchell, 1997).

It is not clear which behavioral mechanisms are responsible for the effects of antecedent aerobic exercise on stereotypy. It is possible that mere fatigue plays a role
(Rapp & Vollmer, 2005). Even so, given that it is important for all humans to experience exercise on a nearly daily basis and given the added value that exercise may serve
to reduce stereotypy for some individuals, it is clearly an evidence-based recommen-
dation as an intervention component for both health and behavioral reasons.

Promising Procedures

Intervention components were considered to be "promising" if initial research results showed favorable effects, but there were not yet enough studies to qualify the component as evidence based (Chambless & Hollon, 1998). In this section, we will review the following procedures: inhibitory stimulus control and stimulus fading, response cost, self-management plus differential reinforcement, assistive technology, and psychotropic medication.

Inhibitory stimulus control and stimulus fading

Rapp et al. (2009) reduced stereotypy via reprimands. Reprimands and response cost were paired with a red card. For one participant, the red card effectively suppressed stereotypy in the absence of reprimands and response cost. This finding suggests that more research should address the possibility of using inhibitory stimulus control to suppress stereotypy. Other studies have shown that stereotypy is suppressed in the presence of the adult who administers the intervention. For example, Athens et al. (2008) demonstrated that a treatment involving noncontingent toys and attention, coupled with contingent effort, effectively suppressed stereotypy only when the adult therapist was in the room. Athens et al. then implemented a procedure to systematically remove the adult from the room while maintaining treatment effects.

Instructional methods

A couple of studies suggest that using sound, predictable instructional routines reduces the frequency of stereotypy. For example, Dib and Sturmey (2007) improved the teacher use of discrete-trial teaching procedures and noted dramatic decreases in stereotypy as instructional integrity improved for three boys with autism. Tustin (1995) implemented a procedure to signal activity changes with a "2-min" warning for transitions. The subject engaged in less stereotypy when the transitions were signaled. Collectively, these two studies suggest that more research should be done on predictable and consistent instructional routines.

Response cost

We found four studies that implemented response cost as treatment for stereotypy (Athens et al., 2008; Bartlett, Rapp, Krueger, & Henrickson, 2010; Falcomata, Roane, Hovanetz, Kettering, & Keeney, 2004; Rapp et al., 2009); however, some of those studies involved treatment packages, and it is difficult to identify the independent role of response cost in the interventions. Response cost makes intuitive sense as a treatment because if the individual is given highly preferred items or activities during environmental enrichment, and those items are taken away contingent on stereotypy, and because the procedure is functionally akin to differential reinforcement (Rolider & Van Houten, 1990), which has a strong evidence base. For now, however, response cost must be categorized as promising but not evidence based.

Self-management plus differential reinforcement

We identified five studies showing favorable results with self-management (Koegel & Koegel, 1990; Moore, 2009; O'Reilly et al., 2002; Shabani et al., 2001; Stahmer & Schreibman, 1992); however, in all cases, the self-management procedure was combined with some sort of differential reinforcement procedure mediated by a therapist. Thus, more research is needed to show that the differential reinforcement component can be faded or otherwise omitted from the self-management intervention.

Assistive technology

Numerous studies have used assistive technology (e.g., devises that activate reinforcers via microswitch). We did not consider this to be a treatment category per se, but because some authors do categorize assistive technology as a treatment modality, we wanted to acknowledge that it is clearly a technology that can assist with differential reinforcement and environmental enrichment (e.g., Lancioni et al., 2008).

Psychotropic medication

The Food and Drug Administration (FDA) has approved the use of risperidone as a treatment for "irritability" in autism (aggression, self-injury, tantrums); however, the randomized clinical trials on which that approval was based also found significant decreases on the stereotypy scale of the Aberrant Behavior Checklist (Research Units on Pediatric Psychopharmacology (RUPP) Autism Network, 2002; Shea et al., 2004; Stigler & McDougle, 2008). Given that the studies utilized scale measurement and not direct behavioral observation, the extent of socially valid behavior change is unclear. Further, the longer-term effects need to be evaluated. Thus, in keeping with our approach with other evidence-based practices, risperidone is viewed as a promising evidence-based treatment component. Some authors have gone so far as to call risperidone evidence based (Soorya, Kiarashi, & Hollander, 2008).

Soorya et al. (2008) also reported that there have been conflicting results for *fluvoxamine* (McDougle et al., 1996), even within the same research team. There appears to be some promise for *fluoxetine*; however, the two studies to date have been published by the same research team so the intervention must be considered not yet evidence based (Buchsbaum et al., 2001; Hollander et al., 2005). Soorya et al. noted that *sertraline* has shown efficacy in two open-label studies, but those studies lacked a control group so the medication should be viewed as perhaps promising but with insufficient evidence base (McDougle et al., 1998; Steingard et al., 1997; and see Miguel et al., 2009). Similar promise has been shown for *citalopram* (Namerow, Thomas, Bostic, Prince, & Monuteaux, 2003), but it is not yet sufficiently evidence based. Currently, the National Institutes of Health is sponsoring a network study on liquid citalopram, so more should be known in coming years (Soorya et al.).

Insufficient or Inadequate Research

Interventions in this category include those where either not enough research has been done to provide an evidence base or the existing research shows that the intervention is not effective. Although numerous interventions are covered, they fall generally in the categories of dietary manipulations, sensory-related therapies, medical therapies, and other (miscellaneous) therapies.

Dietary manipulations

Gluten- and casein-free diet
Mulloy et al. (2010) reviewed the existing literature on the use of the gluten- and casein-free diets in the treatment of autism and concluded that the diets are ineffective. "Given the lack of empirical support, and the adverse consequences often associated with GFCF diets (e.g., stigmatization, diversion of treatment resources, reduced bone cortical thickness), such diets should only be implemented in the event a child with ASD experiences acute behavioral changes, seemingly associated with changes in diet, and/or medical professionals confirm through testing the child has allergies or food intolerances to gluten and/or casein" (Mulloy et al., p. 1).

One subsequent and contradictory study was published by Whiteley et al. (2010), who found support for the diet; however, the study did not employ a placebo condition, and the results were based on parental report. Given that this is the one supportive study and given those methodological shortcomings, the gluten- and casein-free diet remains insufficiently evidence based as treatment for stereotypy; however, as pointed out by Mulloy et al. (2010), any individual with allergies or food intolerances is likely to be sensitive and would not surprisingly display problematic behavior. As with any allergy or food intolerance, such medical complications should always be ruled out when developing comprehensive interventions for individuals with ID.

Essential fatty acids (EFAs)

Essential fatty acids (EFAs) (omega-6 and omega-3) are considered to be crucial for many biochemical processes, such as brain and body development. If
the levels of omega-3 are insufficient relative to omega-6, there can be negative
effects on the body and subsequently behavior. Because some previous research
has shown low levels of omega-3 in autistic individuals, some scientists have
proposed a possible relationship with symptoms of autism, including stereotypic behavior (Bent, Bertoglio, & Hendren, 2009); however, Bent et al. (2009)
reviewed the existing literature and found that there was insufficient evidence
to support an omega-3-rich diet as a treatment for autistic symptoms, including
stereotypy. Bent et al. conducted an exhaustive review and only found six
studies meeting their relatively relaxed inclusion criteria; of the six, only one
study, Amminger et al. (2007), utilized adequate controls and that study showed
insignificant results.

Vitamin and megavitamin therapy

For several decades, researchers have hypothesized a relationship between vitamins
and behavior, particularly B6–magnesium. Nye and Brice (2005) reviewed several
studies and only found three met their criteria for review. Only one of those three
reported "adequate data for analysis." Nye and Brice concluded that further research is
needed. A separate study found improved behavioral ratings for children receiving
ascorbic acid as supplemental therapy for characteristics of autism (Dolske, Spollen,
McKay, Lancashire, & Tolbert, 1993); however, there was no mention whether
stereotypy was one of the target forms of behavior and no individual data were
reported.

Homeopathy

Homeopathy involves giving small doses of substances that cause illness in larger doses,
in order to initiate a self-healing response. Although commonly described on Internet
sites, we found not a single supportive study for treating stereotypy in this manner.

Sensory-related therapies

Auditory integration training

Baranek (2002) reviewed nine studies on auditory integration training (AIT).
Baranek summarized the approach as follows: "AIT is based on the concept that
electronically modulated/filtered music provided through earphones may be helpful
in remediating hypersensitivities and overall auditory processing ability that is
thought to be problematic in children with autism" (p. 409). Baranek concluded that
the studies reviewed showed, at best, mixed results and that any favorable effects
could as well be due to other factors such as increased attention, caregiver expectations, and compliance training.

Sensory integration

Sensory integration is based on improving underlying neurological processing and organization and aims at increasing attention and sensitivity to environmental stimuli (Smith, Press, Koenig, & Kinnealey, 2005). It provides sensory stimulation of all sorts but commonly includes deep pressure through brushing, massage, weighted vests, and toy play. Conceivably, if such stimulation is highly preferred, sensory integration could function like environmental enrichment and differential reinforcement; however, to date, there has been little emphasis on stimulus preference in the sensory integration literature. In addition, there is no demonstrable link to the putative effect of improving neurological processing and organization.

Baranek (2002) reviewed sensory and motor interventions for children with autism and concluded that such procedures have limited empirical support and that most articles ostensibly supporting sensory integration therapies have methodological flaws. Although Baranek's review did not focus on stereotypy per se, the empirical research focusing on stereotypy does in fact show flawed methodology. For example, Lower (2000) tested the effects of vestibular stimulation on stereotypy for one subject. Although Lower concluded that the intervention was effective, visual inspection of the data shows modest improvements at best, and no interobserver agreement data were reported, which brings into question the reliability of the data. Three other studies reporting modest or inconsistent (but favorable) effects of sensory integration include McClure and Holtz-Yotz (1991), Smith et al. (2005), and Zisserman (1992); however, in none of those studies were interobserver agreement data collected. One study published by Mason and Iwata (1990) concluded that any favorable effects of sensory integration are artifactual, insofar as they are limited to the functional properties of the target behavior; however, it should be noted that study focused on SIB rather than stereotypy.

Weighted vests are also a common form of sensory integration. If you walk into virtually any school attended by children with autism or ID, you will see children wearing a weighted vest, a vest with weights placed in small pockets. This therapeutic approach is rooted in sensory integration and is tied to the "deep pressure" component of sensory integration. A recent comprehensive review by Stephenson and Carter (2009) concluded that no evidence exists for use of the weighted vest. We are currently conducting an evaluation of the weighted vest, and we have found that for our subjects to date, it does not decrease stereotypy below baseline levels (Bosch, Philips et al., 2010).

Other medical therapies

Chelation

Meso-2,3-dimercaptosuccinic acid (DMSA, chelation therapy) is commonly used to remove lead and other toxic metals from the bodies of individuals who have been poisoned, and the FDA has approved it for this purpose; however, to date, there is no evidence that the intervention has an effect on stereotypy. Although Adams et al. (2009) reported statistically significant results for changes in autism symptoms, there were some methodological limitations to the study, and, most importantly for our purposes, the study did not directly address stereotypy per se. The Adams et al. study used only rating scales rather than direct behavioral measurement and excluded 16 subjects from the study because they did not display high levels of toxic metals in their urinary secretions. Thus, to date, there is insufficient evidence to support chelation as an intervention component.

Hyperbaric chamber
The use of the hyperbaric treatment for autism and related symptoms has been quite popular in recent years; Rossignol et al. (2009) noted that several uncontrolled studies were published supporting its use. In an attempt to address the limitation of previous research, Rossignol et al. conducted a randomized, double-blind, controlled trial. Hyperbaric treatment involves breathing 100% oxygen in a pressurized chamber and has previously been used to treat carbon monoxide poisoning and to more rapidly heal wounds. The results were promising insofar as statistically significant improvements were made on autism symptoms based on the scales used; however, no direct behavioral measures were taken, and research from additional research groups is needed to qualify this as an evidence-based intervention. Thus, to date, the use of hyperbaric treatments for stereotypy is not evidence based.

Medical marijuana
Medical marijuana as a treatment for autism symptoms was popularized—or at least widely discussed—in some recent media reports; however, no research has been done to evaluate this intervention for stereotypy or any other related problematic behavior.

Other treatments

Floor time
Floor time is a treatment model that focuses on relating, communicating, and thinking; it encourages parents and teachers to get down on the floor with the child and work with the child at their current level of functioning (Greenspan & Wieder, 1997). This approach is widely discussed on the Internet and appears to be popular among many families of individuals with ASD; however, the two large-scale studies that have been published ostensibly supporting the floor time model did not use a control group so it is not clear if the supposed improvements were a result of floor time (see Greenspan & Wieder, 1997; Solomon, Nechels, Ferch, & Bruckman, 2007). There is insufficient evidence supporting this approach.

Holding therapy

Holding therapy has received media attention due initially to the success reported in treating autistic children and then later to several deaths that were reported as a result of the therapy. Holding therapy involves making physical contact with a child, even if the child is fighting against the contact. There is no empirical support for this procedure as a treatment for stereotypy and due to the dangers of the procedure, should not be used.

Art, music, and pet therapy

Whereas environmental enrichment is explicitly arranged such that highly preferred activities are used, therapies such as art, music, and pet therapy are treated as interventions in their own right. It is very possible, if not likely, that some individuals would respond favorably to one or more of these therapies, but we are taking a position that art, music, or pet interaction should have no special status above other potentially highly preferred activities or items. For example, if an individual's stereotypy is suppressed when given access to highly preferred computer games, we should not call the approach "computer therapy." To be clear, we are not saying that art, music, or pet interactions would not be highly reinforcing for some individuals, and, hence, they may very well function like environmental enrichment; however, those activities should be treated like any other preferred activity and possibly taught as replacement behavior via differential reinforcement. Art skills, music skills and music appreciation, and pet interaction skills are clearly all suitable and desirable forms of replacement behavior for stereotypy.

With that general caveat, it is important to recognize that some studies have been published using music as a source of stimulation in an enriched environment, with the effect of reducing stereotypy (e.g., Gunter, Fox, McEvoy, Shores, & Denny, 1993; Lanovaz et al., 2009, 2011). For art therapy, there are some supportive studies, but they are lacking methodological rigor. For example, Epp (2008) showed improvements in stereotypy during art therapy for a group of 44 children diagnosed with ASD, but there was no control group from which to compare. Other studies reported anecdotal outcomes but did not present supportive data (Elkis-Abuhoff, 2008; Henley, 1986). One study has been published supporting the use of pet therapy to decrease stereotypy (Redefer & Goodman, 1989), but more research would be needed to consider it an evidence-based intervention component.

Gentle teaching

According to Jordan et al. (1989), Gentle Teaching is an approach in which the goal is to teach "the reinforcing value of social interaction so that 'bonding' will occur between the client and therapist" (p. 9) and the therapist will develop instructional control. Although some studies have directly evaluated Gentle Teaching and found that it does not reduce stereotypy below baseline levels (Jordan et al.), most studies involved insufficient methodology or no reference to stereotypy. Thus, in relation

to stereotypy, Gentle Teaching must be considered ineffective or at best not sufficiently tested (see Jones & McCaughey, 1992, for a review).

Social stories

Social Stories are written expectations about behavior in particular contexts which
may have a useful role in educating individuals with ID; to date, there is insufficient
evidence that the procedure is a treatment for stereotypy. Although numerous
studies on social stories exist, we found only two that utilized social stories in isolation to address stereotypy. Reynhout and Carter (2007) used a Social Story to
decrease stereotypic tapping in a boy with autism; however, they used an ABC
sequential design with no return to baseline or other control condition. Hence, no
experimental control was demonstrated. Demiri (2004) evaluated Social Stories to
address various target behavior for five children with ASD. For two of the children,
stereotypy was a target response, but no reductions were observed for stereotypy
as a function of Social Stories.

Timeout

Timeout involves the contingent withholding of opportunities to obtain reinforcement. The procedure is especially tricky in relation to stereotypy because when the
person is in timeout, they can automatically obtain reinforcement by engaging in the
stereotypy. On the other hand, if the time in environment is sufficiently enriched, it
is possible that contingent withholding of the time in reinforcers would sufficiently
punish stereotypy. Given this range of possible outcomes and functional properties
of timeout, it is perhaps not surprising that the findings on timeout as treatment for
stereotypy are mixed. We reviewed several studies with methodological shortcomings, but those will not be considered here.

Among those with appropriate experimental control, Pendergrass (1972) showed
that timeout did in fact suppress stereotypy for two individuals with severe ID.
Pendergrass used a timeout booth, which is probably not usable in today's culture in
most schools. Similarly, Solnick, Rincover, and Peterson (1977) showed that timeout
suppressed stereotypy, but only if the time in environment was sufficiently enriched.
Haring and Kennedy (1990) also found that timeout was only effective if it occurred
in the context of leisure time (as opposed to task time). Conversely, Harris and
Wolchik (1979) found that timeout was ineffective in comparison to overcorrection
as treatment for stereotypy. In addition, all functional analysis research showing
high rates of stereotypy in an alone condition calls into question the use of timeout
because it suggests that automatically reinforced behavior would persist *during* the
timeout interval.

Collectively, the data on timeout suggest that it could be considered as a
treatment component *if and only if* the time in context was demonstrably
enriched and, hence, it was punishing to withhold access to that time in environment. Additionally, data should be collected on the target behavior during
timeout to ensure that behavior rates outside of timeout do not falsely deflate
overall rates.

Conclusion

Evidence-based treatments

Based on the standards set by Chambless and Hollon (1998), relatively few of the treatments for stereotypy are evidence based: Environmental enrichment, extinction procedures, differential reinforcement, punishment procedures, and antecedent activity are the only interventions that meet criteria. All other treatments lack sufficient evidence to be called evidence based, and holding therapy should not be used due to potential harm (see Table 7.1 for a list).

Several caveats to the notion of evidence based have been previously noted in the chapter and will be revisited here. Not every case of stereotypy will be appropriate for treatment by each of the evidence-based interventions. First, a particular form of behavior may not be serious enough to warrant an intrusive or time-consuming intervention. In addition, due to the idiosyncratic nature of individual reinforcement histories and behavior maintained by automatic reinforcement, it will likely be the case that not every evidence-based procedure will be effective in reducing each case of stereotypy. For these reasons, interventions must be selected on a case-by-case basis. Hence, we are recommending a model for treating stereotypy that incorporates the interventions identified as evidence based in a sequential and cumulative fashion.

An evidence-based model

Our review of the literature leaves us in a position to suggest the following 11-phase model for intervention, based on evidence or promising research. It is important to note that the preponderance of evidence supports a behavior analytic approach to assessment and treatment. No conclusive studies were found for approaches such as cognitive behavior therapy or counseling:

1. Conduct a functional analysis of behavior to ensure that the behavior is in fact stereotypic (i.e., is maintained by automatic reinforcement). For an overview of functional analysis efficacy, see Hanley, Iwata, and McCord (2003). For an overview of functional analysis methods, see Iwata and Dozier (2008).
2. Establish an effective means of data collection so that you can judge the efficacy of successive intervention components during distinct daily contexts (such as work time, leisure time, before and after exercise). Usually, because stereotypy is high-rate behavior, some type of time sampling procedure is sufficient. For example, the frequency of behavior might be observed during three or four 10-min blocks per day.
3. In conjunction with the individual's physician, implement a daily exercise regimen.
4. Conduct a stimulus preference assessment to identify not only preferred stimuli and activities but hopefully some items that will match the stimulus products of stereotypy in some way.

Table 7.1   Evidence-Based Practice for Stereotypy

Treatment	Evidence of treatment
Environmental enrichment	Effective
Extinction	
Sensory extinction	Effective
Response blocking	Effective
Differential reinforcement	Effective
DRA (of alternative behavior)	Effective
DRO (of other behavior)	Effective
Punishment	Effective
Positive punishment	Effective
Punishment, restraints	Effective
Overcorrection	Effective
Antecedent exercise	Effective
Inhibitory stimulus control	Insufficient evidence
Instructional methods	Insufficient evidence
Three-component multiple schedules	Insufficient evidence
Response cost	Insufficient evidence
Self-management	Insufficient evidence
Assistive technology	Insufficient evidence
Medication	Insufficient evidence
Dietary manipulations	Insufficient evidence
Gluten- and casein-free diet	Insufficient evidence
EFAs	Insufficient evidence
Vitamin treatment and megavitamin therapy	Insufficient evidence
Sensory-related therapies	Insufficient evidence
Auditory integration training	Insufficient evidence
Floor time	Insufficient evidence
Holding therapy	Insufficient evidence, dangerous
Sensory integration	Insufficient evidence
Weighted vest	Insufficient evidence
Medical-related therapies	Insufficient evidence
Chelation	Insufficient evidence
Hyperbaric chamber	Insufficient evidence
Medical Marijuana	Insufficient evidence
Art, music, and pet therapy	Insufficient evidence
Gentle Teaching	Insufficient evidence
Social Stories	Insufficient evidence
Timeout	Insufficient evidence

5. During free time (leisure time), implement environmental enrichment using the items identified in the stimulus preference assessment.

6. If the individual does not engage with the items during environmental enrichment, implement differential reinforcement (such as using primary reinforcers) to reinforce item engagement.

7. During instructional activity, ensure that instructors are using consistent procedures with good integrity (Dib & Sturmey, 2007). Instructional activities should themselves be evidence based.
8. During instructional activity, block the occurrence of stereotypy. For hand stereotypy, consider a brief, hands-down procedure (e.g., 10 s).
9. Pair a mild verbal statement, such as "no" with the blocking. Precede the block with a simple instruction "hands down, please."
10. If stereotypy persists and if it represents a danger to the individual or others in the environment, consider a more intrusive punishment procedure such as contingent effort (i.e., overcorrection), combined with differential reinforcement for the non-occurrence of stereotypy. Also, if medication is used, risperidone is presently the only evidence-based medication, but even that, research has some limitations.
11. Establish inhibitory stimulus control by pairing some salient stimulus with the suppression procedure (hands-down, overcorrection, differential reinforcement), such that eventually the person who intervenes does not need to be present. Systematically fade the use of blocking or even the presence of the person who intervenes.

Future Directions

Unlike when problematic behavior is socially reinforced, stereotypy is especially difficult to treat because the specific source of reinforcement is often unknown. Based on functional analysis outcomes, we know that it is not socially reinforced, but little else is known. Thus, future research should focus on identifying specific establishing operations and contingencies of reinforcement for stereotypy. Further, many of the effective treatments are either labor intensive (e.g., blocking) or intrusive (e.g., overcorrection). Research should explore methods of systematically fading out treatment, transferring inhibitory stimulus control, or both. Finally, given that some sources of automatic reinforcement could be biological, double-blind, placebo-controlled medication studies are warranted using repeated measures of behavior.

References

Adams, J. B., Baral, M., Geis, E., Mitchell, J., Ingram, J., Hensley, A., et al. (2009). Safety and efficacy of oral DMSA therapy for children with autism spectrum disorders: Part B—behavioral results. *BMC Clinical Pharmacology, 9*, 17–25.

Ahearn, W. H., Clark, K. M., DeBar, R., & Florentino, C. (2005). On the role of preference in response competition. *Journal of Applied Behavior Analysis, 38*, 247–250.

Ahearn, W. H., Clark, K. M., Gardenier, N. C., Chung, B. I., & Dube, W. V. (2003). Persistence of stereotypic behavior: Examining the effects of external reinforcers. *Journal of Applied Behavior Analysis, 36*, 439–448.

Ahearn, W. H., Clark, K. M., MacDonald, R. P. F., & Chung, B. I. (2007). Assessing and treating vocal stereotypy in children with autism. *Journal of Applied Behavior Analysis, 40*, 263–275.

Aiken, J. M., & Salzberg, C. L. (1984). The effects of a sensory extinction procedure on ste-
     reotypic sounds of two autistic children. *Journal of Autism and Developmental Disorders,
     14,* 291–299.
Amminger, G. P., Berger, G. E., Schafer, M. R., Klier, C., Friedrich, M. H., & Feucht, M. (2007).
     Omega-3 fatty acids supplementation in children with autism: A double-blind
     randomized, placebo-controlled pilot study. *Biological Psychiatry, 61,* 551–553.
Anderson, C. M., Doughty, S. S., Doughty, A. H., Williams, D. C., & Saunders, K. J. (2010).
     Evaluation of stimulus control over a communication response as an intervention for
     stereotypical responding. *Journal of Applied Behavior Analysis, 43,* 333–339.
Arntzen, E., Tonnessen, I. R., & Brouwer, G. (2006). Reducing aberrant verbal behavior by
     building a repertoire of rational verbal behavior. *Behavioral Interventions, 21,* 177–193.
Athens, E. S., Vollmer, T. R., Sloman, K. N., & St. Peter Pipkin, C. (2008). An analysis of vocal
     stereotypy and therapist fading. *Journal of Applied Behavior Analysis, 41,* 291–297.
Azrin, N. H., Kaplan, S. J., & Foxx, R. M. (1973). Autism reversal: Eliminating stereotyped
     self-stimulation of retarded individuals. *American Journal of Mental Deficiency, 78,*
     241–248.
Bachman, J. E., & Fuqua, R. W. (1983). Management of inappropriate behaviors of trainable
     mentally impaired students using antecedent exercise. *Journal of Applied Behavior
     Analysis, 16,* 477–484.
Bachman, J. E., & Sluyter, D. (1988). Reducing inappropriate behaviors of developmentally
     disabled adults using antecedent aerobic dance exercises. *Research in Developmental
     Disabilities, 9,* 73–83.
Baranek, G. T. (2002). Efficacy of sensory and motor interventions for children with autism.
     Journal of Autism and Developmental Disorders, 32, 397–422.
Barrett, R. P., Staub, R. W., & Sisson, L. A. (1983). Treatment of compulsive rituals with visual
     screening: A case study with long-term follow-up. *Journal of Behavior Therapy and
     Experimental Psychiatry, 14,* 55–59.
Bartlett, S., Rapp, J. T., Krueger, T. K., & Henrickson, M. (2010). The use of response cost to
     treat spitting. *Behavioral Interventions, 26,* 76–83.
Baum, W. M. (1973). The correlation-based law of effect. *Journal of the Experimental Analysis
     of Behavior, 20,* 137–153.
Baumeister, A. A. (1978). Origins and control of stereotyped movements. In C. E. Meyers
     (Ed.), *Quality of life in severely and profoundly retarded people* (pp. 353–384). Washington,
     DC: American Association on Mental Deficiency.
Baumeister, A. A., & MacLean, W. E. (1984). Deceleration of self-injurious responding by
     exercise. *Applied Research in Mental Retardation, 5,* 385–393.
Beare, P. L., Severson, S., & Brandt, P. (2004). The use of a positive procedure to increase engage-
     ment on-task and decrease challenging behavior. *Behavior Modification, 28,* 28–44.
Bent, S., Bertoglio, K., & Hendren, R. L. (2009). Omega-3 fatty acids for autistic spectrum
     disorder: A systematic review. *Journal of Autism and Developmental Disorders, 39,*
     1145–1154.
Berg, W. K., Wacker, D. P., Ringdahl, J. E., Stricker, J., Vinquist, K., Dutt, A. S. K., et al.
     (in press). Assessment of problem behavior maintained by automatic reinforcement
     to select treatments based on noncontingent and differential reinforcement. *Journal
     of Applied Behavior Analysis.*
Berkson, G. (1967). Abnormal stereotyped motor acts. In J. Zubin & H. Hunt (Eds.),
     Comparative psychology (pp. 76–94). New York: Grune and Stratton.

Berkson, G. (1983). Repetitive stereotyped behaviors. *American Journal of Mental Deficiency,* *88*, 239–246.

Bodfish, J. W., Crawford, T. W., Powell, S. B., Parker, D. E., Golden, R. N., & Lewis, M. H. (1995). Compulsion in adults with mental retardation: Prevalence, phenomenology, and comorbidity with stereotypy and self-injury. *American Journal on Mental Retardation,* *100*, 183–192.

Bosch, A., Phillips, C. L., Vollmer, T. R., Zawoyski, A., Broome, D., & Nyman, A. (2010). An evaluation of a common autism treatment: Empirical evidence tips the scales against the weighted vest. In K. Sloman (Chair), *Evaluation of commonly used nonbehavioral interventions for individuals with autism.* Symposium presented at the 36th annual convention of the Association of Behavior Analysis, San Antonio, TX.

Bosch, A., Vollmer, T. R., Breeden, A., Nyman, A., Zawoyski, A., & Broome, D. (2010). An evaluation of repetitive behavior in typically functioning adults and implications for functional analyses. In H. E. Hoch (Chair), *Recent research in the assessment and treatment of stereotypic behavior.* Symposium presented at the 36th annual convention of the Association of Behavior Analysis, San Antonio, TX.

Britton, L. N., Carr, J. E., Landaburu, H. J., & Romick, K. S. (2002). The efficacy of non-contingent reinforcement as treatment for automatically reinforced stereotypy. *Behavioral Interventions, 17*, 93–103.

Buchsbaum, M. S., Hollander, E., Haznedar, M. M., Tang, C., Spiegel-Cohen, J., Wei, T. C., et al. (2001). Effect of fluoxetine on regional cerebral metabolism in autistic spectrum disorders: A pilot study. *International Journal of Neuropsychopharmacology, 4*, 119–125.

Campbell, M., Locascio, J. J., Chorroco, M. C., Spencer, E. K., Malone, R. P., Kafantaris, V., et al. (1990). Stereotypies and Tardive Dyskinesia: Abnormal movements in autistic children. *Psychopharmacology Bulletin, 26*, 260–266.

Carroll, R. A., Rapp, J. T., Richling, S., Sennott, L., Maltese, D., Shrader, L, et al. (2010). The effects of unconditioned and conditioned abolishing operations on stereotypy. In M. Lanovax (Chair), *Innovations in the assessment of stereotypy.* Symposium presented at the annual meeting of the Association for Behavior Analysis International, San Antonio, TX.

Celiberti, D. A., Bobo, H. E., Kelly, K. S., Harris, S. L., & Handleman, J. S. (1997). The differential and temporal effects of antecedent exercise on the self-stimulatory behavior of a child with autism. *Research in Developmental Disabilities, 18*, 139–150.

Chambless, D. L., & Hollon, S. D. (1998). Defining empirically supported therapies. *Journal of Consulting and Clinical Psychology, 66*, 7–18.

Charlop, M. H., Burgio, L. D., Iwata, B. A., & Ivancic, M. T. (1988). Stimulus variation as a means of enhancing punishment effects. *Journal of Applied Behavior Analysis, 21*, 89–95.

Charlop-Christy, M. H., & Haymes, L. K. (1996). Using obsessions as reinforcers with and without mild reductive procedures to decrease inappropriate behaviors of children with autism. *Journal of Autism and Developmental Disorders, 26*, 527–546.

Cipani, E., Brendlinger, J., McDowell, L., & Usher, S. (1991). Continuous vs. intermittent punishment: A case study. *Journal of Developmental and Physical Disabilities, 3*, 147–156.

Cole, G. A., Montgomery, R. W., Wilson, K. M., & Milan, M. A. (2000). Parametric analysis of overcorrection duration effects: Is longer really better than shorter? *Behavior Modification, 24*, 359–378.

Coleman, R. S., Whitman, T. L., & Johnson, M. R. (1979). Suppression of self-stimulatory behavior of a profound retarded boy across staff and settings: An assessment of situational generalization. *Behavior Therapy, 10*, 266–280.

Cuvo, A. J., May, M. E., & Post, T. M. (2001). Effects of living room, Snoezelen room, and outdoor activities on stereotypic behavior and engagement by adults with profound mental retardation. *Research in Developmental Disabilities, 22*, 183–204.

Demiri, V. (2004). *Teaching social skills to children with autism using social stories: An empirical study*, Doctoral dissertation, Hofstra University, California School of Professional Psychology, San Diego, TX. ProQuest Dissertations and Theses.

Dib, N., & Sturmey, P. (2007). Reducing student stereotypy by improving teachers' implementation of discrete-trial teaching. *Journal of Applied Behavior Analysis, 40*, 339–343.

Dolske, M. C., Spollen, J., McKay, S., Lancashire, E., & Tolbert, L. (1993). A preliminary trial of ascorbic acid as supplemental therapy for autism. *Progressive Neuropsychopharmacology & Biological Psychiatry, 17*, 765–774.

Dorsey, M. F., Iwata, B. A., Ong, P., & McSween, T. E. (1980). Treatment of self-injurious behavior using a water mist: Initial response suppression and generalization. *Journal of Applied Behavior Analysis, 13*, 343–353.

Doughty, S. S., Anderson, C. M., Doughty, A. H., Williams, D. C., & Saunders, K. J. (2007). Discriminative control of punished stereotyped behavior in humans. *Journal of the Experimental Analysis of Behavior, 87*, 325–336.

Durand, V. M., & Carr, E. G. (1987). Social influences on "self-stimulatory" behavior: Analysis and treatment application. *Journal of Applied Behavior Analysis, 20*, 119–132.

Elkis-Abuhoff, D. L. (2008). Art therapy applied to an adolescent with Asperger's syndrome. *The Arts in Psychotherapy, 35*, 262–270.

Elliott, R. O., Jr., Dobbin, A. R., Rose, G. D., & Soper, H. V. (1994). Vigorous aerobic exercise versus general motor training activities: Effects on maladaptive and stereotypic behaviors of adults with both autism and mental retardation. *Journal of Autism and Developmental Disorders, 24*, 565–576.

Ellis, D. N., MacLean, W. E., & Gazdag, G. (1989). The effects of exercise and cardiovascular fitness on stereotyped body rocking. *Journal of Behavior Therapy and Experimental Psychiatry, 20*, 251–256.

Epp, K. M. (2008). Outcome-based evaluation of a social skills program using art therapy and group therapy for children on the autism spectrum. *Children & Schools, 30*, 27–36.

Epstein, L. H., Doke, L. A., Sajwaj, T. E., Sorrell, S., & Rimmer, P. (1974). Generality and side effects of overcorrection. *Journal of Applied Behavior Analysis, 7*, 385–390.

Facon, B., Beghin, M., & Riviere, V. (2007). The reinforcing effect of contingent attention on verbal perseverations of two children with severe visual impairment. *Journal of Behavior Therapy and Experimental Psychology, 38*, 23–28.

Falcomata, T. S., Roane, H. S., Hovanetz, A. N., Kettering, T. L., & Keeney, K. M. (2004). An evaluation of response cost in the treatment of inappropriate vocalizations maintained by automatic reinforcement. *Journal of Applied Behavior Analysis, 37*, 83–87.

Favell, J. E., McGimsey, J. F., & Schell, R. M. (1982). Treatment of self-injury by providing alternate sensory activities. *Analysis and Intervention in Developmental Disabilities, 2*, 83–104.

Fisher, W., Piazza, C. C., Bowman, L. G., Hagopian, L. P., Owens, J. C., & Slevin, I. (1992). A comparison of two approaches for identifying reinforcers for persons with severe and profound disabilities. *Journal of Applied Behavior Analysis, 25*, 491–498.

Forehand, R., & Baumeister, A. A. (1973). Body rocking and activity level as a function of prior movement restraint. *American Journal of Mental Deficiency, 74*, 608–610.

Foxx, R. M., & Axrin, N. H. (1973). The elimination of autistic self-stimulatory behavior by overcorrection. *Journal of Applied Behavior Analysis, 6*, 1–14.

Friman, P. C., Cook, J. W., & Finney, J. W. (1984). Effects of punishment procedures on the self-stimulatory behavior of an autistic child. *Analysis and Intervention in Developmental Disabilities, 4*, 39–46.

Gabler-Halle, D., Halle, J. W., & Chung, Y. B. (1993). The effects of aerobic exercise on psychological and behavioral variables of individuals with developmental disabilities: A critical review. *Research in Developmental Disabilities, 14*, 359–386.

Green, V. A., Pituch, K. A., Itchon, J., Choi, A., O'Reilly, M., & Sigafoos, J. (2006). Internet survey of treatments used by parents of children with autism. *Research in Developmental Disabilities, 27*, 70–84.

Greenspan, S. I., & Wieder, S. (1997). Developmental patterns and outcomes in infants and children with disorders in relating and communicating: A chart review of 200 cases of children with autistic spectrum diagnoses. *Journal of Developmental and Learning Disorders, 1*, 87–141.

Gunter, P. L., Fox, J. J., McEvoy, M. A., Shores, R. E., & Denny, R. K. (1993). A case study of the reduction of aberrant, repetitive responses of an adolescent with autism. *Education and Treatment of Children, 16*, 187–197.

Haag, S. S., & Anderson, C. M. (2004). *Establishing stimulus control of self-stimulatory responding by an antecedent stimulus using punishment.* Unpublished doctoral dissertation, West Virginia University, Morgantown, WV.

Hagopian, L. P., & Toole, L. M. (2009). Effects of response blocking and competing stimuli on stereotypic behavior. *Behavioral Interventions, 24*, 117–125.

Hanley, G. P., Iwata, B. A., & McCord, B. E. (2003). Functional analysis of problem behavior: A review. *Journal of Applied Behavior Analysis, 36*, 147–185.

Hanley, G. P., Iwata, B. A., Thompson, R. H., & Lindberg, J. S. (2000). A component analysis of "stereotypy as reinforcement" for alternative behavior. *Journal of Applied Behavior Analysis, 33*, 285–297.

Haring, T. G., & Kennedy, C. H. (1990). Contextual control of problem behavior in students with severe disabilities. *Journal of Applied Behavior Analysis, 23*, 235–243.

Harris, J. (1996). Physical restraint procedures for managing challenging behaviours presented by mentally retarded adults and children. *Research in Developmental Disabilities, 17*, 99–134.

Harris, S. L., & Wolchik, S. A. (1979). Suppression of self-stimulation: Three alternative strategies. *Journal of Applied Behavior Analysis, 12*, 199–210.

Henley, D. (1986). Emotional handicaps in low-functioning children: Art educational/art therapeutic interventions. *The Arts in Psychotherapy, 13*, 35–44.

Hess, K. L., Morrier, M. J., Heflin, L. J., & Ivey, M. L. (2008). Autism treatment survey: Services received by children with autism spectrum disorders in public school classrooms. *Journal of Autism and Developmental Disorders, 38*, 961–971.

Higbee, T. S., Chang, S.-M., & Endicott, K. (2005). Noncontingent access to preferred sensory stimuli as a treatment for automatically reinforced stereotypy. *Behavioral Interventions, 20*, 177–184.

Hollander, E., Phillips, A., Chaplain, W., Zagursky, K., Novotny, S., & Wasserman, S., et al. (2005). A placebo-controlled cross-over trial of liquid fluoxetine on repetitive behaviors in childhood and adolescent autism. *Neuropsychopharmocology, 30*, 582–589.

Horner, R. D. (1980). The effects of an environmental "enrichment" program on the behavior of institutionalized profoundly retarded children. *Journal of Applied Behavior Analysis, 13,* 473–491.

Horton, S. V. (1987). Reduction of maladaptive mouthing behavior by facial screening. *Journal of Behavior Therapy and Experimental Psychiatry, 18,* 185–190.

Iwata, B. A., & Dozier, C. L. (2008). Clinical application of functional analysis methodology. *Behavior Analysis in Practice, 1,* 3–9.

Iwata, B. A., Pace, G. M., Dorsey, M. F., Zarcone, J. R., Vollmer, T. R., Smith, R. G., et al. (1994). The functions of self-injurious behavior: An experimental-epidemiological analysis. *Journal of Applied Behavior Analysis, 27,* 215–240.

Jones, R. S. P., & McCaughey, R. E. (1992). Gentle teaching and applied behavior analysis: A critical review. *Journal of Applied Behavior Analysis, 25,* 853–867.

Jordan, J., Singh, N. N., & Repp, A. C. (1989). An evaluation of gentle teaching and visual screening in the reduction of stereotypy. *Journal of Applied Behavior Analysis, 22,* 9–22.

Kennedy, C. H., Meyer, K. A., Knowles, T., & Shukla, S. (2000). Analyzing the multiple functions of stereotypical behavior for students with autism: Implications for assessment and treatment. *Journal of Applied Behavior Analysis, 33,* 559–571.

Kern, L., Koegel, R. L., & Dunlap, G. (1984). The influence of vigorous versus mild exercise on autistic stereotyped behaviors. *Journal of Autism and Developmental Disorders, 14,* 57–67.

Kern, L., Koegel, R. L., Dyer, K., Blew, P A., & Fenton, L. R. (1982). The effects of physical exercise on self-stimulation and appropriate responding in autistic children. *Journal of Autism and Developmental Disorders, 12,* 399–419.

Koegel, R. L., & Koegel, L. K. (1990). Extended reductions in stereotypic behavior of students with autism through a self-management treatment package. *Journal of Applied Behavior Analysis, 23,* 119–127.

Lancioni, G. E., Singh, N. N., O'Reilly, M. F., Sigafoos, J., Didden, R., Smaldone, A., et al. (2008). Helping a man with multiple disabilities increase object-contact responses and reduce hand stereotypy via a microswitch cluster program. *Journal of Intellectual and Developmental Disability, 33,* 349–353.

Lang, R., O'Reilly, M., Sigafoos, J., Machalicek, W., Rispoli, M., Lancioni, G. E., et al. (2010). The effects of an abolishing operation intervention component on play skills, challenging behavior, and stereotypy. *Behavior Modification, 34,* 267–289.

Lanovaz, M. J., & Argumedes, M. (2009). Using the three-component multiple-schedule to examine the effects of treatments on stereotypy. *Journal on Developmental Disabilities, 15,* 64–68.

Lanovaz, M. J., & Argumedes, M. (2010). Immediate and subsequent effects of differential reinforcement of other behavior and noncontingent matched stimulation on stereotypy. *Behavioral Interventions, 25,* 229–238.

Lanovaz, M. J., Fletcher, S. E., & Rapp, J. T. (2009). Identifying stimuli that alter immediate and subsequent levels of vocal stereotypy: A further analysis of functionally matched stimulation. *Behavior Modification, 33,* 682–704.

Lanovaz, M. J., Sladeczek, I. E., & Rapp, J. T. (2011). Effects of music on vocal stereotypy in children with autism. *Journal of Applied Behavior Analysis, 44,* 647–651.

Lerman, D. C., & Iwata, B. A. (1996). A methodology for distinguishing between extinction and punishment effects associated with response blocking. *Journal of Applied Behavior Analysis, 29,* 231–233.

Lerman, D. C., Kelley, M. E., Vorndran, C. M., & Van Camp, C. M. (2003). Collateral effects of response blocking during the treatment of stereotypic behavior. *Journal of Applied Behavior Analysis, 36,* 119–123.

Lewis, M. H., & Baumeister, A. A. (1982). Stereotyped mannerisms in mentally retarded persons: Animal models and theoretical. *International Review of Research in Mental Retardation, 11*, 123–161.

Lindberg, J. S., Iwata, B. A., & Kahng, S. (1999). On the relation between object manipulation and stereotypic self-injurious behavior. *Journal of Applied Behavior Analysis, 32*, 51–62.

Lovaas, I., Newsom, C., & Hickman, C. (1987). Self-stimulatory behavior and perceptual reinforcement. *Journal of Applied Behavior Analysis, 20*, 45–68.

Lower, T. A. (2000). The effect of rotary vestibular stimulation on a stereotypic behavior: A case study. *Journal of Developmental and Physical Disabilities, 12*, 377–385.

Luiselli, J. K., Pemberton, B. W., & Helfen, C. S. (1978). Effects and side effects of a brief overcorrection procedure in reducing multiple self-stimulatory behavior: A single case analysis. *Journal of Mental Deficiency Research, 22*, 287–293.

Mason, S. A., & Iwata, B. A. (1990). Artifactual effects of sensory-integrative therapy on self-injurious behavior. *Journal of Applied Behavior Analysis, 23*, 361–370.

Mason, S. A., & Newsom, C. D. (1990). The application of sensory change to reduce stereotyped behavior. *Research in Developmental Disabilities, 11*, 257–271.

Mazaleski, J. L., Iwata, B. A., Rodgers, T. A., Vollmer, T. R., & Zarcone, J. R. (1994). Protective equipment as treatment for stereotypic hand mouthing: Sensory extinction or punishment effects? *Journal of Applied Behavior Analysis, 27*, 345–355.

McClure, M. K., & Holtz-Yotz, M. (1991). The effects of sensory stimulatory treatment on an autistic child. *American Journal of Occupational Therapy, 45*, 1138–1142.

McDougle, C. J., Brodkin, E. S., Naylor, S. T., Carlson, D. C., Cohen, D. J., & Price, L. H. (1998). Sertraline in adults with pervasive developmental disorders: A prospective open-label investigation. *Journal of Clinical Psychopharmacology, 18*, 62–66.

McDougle, C. J., Naylor, S. T., Cohen, D. J., Volkmar, R., Heninger, G. R., & Price, L. H. (1996). A double-blind, placebo-controlled study of fluvoxamine in adults with autistic disorder. *Archives of General Psychiatry, 53*, 1001–1008.

Michael, J. (1982). Distinguishing between discriminative and motivational functions of stimuli. *Journal of the Experimental Analysis of Behavior, 37*, 149–155.

Miguel, C. F., Clark, K., Tereshko, L., & Ahearn, W. H. (2009). The effects of response interruption and redirection and sertraline on vocal stereotypy. *Journal of Applied Behavior Analysis, 42*, 883–888.

Miltenberger, R. G., & Fuqua, R. W. (1981). Overcorrection: A review and critical analysis. *The Behavior Analyst, 4*, 123–141.

Moore, T. R. (2009). A brief report on the effects of a self-management treatment package on stereotypic behavior. *Research in Autism Spectrum Disorders, 3*, 695–701.

Morrison, H., Roscoe, E. M., & Atwell, A. (2011). An evaluation of antecedent exercise on behavior maintained by automatic reinforcement using a three-component multiple-schedule procedure. *Journal of Applied Behavior Analysis, 44*, 523–541.

Morrissey, P. A., Franzini, L. R., & Karen, R. L. (1992). The salutary effects of light calisthenics and relaxation training on self-stimulation in the developmentally disabled. *Behavioral Residential Treatment, 7*, 373–389.

Mulloy, A., Lang, R., O'Reilley, M., Sigafoos, J., Lancioni, G., & Rispoli, M. (2010). Gluten-free and casein-free diets in the treatment of autism spectrum disorders: A systematic review. *Research in Autism Spectrum Disorders, 4*, 328–339.

Namerow, L. B., Thomas, P., Bostic, J. Q., Prince, J., Monuteaux, M. C. (2003). Use of citalopram in pervasive developmental disorders. *Journal of Developmental Behavioral Pediatrics, 24*, 104–108.

Newell, K. M., & Bodfish, J. W. (2007). Dynamical origins of stereotypy: Relation of postural movements during sitting to stereotyped movements during body-rocking. *American Journal on Mental Retardation, 112,* 66–75.

Nuzzolo-Gomez, R., Leonard, M. A., Ortiz, E., Rivera, C. M., & Greer, R. D. (2002). Teaching children with autism to prefer books or toys over stereotypy or passivity. *Journal of Positive Behavior Interventions, 4,* 80–87.

Nye, C., & Brice, A. (2005). Combined vitamin B6-magnesium treatment in autism spectrum disorder. *Cochrane Database of Systematic Reviews,* (4), CD003497. doi:10.1002/14651858. CD003497.pub2.

O'Reilly, M., Tiernan, R., Lancioni, G., Lacey, C., Hillery, J., & Gardiner, M. (2002). Use of self-monitoring and delayed feedback to increase on-task behavior in a post-institutionalized child within regular classroom settings. *Education and Treatment of Children, 25,* 91–102.

Pendergrass, V. E. (1972). Timeout from positive reinforcement following persistent, high-rate behavior in retardates. *Journal of Applied Behavior Analysis, 5,* 85–91.

Piazza, C. C., Adelinis, J. D., Hanley, G. P., Goh, H., & Delia, M. D. (2000). An evaluation of the effects of matched stimuli on behaviors maintained by automatic reinforcement. *Journal of Applied Behavior Analysis, 33,* 13–27.

Power, S., Thibadeau, S., & Rose, K. (1992). Antecedent exercise and its effects on self-stimulation. *Behavioral Residential Treatment, 7,* 15–22.

Prupas, A., & Reid, G. (2001). Effects of exercise frequency on stereotypic behaviors of children with developmental disabilities. *Education and Training in Mental Retardation and Developmental Disabilities, 36,* 196–206.

Rapp, J. T. (2004). Effects of prior access and environmental enrichment on stereotypy. *Behavioral Interventions, 19,* 287–295.

Rapp, J. T. (2005). Some effects of audio and visual stimulation on multiple forms of stereotypy. *Behavioral Interventions, 20,* 255–272.

Rapp, J. T. (2006). Toward an empirical method for identifying matched stimulation for automatically reinforced behavior: A preliminary investigation. *Journal of Applied Behavior Analysis, 39,* 137–140.

Rapp, J. T. (2007). Further evaluation of methods to identify matched stimulation. *Journal of Applied Behavior Analysis, 40,* 73–88.

Rapp, J. T., Dozier, C. L., Carr, J. E., Patel, M. R., & Enloe, K. A. (2000). Functional analysis of hair manipulation: A replication and extension. *Behavioral Interventions, 15,* 121–133.

Rapp, J. T., Miltenberger, R. G., Galensky, T. L., Ellingson, S. A., & Long, E. S. (1999). A functional analysis of hair pulling. *Journal of Applied Behavior Analysis, 32,* 329–337.

Rapp, J. T., Patel, M. R., Ghezzi, P. M., O'Flaherty, C. H., & Titterington, C. J. (2009). Establishing stimulus control of vocal stereotypy displayed by young children with autism. *Behavioral Interventions, 24,* 85–105.

Rapp, J. T., & Vollmer, T. R. (2005). Stereotypy I: A review of behavioral assessment and treatment [Literature Review]. *Research in Developmental Disabilities, 26,* 527–547.

Rapp, J. T., Vollmer, T. R., St. Peter, C., Dozier, C. L., & Cotnoir, N. M. (2004). Analysis of response allocation in individuals with multiple forms of stereotyped behavior. *Journal of Applied Behavior Analysis, 37,* 481–501.

Redefer, L. A., & Goodman, J. F. (1989). Brief report: Pet facilitated therapy with autistic children. *Journal of Autism and Developmental Disorders, 19,* 461–467.

Research Units on Pediatric Psychopharmacology (RUPP) Autism Network. (2002). Risperidone in children with autism and serious behavioral problems. *The New England Journal of Medicine, 347,* 314–321.

Reynhout, G., & Carter, M. (2007). Social Story™ efficacy with a child with autism spectrum disorder and moderate intellectual disability. *Focus on Autism and Other Developmental Disabilities, 22,* 173–182.

Richmond, G. (1983). Evaluation of a treatment for a hand-mouthing stereotypy. *American Journal of Mental Deficiency, 87,* 667–669.

Rincover, A. (1978). Sensory extinction: A procedure for eliminating self-stimulatory behavior in developmentally disabled children. *Journal of Abnormal Child Psychology, 6,* 299–310.

Rincover, A., Cook, R., Peoples, A., & Packard, D. (1979). Sensory extinction and sensory reinforcement principles for programming multiple adaptive behavior change. *Journal of Applied Behavior Analysis, 12,* 221–233.

Ringdahl, J. E. (2011). Rituals, stereotypies, and obsessive compulsive behavior. In J. L. Matson & P. Sturmey (Eds.), *International handbook of autism and pervasive developmental disorders* (pp. 479–490). New York: Springer.

Ringdahl, J. E., Andelman, M. S., Kitsukawa, K., Winborn, L. C., Barretto, A., & Wacker, D. P. (2002). Evaluation and treatment of covert stereotypy. *Behavioral Interventions, 17,* 43–49.

Ringdahl, J. E., Vollmer, T. R., Marcus, B. A., & Roane, H. S. (1997). An analogue evaluation of environmental enrichment: The role of stimulus preference. *Journal of Applied Behavior Analysis, 30,* 203–216.

Rolider, A., & Van Houten, R. (1990). The role of reinforcement in reducing inappropriate behavior: Some myths and misconceptions. In A. C. Repp & N. N. Singh (Eds.), *Perspectives on the use of nonaversive and aversive interventions for persons with developmental disabilities.* Sycamore, IL: Sycamore Press.

Rollings, J. P., & Baumeister, A. A. (1981). Stimulus control of stereotypic responding: Effects on target and collateral behavior. *American Journal of Mental Deficiency, 86,* 67–77.

Rosenthal-Malek, A., & Mitchell, S. (1997). Brief report: The effects of exercise on the self-stimulatory behaviors and positive responding of adolescents with autism. *Journal of Autism and Developmental Disorders, 27,* 193–202.

Rossignol, D. A., Rossignol, L. W., Smith, S., Schneider, C., Logerquist, S., Usman, A., et al. (2009). Hyperbaric treatment for children with autism: A multicenter randomized double-blind, controlled trial. *BMC Pediatrics, 9,* 21.

Sackett, G. P. (1978). Measurement in observational research. In G. P. Sackett (Ed.), *Observing behavior.* Baltimore: University Park Press.

Saunders, M. D., Saunders, R. R., & Marquis, J. G. (1998). Comparison of reinforcement schedules in the reduction of stereotypy with supported routines. *Research in Developmental Disabilities, 19,* 99–122.

Schumacher, B. I., & Rapp, J. T. (2011). Evaluation of the immediate and subsequent effects of response interruption and redirection on vocal stereotypy. *Journal of Applied Behavior Analysis, 44,* 681–685.

Shabani, D. B., Wilder, D. A., & Flood, W. A. (2001). Reducing stereotypic behavior through discrimination training, differential reinforcement of other behavior, and self-monitoring. *Behavioral Interventions, 16,* 279–286.

Shea, S., Turgay, A., Carroll, A., Schultz, M., Orlik, H., Smith, I., et al. (2004). Risperidone in the treatment of disruptive behavioral symptoms in children with autistic and other pervasive developmental disorders. *Pediatrics, 114,* 634–641.

Sidener, T. M., Carr, J. E., & Firth, A. M. (2005). Superimposition and withholding of edible consequences as treatment for automatically reinforced stereotypy. *Journal of Applied Behavior Analysis, 38,* 121–124.

Simmons, J. N., Smith, R. G., & Kliethermes, L. (2003). A multiple-schedule evaluation of immediate and subsequent effects of fixed-time food presentation on automatically maintained mouthing. *Journal of Applied Behavior Analysis, 36,* 541–544.

Singh, N. N., Landrum, T. J., Ellis, C. R., & Donatelli, L. S. (1993). Effects of thioridazine and visual screening on stereotypy and social behavior in individuals with mental retardation. *Research in Developmental Disabilities, 14,* 163–177.

Singh, N. N., & Millichamp, C. J. (1987). Independent and social play among profoundly mentally retarded adults: Training, maintenance, generalization, and long-term follow-up. *Journal of Applied Behavior Analysis, 20,* 23–34.

Singh, N. N., & Winton, A. S. (1984). Effects of a screening procedure on pica and collateral behaviors. *Journal of Behavior Therapy and Experimental Psychiatry, 15,* 59–65.

Smith, R. G., Russo, L., & Le, D. D. (1999). Distinguishing between extinction and punishment effects of response blocking: A replication. *Journal of Applied Behavior Analysis, 32,* 367–370.

Smith, S. A., Press, B., Koenig, K. P., & Kinnealey, M. (2005). Effects of sensory integration intervention on self-stimulating and self-injurious behaviors. *American Journal of Occupational Therapy, 59,* 418–425.

Solnick, J. V., Rincover, A., & Peterson, C. R. (1977). Some determinants of the reinforcing and punishing effects of timeout. *Journal of Applied Behavior Analysis, 10,* 415–424.

Solomon, R., Nechels, J., Ferch, C., & Bruckman, D. (2007). Pilot study of a parent training program for young children with autism. The PLAY Project Home Consultation Program. *SAGE Publications and the National Autistic Society, 11,* 205–224.

Soorya, L., Kiarashi, J., & Hollander, E. (2008). Psychopharmacologic interventions for repetitive behaviors in autism spectrum disorders. *Child and Adolescent Psychiatric Clinics of North America, 17,* 753–771, viii.

Stahmer, A. C., & Schreibman, L. (1992). Teaching children with autism appropriate play in unsupervised environments using a self-management treatment package. *Journal of Applied Behavior Analysis, 25,* 447–459.

Steingard, R. J., Zimnitzky, B., DeMaso, D. R., Bauman, M. L., & Bucci, J. P. (1997). Sertraline treatment of transition-associated anxiety and agitation in children with autistic disorder. *Journal of Child and Adolescent Psychopharmacology, 7,* 9–15.

Stephenson, J., & Carter, M. (2009). The use of weighted vests with children with autism spectrum disorders and other disabilities. *Journal of Autism and Developmental Disorders, 39,* 105–114.

Stigler, K. A., & McDougle, C. J. (2008). Pharmacotherapy of irritability in pervasive developmental disorders. *Child and Adolescent Psychiatric Clinics of North America, 17,* 739–752.

Tarbox, R. S. F., Tarbox, J., Ghezzi, P. M., Wallace, M. D., & Yoo, J. H. (2007). The effects of blocking mouthing of leisure items on their effectiveness as reinforcers. *Journal of Applied Behavior Analysis, 40,* 761–765.

Taylor, B. A., Hoch, H., & Weissman, M. (2005). The analysis and treatment of vocal stereotypy in a child with autism. *Behavioral Interventions, 20,* 239–253.

Tustin, R. D. (1995). The effects of advance notice on activity transitions on stereotypic behavior. *Journal of Applied Behavior Analysis, 28,* 91–92.

Vollmer, T. R., Marcus, B. A., & LeBlanc, L. (1994). Treatment of self-injury and hand mouthing following inconclusive functional analyses. *Journal of Applied Behavior Analysis, 27,* 331–344.

Watters, R. G., & Watters, W. E. (1980). Decreasing self-stimulatory behavior with physical exercise in a group of autistic boys. *Journal of Autism and Developmental Disorders, 10,* 379–387.

Whiteley, P. Haracopos, D., Knivsberg, A., Reichelt, K. L., Parlar, S., Jacobsen, J., et al. (2010). The ScanBrit randomised, controlled, single-blind study of a gluten- and casein-free dietary intervention for children with autism spectrum disorders. *Nutritional Neuroscience, 13,* 87–100.

Wolf, M. M. (1978). Social validity: The case for subjective measurement or how applied behavior analysis is finding its heart. *Journal of Applied Behavior Analysis, 11,* 203–214.

Zissermann, L. (1992). Case report: The effects of deep pressure on self-stimulating behaviors in a child with autism and other disabilities. *American Journal of Occupational Therapy, 46,* 547–551.

8

Feeding Problems

Keith E. Williams, Laura J. Seiverling,
and Douglas G. Field

The term "feeding problem" has been most often reserved to describe the eating behavior of young children and, sometimes more specifically, difficulties in mealtime interaction between a parent and child; however, in this chapter, the term will be used to describe a range of ingestive behaviors in persons with intellectual disabilities (ID). This chapter will focus on evidence-based practice (EBP) for food refusal, pica, and rumination. The evidence for other feeding problems will also be discussed.

Arguably, the most important activity of daily living, eating has been shown to be an area of considerable difficulty for the entire age spectrum of persons with ID. In a heterogeneous group of children with ID, approximately 30% had feeding problems that could be described as food refusal or selectivity (Thommessen, Riis, Kase, Larsen, & Heiberg, 1991), while a more recent review of eating disorders found a similar prevalence rate of feeding problems among adults with ID (Gravestock, 2000).

For this chapter, the literature for feeding problems in persons with ID was reviewed by searching both Medline and Psychlit databases using the search terms "mental retardation" or "intellectual disabilities" combined with "feeding problems," "eating problems," "food refusal," "pica," and "rumination." The studies describing treatments for the feeding problems in this population were examined to determine if any of the treatments met the Chambless and Hollon (1998) criteria for EBP.

Evidence-Based Practice and Intellectual Disabilities, First Edition.
Edited by Peter Sturmey and Robert Didden.
© 2014 John Wiley & Sons, Ltd. Published 2014 by John Wiley & Sons, Ltd.

Food Refusal

Food refusal has been defined as the refusal to eat all or most foods presented, resulting in the person not getting enough food to meet caloric or nutritional needs (Field, Garland, & Williams, 2003). While there is currently not a universally accepted classification system for childhood feeding disorders (Kedesdy & Budd, 1998), similar definitions of food refusal are prevalent in the treatment literature for children. Food refusal is associated with malnutrition, often resulting in the dependency upon either tube feeding or oral supplements and is also typically comorbid with one or more medical conditions related to the etiology of the food refusal (Field et al., 2003). It has been hypothesized that food refusal could be the result of a conditioned aversion related to these comorbid medical problems. For example, gastroesophageal reflux causes frequent vomiting and regurgitation, which results in esophagitis or an inflamed esophagus, making swallowing painful (Mathisen, Worrall, Masel, Wall, & Shepard, 1999). Thus, eating may become associated with vomiting and pain, which leads to the person learning to avoid the pain by refusing to eat. Environmental variables, such as caregiver mealtime actions, can also affect the etiology and maintenance of feeding problems. Williams, Hendy, and Knecht (2008) found that when parents of children with feeding problems were asked the type and frequency of mealtime actions they used (e.g., preparing special meals, rewarding eating), parent mealtime actions were found to be related to both child diet variety and behavior problems during meals. While no research exists which specifies which parent behaviors, such as allowing their children to avoid eating contingent upon maladaptive behavior or provision of high-calorie supplements that impair children's appetites, result in food refusal, it is clear that both biological and environmental variables are involved in the etiology and maintenance of food refusal.

The prevalence of food refusal in children with ID is unclear; however, Field et al. (2003) found that 34% of 349 children, many of whom had special needs, evaluated for feeding problems at a hospital-based feeding program met the criteria for food refusal. Of the children with food refusal, 69% also had gastroesophageal reflux. It is also unclear the extent to which food refusal exists in *adults* with ID as the definitions used for food refusal have not been applied to adult populations. In addition to the studies reporting eating disorders as common among adults with ID, (see Gravestock, 2000 and Jones & Samuel, 2010 for reviews), there is evidence that the behaviors associated with food refusal in children exist in adults with ID. In order to assess feeding problems in those with ID, Matson and Kuhn (2001) developed the Screening Tool of Feeding Problems (STEP). A large sample ($N = 570$) of adults with ID living in an institution was utilized. The most highly endorsed item for the entire sample was a question concerning insufficient intake. In a subsequent study using the STEP with 60 adults with ID, 25% were reported to refuse food (Fodstad & Matson, 2008).

To date, there are no consensus panel reports or controlled group studies which provide evidence for effective interventions for food refusal. There are, however, a growing number of treatment studies which use single-subject designs. For example, a recent review of the food refusal in children included 38 intervention studies (Williams, Field, & Seiverling, 2010), of which 11 included children with ID. All 11 studies described interventions with several behavioral components. One component common to all of these studies was some form of positive reinforcement, often provided in the form of delivery of a preferred item or activity and/or praise contingent upon acceptance of bites of food. Despite the widespread use of positive reinforcement in the treatment of food refusal, studies examining the effectiveness of various treatment components have shown positive reinforcement alone is insufficient to treat food refusal (Hoch, Babbitt, Coe, Krell, & Hackbert, 1994; Patel, Piazza, Martinez, Volkert, & Santana, 2002). These two studies both found that escape extinction, or presentation of food until it is accepted, was necessary to increase food intake. Nine of the eleven studies described the use of an extinction component either in the form of presenting the bite until it was accepted or physical guidance, which involves physically prompting the child's mouth open. In the other two studies, one combined reinforcement and texture fading (Gutentag & Hammer, 2000), while another combined reinforcement and response cost, which involved removing a preferred object if the child refused to take a bite (Kahng, Tarbox, & Wilke, 2001).

Nine small *N* experiments involving 23 children with ID used reinforcement and escape extinction in the successful treatment of food refusal, meeting the Chambless and Hollon (1998) criteria for determining empirically supported therapies. These studies all involved multicomponent treatments with slight variations in their treatment packages utilized; but it is not yet possible to determine the role of each individual treatment component in the overall success of the intervention as extensive component analyses have not been conducted. While reinforcement and escape extinction were used in nine studies, two other studies used reinforcement with other treatment components, one utilizing response cost and the other using texture fading. As each of these small *N* studies only included a single participant, it is not possible to determine if either of these treatment packages is effective in the treatment of food refusal.

While there is evidence that food refusal exists in adults with ID, there is only one study that described interventions. One exception is a small *N* study which described the treatment of food refusal in a 22-year-old woman with ID and severe self-injurious behavior (Kitfield & Masalsky, 2000). The treatment components included negative reinforcement in the form of allowing the woman to leave the eating environment contingent upon consumption of food and positive reinforcement in the form of preferred edibles for consumption of her meal. As with the literature on food refusal in children, the evidence is too limited to provide empirical support for any interventions for the treatment of food refusal in adults with ID. Thus, there are currently no EBP for food refusal in adults with ID.

Conclusions

Depending upon the individual circumstances, behavioral intervention to address food refusal may be only one component of a broader treatment. Medical problems commonly associated with food refusal may require the involvement of medical providers, while changes in diet or tube feedings may require consultation from a nutrition specialist. Some children with food refusal may have oral motor deficits or problems swallowing that may require consultation or treatment from other allied health professionals such as speech pathologists or occupational therapists.

Although interventions using reinforcement and escape extinction have been used successfully with children with ID, there is still much to be learned about the treatment of food refusal in both children and adults. In the review of food refusal previously cited, the majority of interventions for food refusal contained either escape extinction or appetite manipulation, with some interventions using both components (Williams et al., 2010). The motivation to eat is directly related to caloric intake and appetite manipulation and is often achieved by reducing tube feedings or restricting intake of oral supplements. Increasing motivation to eat through appetite manipulation has been identified as a crucial component in the treatment of food refusal (Linscheid, 2006). Despite the fact that the outcomes of many studies utilizing escape extinction include reduction of tube feedings and increases in oral intake, the process of the reduction in tube feedings has often not been described, and there is no discussion of the possible effects of tube feed reductions as a treatment component. Reducing either tube feedings, oral supplements, or access to preferred foods in the treatment of food refusal could serve as a motivating operation that can positively influence the effects of the intervention. Although research describing interventions which utilize appetite manipulation without extinction procedures has been conducted (Levin & Carr, 2001), it has not been extended to children and adults with ID. The role of appetite manipulation is unclear but should be considered when developing a comprehensive treatment for food refusal.

Of the 11 studies of food refusal in children with ID, only one took place in a nonmedical setting (Gutentag & Hammer, 2000). It is noteworthy that this study did not report using escape extinction, but rather used reinforcement and texture fading to treat a child's food refusal in both home and school settings. While two additional studies involved outpatient therapy in which initial treatment sessions were conducted in a therapy room at a rehabilitation center (DeMoor, Didden, & Tolboom, 2005; Didden, Seys, & Schouwink, 1999), the remainder of the studies were conducted in either inpatient or hospital-based day treatment settings. Even though a select group of children may require more intensive treatment in some form of medical setting to allow for medical oversight when tube feedings are being manipulated, it is not clear if this setting is required for all children with ID who present with food refusal. The feasibility of conducting interventions for food refusal that involve escape extinction in the home setting or other community settings has not yet been evaluated.

Pica

Pica, described as the consumption of inedible or nonnutritive materials which persists beyond infancy, is common among persons with ID. In samples of institutionalized adults with ID, the prevalence ranges from 5.7% (Matson & Bamburg, 1999) to 26% (Danford & Huber, 1982). In a community-based sample, the prevalence was 2.9% (Hove, 2004). While there could be several reasons why the persons living in institutional settings demonstrate a greater prevalence of pica, persons living in institutional settings could have more comorbid psychiatric diagnoses and/or behavior problems, both of which have been shown to be positively correlated with the prevalence of pica (Joyce, Ditchfield, & Harris, 2001).

Pica can be an extremely dangerous problem to the affected individual. It is associated with intestinal blockage, parasites, surgeries to remove ingested items, lead poisoning (Piazza et al., 1998), and, in some cases, death (Foxx & Livesay, 1984).

Pica has been described being both reinforced by oral stimulation and resistant to treatment (Piazza et al., 1998). Research focusing on the function of pica indicates pica is maintained primarily by automatic reinforcement rather than aspects of the social environment such as attention or escape (Applegate, Matson, & Cherry, 1999). Because the pica is often automatically reinforced by the sensory stimulation of the objects being mouthed and ingested, in most cases, a successful intervention must compete with the continuous schedule of reinforcement associated with automatic reinforcement. While automatic reinforcement is often an important maintaining variable for pica, social factors have also been found to maintain pica.

Mace and Knight (1986) demonstrated that varying amounts of social interaction affected the rates of pica in an adolescent with pica, while Piazza and her colleagues (1998) found that social attention reduced the occurrence of pica in another individual with pica.

Both behavioral and nutritional interventions have been used in the treatment of pica, with behavioral interventions being the most commonly researched form of treatment. All of the empirical studies, to date, have utilized single-subject experimental designs.

Discrimination training

Discrimination training, in which persons learn to discriminate between inedible objects and safe food items, has been combined with punishment procedures, which the authors of these studies have termed negative consequences. In one of these studies, two adolescents with ID who exhibited pica were taught to eat only foods that were placed on a specific placement and communicate with gestures to obtain more food. The adolescents were praised for selecting foods from the placement and communicating but punished for attempting to eat anything not on the placement by having them wash their faces for 15 s (Johnson, Hunt, & Siebert, 1994). This intervention was effective in reducing pica in different settings including the adolescents' natural settings. In two additional studies, discrimination training combined with punishment in the form of facial screening was used to treat pica in persons with ID (Bogart, Piersel, & Gross, 1995; Fisher et al., 1994). Both of these studies had positive outcomes and demonstrated maintenance over long periods of time.

While discrimination training and punishment appears to be a promising treatment for pica among persons with ID, because the three small N studies involving persons with ID include only seven participants, this intervention does not yet meet the criteria for an effective treatment. It should be mentioned that discrimination training combined with punishment has also been used to success-fully treat pica among children hospitalized for lead poisoning (Finney, Russo, & Cataldo, 1982; Madden, Russo, & Cataldo, 1981).

In a nonexperimental study that examined the long-term treatment and follow-up of 41 individuals with ID treated for pica in a residential facility, a combination of behavioral interventions and environmental controls was effective in eliminating the need for surgeries to remove foreign objects, and 85% of participants demon-strated a decrease in pica of 75% or greater over a 9-year period (Williams, Kirkpatric-Sanchez, Enzinna, & Dunn, 2009). Of these participants, 16 of 41 required long-term use of restrictive procedures including oral hygiene, overcorrection, contingent restraint, and visual screening. This finding highlights the need for effective behavior reduction procedures.

Noncontingent reinforcement

While behavior reduction procedures have been widely used to treat pica among persons with ID, other less intrusive approaches have also been used with success. The noncontingent presentation of attention or preferred objects is an intervention that has also met the criteria of an effective treatment for pica in persons with ID. In five studies using noncontingent presentation, five of the nine participants involved were presented with preferred food items. It has been suggested that food presenta-tion provided an alternate form of oral stimulation by allowing the child to ingest food rather than inedible objects (McAdam, Sherman, Sheldon, & Napolitano, 2004). Four of the five studies using noncontingent presentation of attention or preferred objects were based upon functional analyses. One study involved a 19-year-old man required to wear a helmet with a face shield prior to treatment in an attempt to prevent his high rates of pica (Mace & Knight, 1986). A functional analysis showed the pica to be maintained by attention, and the treatment consisting of increased interaction resulted in low rates of the behavior and elimination of the helmet with face shield.

While the noncontingent presentation of attention or preferred objects met the criteria for an effective intervention for pica, one study found that noncontingent access to preferred items was unsuccessful in the treatment of cigarette pica for four adults with ID (Goh, Iwata, & Kahng, 1999). In this study, preference assessments were used both to develop alternatives to cigarette pica and to examine the role of the cigarette in maintaining the pica. In one of the assessments, three of the four persons chose edibles over cigarette products including the unsmoked filter, the unsmoked cigarette, and cigarette butts, while one person consistently choose the cigarette products. The initial treatment involved noncontingent access to preferred food items, but this did not prove effective when thinning the schedule of when the preferred items were offered. A treatment consisting of differential reinforcement of alternative behavior was successful for three of the four participants, but was not successful for the participant who had previously chosen cigarette products rather than edibles during a preference assessment. This study also demonstrated the use of behavioral assessment in the development of an effective treatment as well as limitations of reinforced-based procedures for some persons.

Differential reinforcement

Other studies have also used differential reinforcement (Donnelly & Olczak, 1990; Goh et al., 1999; Smith, 1987) to treat pica. In one of these studies, cigarette pica was reduced through the use of an alternative edible reinforcer provided when the participants handed the cigarette to a therapist rather than consuming the cigarette (Goh et al., 1999). Despite the positive outcomes in the studies that have used differential reinforcement, there is not yet sufficient evidence for this procedure as the three studies in which it was described involved only six participants who responded to the treatment. While differential reinforcement for the treatment of pica failed to meet the Chambless and Hollon criteria of an EBP, it is a promising treatment, and future research may provide the additional evidence required.

Nutritional interventions

While automatic positive reinforcement in the form of oral stimulation has been hypothesized to be a maintaining variable for pica in many cases, nutrient deficiencies have also been suggested as both etiological and maintaining factors for pica (Lofts, Schroeder, & Maier, 1990). Studies involving both persons with and without ID have demonstrated deficits in nutrients including iron and zinc (Blinder & Salama, 2008). One study showed decreases in pica among institutionalized persons with ID who were provided zinc supplementation (Lofts et al., 1990), while another study which used a single-subject design showed that pica decreased in a girl with ID who was provided with a multivitamin (Pace & Troyer, 2000). Even though there is not sufficient evidence to suggest that nutritional supplementation is an effective treatment for pica, persons with ID who have demonstrated nutritional deficiencies should have these deficiencies corrected to avoid the adverse effects on the health of these individuals.

Positive punishment

A range of punishment procedures, especially common among earlier studies, have been used to address pica. In one study, the pica of a 4-year-old girl with profound ID was treated with physical restraint contingent upon each instance of pica and differential reinforcement of other behavior for the absence of pica (Paniagua, Braverman, & Capriotti, 1986). In another study, the pica of a 33-year-old woman with ID and Prader–Willi syndrome was almost completely eliminated using negative practice (Duker & Nielen, 1993). This procedure consisted of taking the object this person was chewing and holding it to her lips for 2 min, but not allowing her to bite the object. In addition to physical restraint and negative practice, other punishment procedures have included the contingent presentation of aversives (squirt of lemon juice in the mouth, water mist, or sniff of ammonia) and overcorrection (McAdam et al., 2004). Of all the punishment procedures, the effectiveness of overcorrection was demonstrated in six single-subject experimental studies that included nine participants, meeting the criteria for effective treatment. While older studies involving overcorrection frequently involved having the participant brush his/her teeth or wash his/her mouth contingent upon engaging in pica (Foxx & Martin, 1975; Mulick, Barbour, Schroeder, & Rojahn, 1980), a recent study incorporated overcorrection in the form of having a child with autism practice throwing away objects contingent upon actual or attempted pica (Ricciardi, Luiselli, Terrill, & Reardon, 2003). While it may not be possible or feasible to use toothbrushing or mouth washing in all settings, the study by Ricciardi and colleagues did show that overcorrection continues to be an effective and viable treatment component for pica.

While the comparative effectiveness of restrictive procedures is typically not explored, one study did develop a procedure for empirically deriving consequences for the treatment of pica (Fisher et al., 1994). Fisher and his colleagues assessed the effectiveness of various punishers for three children with ID referred for inpatient treatment of their severe pica. The resulting interventions involved discrimination training with an empirically derived punisher contingent upon attempts to engage in pica and produced low rates of pica through 9-month follow-up. This study suggests that behavioral assessment that involves all aspects of intervention development may enhance the treatment efficacy.

Response blocking

Response blocking, or not allowing the person to engage in a maladaptive behavior by blocking attempts at engaging in the behavior, has been used with various automatically maintained behaviors, including pica. A study that compared response blocking to restraint for the treatment of pica found that response blocking was as effective as restraint in reducing pica (LeBlanc, Piazza, & Krug, 1997). Response blocking has also been shown to increase collateral behaviors such as aggression (Rapp, Dozier, & Carr, 2001); however, one study utilizing response blocking found that the aggression associated with the intervention was eliminated when response blocking was paired with redirection to a preferred food item (Hagopian & Adelinis, 2001).

One research study examined two parameters of the response blocking intervention, whether the intervention was initiated either early or late in the response chain, leading to pica and distance between the person engaging in pica and the therapist (McCord, Grosser, Iwata, & Powers, 2005). The results showed that in order for response blocking to be effective, the therapist had to implement the procedure early in the chain of responses and had to implement the response blocking with a high degree of consistency.

Response blocking has been used in four studies but with only six participants to date. Thus, response blocking does not meet the criteria for an EBP. Response blocking also requires considerable effort on the part of the therapist or person implementing the intervention, and studies to date have not demonstrated methods of fading presence of the person(s) implementing the treatment. One study suggested that blocking may be effective in preventing pica but only when initiated early in its response chain and when conducted with a high degree of consistency (McCord et al., 2005).

Conclusion

A wide range of behavioral interventions have been used in the treatment of pica among persons with ID. While positive outcomes have been demonstrated in many studies, only overcorrection and noncontingent presentation of preferred items meet the Chambless and Hollon criteria for EBP. Several interventions such as discrimination training and differential reinforcement are promising, and future research may produce the level of evidence needed for them to be considered effective using these criteria.

One of the significant changes in the development of interventions for pica is the increased use of behavioral interventions. Stimulus preference assessments, functional assessments, and even punisher assessments have been used to make interventions for pica more effective and, in general, less intrusive. Functional analyses have shown that maintaining variables have included attention, automatic reinforcement, and, in the case of persons with cigarette butt pica, nicotine. A better understanding of the maintaining variables for pica has allowed, and will allow, the development of interventions that are less restrictive yet still effective in eliminating pica.

Rumination

Rumination has been described as the chronic, effortless regurgitation of recently ingested food, followed by remastication, reswallowing, or expulsion (Rommel et al., 2010). While rumination is found in persons with and without ID, it is more common among persons with ID with the prevalence of rumination in institution-alized adults with ID ranging from 6% to 10% (Johnston & Greene, 1992; Rogers, Stratton, Victor, Kennedy, & Andres, 1992). Rumination may lead to significant medical problems including dehydration, weight loss, malnutrition, and aspiration (Feldman, 1983). Rumination is also the primary contributing factor of death in 10% of those who exhibit rumination over an extended period of time (Rast, Johnston, Drum, & Conrin, 1981). Additionally, surgery to prevent rumination also carries a significant risk of death (Starin & Fuqua, 1987).

While the etiology of rumination is unclear, it has been associated with impaired gastric relaxation with gastric distension, gastroesophageal reflux, and hiatal hernia (Rommel et al., 2010). In a study of the prevalence of gastroesophageal reflux disease (GERD) in a large sample of institutionalized adults with ID, rumination was found significantly more often among persons diagnosed with GERD than among persons without GERD (Böhmer et al., 1999). In other research, 91% of persons with ID exhibiting rumination had gastrointestinal (GI) abnormalities (Rogers et al., 1992), and in another study, 50% of persons with ID exhibiting rumination were found to have GERD and esophagitis (Kuruvilla & Trewby, 1989). Due to the frequency of which GI and other medical problems are correlated with rumination, it has been recommended that a complete medical evaluation, often including diagnostic testing such as pH probe, endoscopy, or upper GI series, be completed prior to the development of an intervention (Fredricks, Carr, & Williams, 1998).

For some people, even though GERD or other GI issues may be related to the etiology of rumination, other variables have been identified as maintaining the behavior. Self-stimulation has most often been described as the variable that main-tains rumination (Rast, Johnston, Allen, & Drum, 1985); however, socially mediated factors such as attention have also been suggested (Toister, Condrin, Worley, & Arthur, 1975).

Consequence-based approaches

There have been two major approaches to the treatment of rumination—consequence-based behavioral treatments and antecedent-based dietary inter-ventions. Consequence-based behavioral treatments have included a variety of punishers as well as reinforcement strategies. Punishment procedures have included contingent pinches (Minness, 1980), noxious tastes (Hogg, 1982), oral hygiene (Foxx, Snyder, & Schroeder, 1979), overcorrection (Duker & Seys, 1977), and electric shock (Kohlenberg, 1970). While numerous small *N* studies have demonstrated the successful use of punishment procedures, no specific punishment procedure has met the Chambless and Hollon criteria for an EBP. Other small *N* studies have utilized either differential reinforcement of other behavior or differential reinforcement of incompatible behavior (Mulick, Schroeder, & Rojahn, 1980). There was also insufficient data for these procedures to meet the criteria for an EBP.

Dietary interventions

Dietary interventions, such as satiation and liquid rescheduling, could be considered antecedent interventions as the dietary intervention occurs prior to the rumination. Satiation involves providing persons with rumination with large amounts of food, often starches, after meals (Rast et al., 1981), while liquid rescheduling involves reducing fluid intake during and surrounding meals to make it more difficult to ruminate (Barton & Barton, 1985). One study that directly examined liquid rescheduling and satiation found that satiation in the form of offering food every 20 s for 30 min after a meal was more effective at decreasing rumination compared to liquid rescheduling (Wilder, Draper, Williams, & Higbee, 1997). Additionally, positive outcomes have been shown for liquid rescheduling, but not enough research has been accumulated to demonstrate that it meets the criteria for EBP. With nine single-subject experimental studies involving 16 participants, satiation is the only treatment for rumination which meets the Chambless and Hollon criteria for EBP.

Satiation has been used alone and in combination with other behavioral treatments such as an oral hygiene punishment program (Foxx et al., 1979) and noncontingent reinforcement (Wilder et al., 1997). There is also support for satiation being used to suppress rumination for periods of up to 7 years (Dunn, Lockwood, Williams, & Peacock, 1997); however, the way in which satiation interventions were implemented varies. In some interventions, unlimited quantities of food were provided at meals (Clauser & Scibak, 1990); in others, additional foods were provided at the end of meals (Dudley, Johnson, & Barnes, 2002). One study that compared these approaches found that supplemental feedings after the meal were more effective than larger portions during the meal (Kenzer & Wallace, 2007). While it has been suggested that starches are the most effective foods for satiation procedures (Rast et al., 1981), one study that used peanut butter suggested that the caloric density of the food is the most significant factor (Greene et al., 1991). While thicker, more calorically dense starches have been used in many studies, even fruit juice has been shown to decrease rumination (Lyons, Rue, Luiselli, & DiGennaro, 2007). One of the significant concerns expressed with the use of satiation is the potential of weight gain. This concern was addressed in a study which did not increase the amount of food presented at meals, but presented the food in small bites over an extended period of time (McKeegan, Estill, & Campbell, 1987). Their results demonstrated that rumination could be decreased with an intervention that does not increase overall caloric intake.

Nine small *N* studies involving 16 participants with ID have demonstrated that satiation meets the criteria for an effective intervention for rumination. To date, four small *N* studies involving seven participants with ID have demonstrated the effectiveness of liquid rescheduling. While this does not meet the criteria for an effective treatment, it is a promising treatment.

Conclusion

While consequence-based interventions have been shown to decrease rumination, satiation has also been shown to be an effective treatment for rumination without the use of restrictive procedures. It is not clear that satiation will be effective for all persons with rumination, but it has been successfully used with a wide range of persons with ID. Further, more evidence exists supporting the efficacy of this intervention than any other intervention for rumination.

Even though there are several medical issues that are commonly associated with rumination, intervention research typically discusses the behavioral or dietary aspects of the intervention and excludes discussion of the role of medical issues or the integration of medical treatment into an overall treatment of the rumination. One exception was a study which described a multidisciplinary treatment of ruminative vomiting (Luiselli, Haley, & Smith, 1993). This study described the treatment of a 13-year-old adolescent with ID who was diagnosed with gastroesophageal reflux and esophageal dysmotility along with the diagnosis of rumination. The intervention included not only behavioral components but medications to address the reflux and dysmotility. While there may be persons with ID who exhibit rumination who have no comorbid medical issues, there are many persons with rumination that do have associated medical problems. Treating these medical issues may increase the effectiveness of the overall intervention. GI conditions such as GERD or motility problems make it easier to regurgitate or ruminate food; medications used to treat these problems may lead to a reduction in rumination by improving motility and making it more difficult for the individual to engage in the behavior. Thus, if the response effort of engaging in rumination is increased by medication and the reinforcing function of the rumination is replaced with a satiation procedure, the probability that the treatment will be effective is increased. Medical treatment alone will probably not be an intervention for rumination, but medical treatment may prove to be a useful component in a successful treatment for rumination.

Other Feeding Issues

Food selectivity

Food selectivity involves eating a narrow range of food and is the most commonly reported feeding problem among those with autism spectrum disorder (ASD) (Williams & Seiverling, 2010). There is a high comorbidity between ASD and ID, and those with both ID and ASD may be likely to exhibit selective eating patterns. Supporting this notion, Fodstad and Matson (2008) found that adults with ASD and ID exhibited more food selectivity- and refusal-related difficulties compared to adults with ID alone when administering the STEP (Matson & Kuhn, 2001). There is a growing literature on treating food selectivity in children with ASD in both home and clinical settings with treatment components often involving reinforcement for taking bites of new or nonpreferred foods, extinction procedures, as well as gradually increasing portion size or number of bites presented. These studies were described in a recent review (Williams & Seiverling, 2010).

Rapid eating

Rapid eating, which involves eating at a pace that does not allow for proper chewing and swallowing, has been reported as a problem among persons with ID (Matson, Gardner, Coe, & Sovner, 1991) but has received minimal research attention compared to other feeding problems in this population. Two studies that have targeted this behavior in adults and adolescents with ID (Lennox, Miltenberger, & Donnelly,1987; Wright & Vollmer, 2002) implemented differential reinforcement of low responding (DRL), response blocking, and prompting procedures to reduce rapid eating in adults and one teenager with ID. In a recent study conducted with three teenage boys with ASD, Anglesea, Hoch, and Taylor (2008) taught students to take bites when a pager vibrated at varying time intervals. All students slowed consumption of food during mealtimes and increased total mealtime duration.

Adipsia

The refusal to drink has been noted in pair studies involving persons with ID (Babbitt, Shore, Smith, Williams, & Coe, 2001; Frieden, Borakove, & Fox, 1982). These studies both used stimulus fading procedures to increase consumption of fluids. One study used a spoon to cup fading procedure in which two children with Down syndrome were initially taught to drink from a spoon, and then a cup was taped to the spoon and systematically faded toward the children's faces until the children were drinking from the cup (Babbitt et al., 2001). In the other study, milk consumption was increased by teaching a child with multiple handicaps to drink from progressively larger measuring spoons and then fading to a variety of other fluids (Frieden et al., 1982). Adipsia was also the target of intervention in a child with autism dependent upon gastrostomy tube feeds (Patel, Piazza, Kelley, Ochsner, & Santana, 2001). This study also used a fading intervention in which the child's water consumption was first increased, then instant breakfast powder was faded into the water, and finally the water was systematically replaced with milk.

Conclusions

Due to the paucity of intervention studies targeting food selectivity, rapid eating, and adipsia in persons with ID, the treatments developed to date for these feeding problems do not yet meet the criteria for EBP. It should be mentioned, however, that there is a rapidly growing body of research involving interventions for food selectivity among children with ASD. Several recent reviews have summarized the intervention literature for those with ASD and food selectivity (Matson & Fodstad, 2009; Seiverling, Williams, Ward-Horner, & Sturmey, 2011; Volkert & Vaz, 2010; Williams & Seiverling, 2010). Clinicians may have success implementing similar procedures to target food selectivity in children and adults with ID. While the few published studies involving the treatment of rapid eating and adipsia have demonstrated positive outcomes, these problems are not as commonly reported as other problems such as food refusal and have not been well researched.

General Discussion

There is currently evidence for EBP for food refusal, pica, and rumination. Additionally, there are promising treatments for these problems as well as other feeding problems among persons with ID such as food selectivity, rapid eating, and adipsia. As the research literature on feeding interventions continues to grow, it is expected that the range and number of empirically supported treatments will also grow. Despite the increasing number of studies with positive outcomes, there are significant limitations to the intervention literature.

One of the major limitations of the literature of feeding interventions is one of definition. In studies in which the participants are adults, and even adolescents, it is often difficult to determine whether the participants have ID. Among younger children, especially in the United States, it is often not clear if participants in interventions studies have ID because many studies describing feeding interventions with young children use the terms *developmental disabilities* or *special needs* to describe any delay in development. These terms may be used to describe both a mild delay and a more significant delay that would meet the criteria for ID. When these terms are used, it is difficult to determine if the study should be included in the literature for those with ID because it is not possible to determine the extent of

Table 8.1   EBP for Specific Feeding Problems

Feeding problem	Evidence of treatment
Food refusal	
Escape extinction and reinforcement	Effective
Response cost and reinforcement	Insufficient evidence
Texture fading and reinforcement	Insufficient evidence
Pica	
Overcorrection	Effective
Reinforcement/environmental enrichment	Effective
Discrimination training and punishment	Insufficient evidence
Contingent aversive stimulation	Insufficient evidence
Response blocking	Insufficient evidence
Rumination	
Satiation	Effective
Liquid rescheduling	Insufficient evidence
Contingent pinches	Insufficient evidence
Noxious tastes	Insufficient evidence
Oral hygiene	Insufficient evidence
Overcorrection	Insufficient evidence
Electric shock	Insufficient evidence
Differential reinforcement	Insufficient evidence
Rapid eating	
DRL, response blocking, and prompting	Insufficient evidence
Food selectivity	
No studies involving persons with ID	
Adipsia	
Stimulus fading	Insufficient evidence

the child's developmental issues. Using these terms also makes it harder to estimate the generalizability of the results of these studies. The terms *autism* and *autism spectrum disorder* are similarly problematic as an increasing number of children are diagnosed with some form of autism, but their level of cognitive functioning is not specified, so it is not possible to determine whether these children also meet the criteria for ID, which is often comorbid with ASD.

Another issue is that the research for interventions for specific feeding problems has not been conducted across the age span. For example, studies involving interventions for food refusal almost exclusively describe participants who are young children despite the fact that there is evidence that adults with ID commonly exhibit food refusal. The extinction procedures described in many of the food refusal studies may be difficult to adapt to adults. Inversely, the recent studies involving rumination involve mostly adolescents and adults, with a few school-aged children and no young children.

A range of behavioral interventions have been used for the treatment of feeding problems in persons with ID. While none of these interventions meet the Chambless and Hollon criteria for group designs, several of these interventions have been shown to be empirically supported treatments through the use of single-subject methodology. A summary of the interventions used for the treatment of feeding problems and the level of evidence is shown in Table 8.1. As research on the feeding problems of persons with ID continues to amass, it is expected that more behavioral interventions will meet the criteria for EBP.

References

Anglesea, M. M., Hoch, H., & Taylor, B. A. (2008). Reducing rapid eating in teenagers with autism: Use of a pager prompt. *Journal of Applied Behavior Analysis, 41*, 107–111.

Applegate, H., Matson, J., & Cherry, K. (1999). An evaluation of functional variables affecting severe problem behaviors in adults with mental retardation by using the questions about behavioral function scale (QABF). *Research in Developmental Disabilities, 20*, 229–237.

Babbitt, R. L., Shore, B. A., Smith, M., Williams, K. E., & Coe, D. A. (2001). Stimulus fading in the treatment of fading. *Behavior Interventions, 16*, 197–207.

Barton, L. E., & Barton, C. L. (1985). An effective and benign treatment of rumination. *Journal of the Association for Persons with Severe Handicaps, 10*, 168–171.

Blinder, B. J., & Salama, C. (2008, May). An update on pica. *Psychiatric Times*, pp. 66–73.

Bogart, L. C., Piersel, W. C., & Gross, E. J. (1995). The long-term treatment of life-threatening pica: A case study of a woman with profound mental retardation living in an applied setting. *Journal of Developmental and Physical Disabilities, 14*, 445–456.

Böhmer, C. J. M., Niezen-de Boer, M. C., Klinkenberg-Knol, E. C., Deville, W. L. J. M., Nadorp, J. H. S. M., & Meuwissen, S. G. M. (1999). The prevalence of gastroesophageal reflux disease in institutionalized intellectually disabled individuals. *The American Journal of Gastroenterology, 94*, 804–810.

Chambless, D. L., & Hollon, S. D. (1998). Defining empirically supported therapies. *Journal of Consulting and Clinical Psychology, 66*, 7–18.

Clauser, B., & Scibak, J. W. (1990). Direct and generalized effects of food satiation in reducing rumination. *Research in Developmental Disabilities, 11*, 23–36.

Danford, D. E., & Huber, A. E. (1982). Pica among mentally retarded adults. *American Journal of Mental Deficiency, 87*, 141–146.

DeMoor, J., Didden, R., & Tolboom, J. (2005). Severe feeding problems secondary to anatomical disorders: Effectiveness of behavioural treatment in three school-aged children. *Educational Psychology, 25*, 325–340.

Didden, R., Seys, D., & Schouwink, D. (1999). Treatment of chronic food refusal in a young developmentally disabled child. *Behavioral Interventions, 14*, 213–222.

Donnelly, D. R., & Olczak, P. V. (1990). The effect of differential reinforcement of incompatible behaviors (DRI) on pica for cigarettes in persons with intellectual disability. *Behavior Modification, 14*, 81–96.

Dudley, L. J., Johnson, C., & Barnes, R. S. (2002). Decreasing rumination using a starchy food satiation procedure. *Behavioral Interventions, 17*, 21–29.

Duker, P., & Nielen, M. (1993). The use of negative practice for the control of pica behavior. *Journal of Behavior Therapy and Experimental Psychiatry, 24*, 249–253.

Duker, P., & Seys, D. (1977). A quasi-experimental study on the effect of electrical aversion treatment on imposed mechanical restraint for severe self-injurious behavior. *Research in Developmental Disabilities, 21*, 235–242.

Dunn, J., Lockwood, K., Williams, D., & Peacock, S. (1997). A seven year follow-up of treating rumination with dietary satiation. *Behavioral Interventions, 12*, 163–172.

Feldman, M. (1983). Nausea and vomiting. In M. H. Sliesenger & J. S. Fordtran (Eds.), *Gastrointestinal disease: Pathology, diagnosis, management* (3rd ed., pp. 160–177). Philadelphia: W. B. Saunders Co.

Field, D., Garland, M., & Williams, K. (2003). Correlates of specific childhood feeding problems. *Journal of Pediatrics and Child Health, 39*, 299–304.

Finney, J. W., Russo, D. C., & Cataldo, M. F. (1982). Reduction of pica in young children with lead poisoning. *Journal of Pediatric Psychology, 7*, 197–207.

Fisher, W. W., Piazza, C., Bowman, L. G., Kurtz, P. F., Sherer, M. R., & Lachman, S. R. (1994). A preliminary evaluation of empirically derived consequences for the treatment of pica. *Journal of Applied Behavior Analysis, 26*, 23–36.

Fodstad, J. C., & Matson, J. L. (2008). A comparison of feeding and mealtime problems in adults with intellectual disabilities with and without autism. *Journal of Developmental and Physical Disabilities, 20*, 541–550.

Foxx, R. M., & Livesay, J. (1984). Maintenance of response suppression following overcorrection: A 10-year retrospective analysis of eight cases. *Analysis and Intervention in Developmental Disabilities, 4*, 65–79.

Foxx, R. M., & Martin, E. D. (1975). Treatment of scavenging behavior (coprophagy and pica) by overcorrection. *Behaviour, Research and Therapy, 13*, 153–162.

Foxx, R. M., Snyder, M. S., & Schroeder, F. (1979). Food satiation and oral hygiene punishment program to suppress chronic rumination by retarded persons. *Journal of Autism and Developmental Disorders, 9*, 399–411.

Fredricks, D. W., Carr, J. E., & Williams, W. L. (1998). Overview of the treatment of rumination disorder for adults in a residential setting. *Journal of Behavior Therapy and Experimental Psychiatry, 29*, 31–40.

Frieden, B. D., Borakove, L. S., & Fox, K. T. (1982). Treatment of an abnormal avoidance of fluid consumption. *Journal of Behavioral Therapy and Experimental Psychiatry, 13*, 85–87.

Goh, H. L., Iwata, B. A., & Kahng, S. W. (1999). Multicomponent assessment and treatment of cigarette pica. *Journal of Applied Behavior Analysis, 32*, 297–315.

Gravestock, J. (2000). Eating disorders in adults with intellectual disability. *Journal of Intellectual Disability Research, 44*, 625–637.

Greene, K. S., Johnston, J. M., Rossi, M., Rawal, A., Winston, M., & Barron, S. (1991). Effects of peanut butter on ruminating. *American Journal on Mental Retardation, 95*, 631–645.

Gutentag, S., & Hammer, D. (2000). Shaping oral feeding in a gastrostomy tube-dependent child in natural settings. *Behavioral Modification, 24*, 395–410.

Hagopian, L. P., & Adelinis, J. D. (2001). Response blocking with and without redirection for the treatment of pica. *Journal of Applied Behavior Analysis, 34*, 527–530.

Hoch, T., Babbitt, R., Coe, D., Duncan, A., & Trusty, E. (1995). A swallow induction avoidance procedure to establish eating. *Journal of Behavioral Therapy & Experimental Psychiatry, 26*, 41–50.

Hoch, T., Babbitt, R., Coe, D., Krell, D., & Hackbert, L. (1994). Contingency contacting: Combining positive reinforcement and escape extinction procedures to treat persistent food refusal. *Behavior Modification, 18*, 106–128.

Hogg, J. (1982). Reduction of self-induced vomiting in a multiply handicapped girl by "lemon juice therapy" and concomitant changes in social behavior. *British Journal of Clinical Psychology, 21*, 227–228.

Hove, O. (2004). Prevalence of eating disorders in adults with mental retardation living in the community. *American Journal on Mental Retardation, 109*, 501–506.

Johnson, C., Hunt, F., & Siebert, M. (1994). Discrimination training in the treatment of pica and food scavenging. *Behavior Modification, 18*, 214–229.

Johnston, J. M., & Greene, K. S. (1992). Relation between ruminating and quantity of food consumed. *Mental Retardation, 30*, 7–11.

Jones, C. J., & Samuel, J. (2010). The diagnosis of eating disorders in adults with learning disabilities: Conceptualisation and implications for clinical practice. *European Eating Disorders Review, 18*, 352–366.

Joyce, T., Ditchfield, H., & Harris, P. (2001). Challenging behaviour in community services. *Journal of Intellectual Disability Research, 45*, 130–138.

Kahng, S., Tarbox, J., & Wilke, A. (2001). Use of a multicomponent treatment for food refusal. *Journal of Applied Behavior Analysis, 34*, 93–96.

Kedesdy, J. H., & Budd, K. (1998). *Childhood feeding disorders*. Baltimore: Brookes.

Kenzer, A. L., & Wallace, M. D. (2007). Treatment of rumination maintained by automatic reinforcement: A comparison of extra portions during a meal and supplemental post-meal feedings. *Behavioral Interventions, 22*, 297–304.

Kitfield, E. B., & Masalsky, C. (2000). Negative reinforcement-based treatment to increase food intake. *Behavior Modification, 24*, 600–608.

Kohlenberg, R. J. (1970). The punishment of persistent vomiting: A case study. *Journal of Applied Behavior Analysis, 3*, 241–245.

Kuruvilla, J., & Trewby, P. N. (1989). Gastro-esophageal disorders in adults with severe mental impairment. *British Medical Journal, 299*, 95–96.

LeBlanc, L. A., Piazza, C. C., & Krug, M. A. (1997). Comparing methods for maintaining the safety of a child with pica. *Research in Developmental Disabilities, 18*, 215–220.

Lennox, D. B., Miltenberger, R. G., & Donnelly, D. R. (1987). Response interruption and DRL for the reduction of rapid eating. *Journal of Applied Behavior Analysis, 20*, 279–284.

Levin, L., & Carr, E. G. (2001). Food selectivity and problem behavior in children with developmental disabilities: Analysis and intervention. *Behavior Modification, 25*, 443–470.

Linscheid, T. (2006). Behavioral treatments for pediatric feeding disorders. *Behavior Modification, 30*, 6–23.

Lofts, R. H., Schroeder, S. R., & Maier, R. H. (1990). Effects of serum zinc supplementation of pica behavior of persons with mental retardation. *American Journal of Mental Retardation, 95*, 105–109.

Luiselly, J., Haley, S., & Smith, A. (1993). Evaluation of a behavioral medicine consultative treatment for chronic, ruminative vomiting. *Journal of Behavior Therapy and Experimental Psychiatry, 24*, 27–35.

Lyons, E. A., Rue, H. C., Luiselli, J. K., & DiGennaro, F. D. (2007). Brief functional analysis and supplemental feeding for postmeal rumination in children with developmental disabilities. *Journal of Applied Behavior Analysis, 40,* 743–747.

Mace, F. C., & Knight, D. (1986). Functional analysis and treatment of severe pica. *Journal of Applied Behavior Analysis, 19,* 411–416.

Madden, N. A., Russo, D. C., & Cataldo, M. F. (1981). Behavioral treatment of pica in children with lead poisoning. *Child & Family Behavior Therapy, 2,* 67–81.

Mathisen, B., Worrall, L., Masel, J., Wall, C., & Shepard, R. W. (1999). Feeding problems in infants with gastroesophageal reflux disease: A controlled study. *Journal of Pediatrics and Child Health, 35,* 63–69.

Matson, J. L., & Bamburg, J. W. (1999). A descriptive study of pica behavior in persons with mental retardation. *Journal of Developmental and Physical Disabilities, 11,* 353–361.

Matson, J., & Kuhn, D. (2001). Identifying feeding problems in mentally retarded persons: Development and reliability of the screening tool of eating problems (STEP). *Research in Developmental Disabilities, 21,* 165–172.

Matson, J. L., & Fodstad, J. C. (2009). The treatment of food selectivity and other feeding problems in children with autism spectrum disorders. *Research in Autism Spectrum Disorders, 3,* 455–461.

Matson, J. L., Gardner, W. I., Coe, D. A., & Sovner, R. (1991). A scale for evaluating emotional disorders in severely and profoundly mentally retarded persons: Development of the Diagnostic Assessment of the Severely Handicapped (DASH) Scale. *British Journal of Psychiatry, 159,* 404–409.

McAdam, D. B., Sherman, J. A., Sheldon, J. B., & Napolitano, D. A. (2004). Behavioral interventions to reduce the pica of persons with developmental disabilities. *Behavior Modification, 28,* 45–72.

McCord, B. E., Grosser, J. W., Iwata, B. A., & Powers, L. A. (2005). An analysis of response blocking parameters in the treatment of pica. *Journal of Applied Behavior Analysis, 38,* 391–394.

McKeegan, G., Estill, K., & Campbell, B. (1987). Elimination of rumination by controlled eating and differential reinforcement. *Journal of Behavior Therapy and Experimental Psychiatry, 18,* 143–148.

Minness, P. M. (1980). Treatment of compulsive hand in mouth behavior in a profoundly retarded child using a sharp pinch as the aversive stimulus. *Australian Journal of Developmental Disabilities, 6,* 5–10.

Mulick, J. A., Barbour, R., Schroeder, S. R., & Rojahn, J. (1980a). Overcorrection of pica in two profoundly retarded adults: Analysis of setting effects, stimulus, and response generalization. *Applied Research in Mental Retardation, 1,* 241–252.

Mulick, J. A., Schroeder, S. R., & Rojahn, J. (1980b). Chronic ruminative vomiting: A comparison of four treatment procedures. *Journal of Autism and Developmental Disabilities, 10,* 203–213.

Pace, G., & Toyer, E. (2000). The effects of a vitamin supplement on the pica of a child with severe mental retardation. *Journal of Applied Behavior Analysis, 33,* 619–622.

Paniagua, F. A., Braverman, C., & Capriotti, R. M. (1986). Use of a treatment package in the management of a profoundly mentally retarded girl's pica and self-stimulation. *American Journal of Mental Deficiency, 90,* 550–557.

Patel, M., Piazza, C., Kelley, M., Ochsner, C., & Santana, C. (2001). Using a fading procedure to increase fluid consumption in a child with feeding problems. *Journal of Applied Behavior Analysis, 34*, 357–360.

Patel, M., Piazza, C., Martinez, C., Volkert, V., & Santana, C. (2002). An evaluation of two differential reinforcement procedures with escape extinction to treat food refusal. *Journal of Applied Behavior Analysis, 35*, 363–374.

Piazza, C., Fisher, W., Hanley, G., LeBlanc, L., Wordsell, A., Lindauer, S., et al. (1998). Treatment of pica through multiple analyses of its reinforcing functions. *Journal of Applied Behavior Analysis, 31*, 165–189.

Rapp, J. T., Dozier, C. L., & Carr, J. E. (2001). Functional assessment and treatment of pica: A single-case experiment. *Behavioral Interventions, 16*, 111–125.

Rast, J., Johnston, J. M., Allen, J. E., & Drum, C. (1985). Effects of nutritional and mechanical properties of food on ruminative behavior. *Journal of the Experimental Analysis of Behavior, 44*, 195–206.

Rast, J., Johnston, J. M., Drum, C., & Conrin, J. (1981). A parametric analysis of the relationship between food quantity and rumination. *Journal of the Experimental Analysis of Behavior, 41*, 125–134.

Ricciardi, J. N., Luiselli, J. K., Terrill, S., & Reardon, K. (2003). Alternate response training with contingent practice as intervention for pica in a school setting. *Behavioral Interventions, 18*, 219–226.

Rogers, B., Stratton, P., Victor, J., Kennedy, B., & Andres, M. (1992). Chronic rumination among persons with mental retardation: A need for combined medical and interdisciplinary strategies. *American Journal of Mental Retardation, 96*, 522–527.

Rommel, N., Tack, J., Arts, J., Caenepeel, P., Bisschops, R., & Sifrim, D. (2010). Rumination or belching-regurgitation? Differential diagnosis using oesophageal impedance-manometry. *Neurogastroenterology & Motility, 22*, e97–e104.

Seiverling, L. J., Williams, K. E., Ward-Horner, J. C., & Sturmey, P. (2011). Feeding problems in those with autism spectrum disorders: A comprehensive review. In J. L. Matson & P. Sturmey (Eds.), *International handbook of autism and pervasive developmental disorders* (pp. 491–507). New York: Springer.

Smith, M. D. (1987). Treatment of pica in an adult disabled by autism by differential reinforcement of incompatible behavior. *Journal of Behavior Therapy and Experimental Psychiatry, 18*, 285–288.

Starin, S. P., & Fuqua, R. W. (1987). Rumination and vomiting in the developmentally disabled: A critical review of the behavioral, medical, and psychiatric treatment research. *Research in Developmental Disabilities, 8*, 575–605.

Thommessen, M., Riis, G., Kase, B. F., Larsen, S., & Heiberg, A. (1991). Energy and nutrient intakes of disabled children: Do feeding problems make a difference? *Journal of the American Dietetic Association, 91*, 1522–1525.

Toister, R. P., Condrin, J., Worley, L. M., & Arthur, D. (1975). Faradic therapy of chronic vomiting in infancy: A case study. *Journal of Behavior Therapy and Experimental Psychiatry, 6*, 55–59.

Volkert, V. M., & Vaz, P. C. (2010). Recent studies of feeding problems in children with autism. *Journal of Applied Behavior Analysis, 43*, 155–159.

Wilder, D. A., Draper, R., Williams, W. L., & Higbee, T. S. (1997). A comparison of noncontingent reinforcement, other competing stimulation, and liquid rescheduling for the treatment of rumination. *Behavioral Interventions, 12*, 55–64.

Williams, D., Kirkpatrick-Sanchez, S., Enzinna, C., & Dunn, J. (2009). The clinical management and prevention of pica: A retrospective follow-up of 41 individuals with intellectual disabilities and pica. *Journal of Applied Research in Intellectual Disabilities, 22*, 210–215.

Williams, K. E., Field, D. G., & Seiverling, L. (2010). Food refusal in children: A review of the literature. *Research in Developmental Disabilities, 31*, 625–633.

Williams, K. E., Hendy, H., & Knecht, S. (2008). Parent feeding practices and child variables associated with childhood feeding problems. *Journal of Developmental and Physical Disabilities, 20*, 231–242.

Williams, K. E., & Seiverling, L. J. (2010). Eating problems in children with autism spectrum disorders. *Topics in Clinical Nutrition, 25*, 27–37.

Wright, C. S., & Vollmer, T. R. (2002). Evaluation of a treatment package to reduce rapid eating. *Journal of Applied Behavior Analysis, 35*, 89–93.

9

Sleep Problems

Robert Didden, Wiebe Braam, Anneke Maas,
Marcel Smits, Peter Sturmey, Jeff Sigafoos,
and Leopold Curfs

Introduction

Types of sleep problems

Although over 80 different sleep disorders are listed in the *International Classification of Sleep Disorders* (American Academy of Sleep Medicine, 2005), three main types of sleep problems may be distinguished: (a) sleeplessness (insomnia), (b) excessive sleep (hypersomnia), and (c) unusual behaviors during sleep (parasomnias). Most of the literature on sleep in individuals with intellectual disabilities (ID) does not distinguish between sleep disorders and sleep problems. Many sleep studies present data only on "symptoms" or sleep problems and not on "underlying" sleep disorders. For example, sleeplessness may be caused by a variety of sleep disorders such as limit-setting problems or a delayed sleep phase disorder. This distinction is essential in interpreting results of studies on the effectiveness of intervention strategies for addressing sleep problems in individuals with ID.

Prevalence

Sleep problems are highly prevalent in individuals at all levels of ID. Surveys have revealed that sleep problems are more common in children and adults with intellectual and/or other developmental disabilities (autism spectrum disorder (ASD)) than in their nondisabled peers. Prevalence rates for individuals with ID range from 15% to 85% depending on study design, instrument with which the sleep

Evidence-Based Practice and Intellectual Disabilities, First Edition.
Edited by Peter Sturmey and Robert Didden.

problem is measured, participant characteristics, and definition of the sleep problem (Didden & Sigafoos, 2001; Van de Wouw, Evenhuis, & Echteld, 2012).

Adverse consequences

Sleep problems often have adverse consequences for the person involved and his or her caregivers. For example, children with ID who have sleep problems exhibit more daytime problem behaviors than children with ID but without a sleep problem (e.g., Didden, Korzilius, van Aperlo, van Overloop, & de Vries, 2002; Lenjavi, Ahuja, Touchette, & Sandman, 2010). Although the causal relationship is not clear, it may be assumed that sleep problems such as insomnia result in daytime irritability and challenging behavior. Schreck, Mulick, and Smith (2004) have investigated the relationship between ASD symptoms and sleep problems in 55 children with ASD who were between 5 and 12 years old. Results showed that fewer hours of sleep per night predicted overall autism symptomatology (e.g., stereotypic behaviors) and social skills deficits. Further, sleep deprivation may lead to daytime fatigue and stress in both the individual involved and his or her caretakers, and diminished cognitive functioning and impaired learning (Didden, Korzilius et al., 2002; Richdale, Gavidia-Payne, Francis, & Cotton, 2000; Wiggs & Stores, 2001).

Risk factors

There are relatively many risk factors that increase the probability that a child or adult with ID may develop a sleep problem (see Didden & Sigafoos, 2001; Richdale & Wiggs, 2005; Van de Wouw et al., 2012; Wiggs, 2007). A range of somatic factors may cause a sleep problem, such as (nighttime) epileptic seizures, gastroesophageal reflux, sleep apnea (breathing difficulties), and blindness. The ID itself may also be a risk factor. Because of the ID, it may be difficult to teach the child or adult to develop and maintain adequate sleep–wake behavior and circadian rhythm. Sleep problems are frequently occurring in genetic disorders, such as in Angelman syndrome, Smith–Magenis syndrome, Prader–Willi syndrome, Down syndrome, and fragile X syndrome and in ASD. The genotype is then linked to a sleep problem although causal pathways are not always clear (Cotton & Richdale, 2010).

Evidence-based practice

The aim of the present chapter is to review the evidence base for treatments to reduce sleep problems in individuals with ID using the criteria set by Chambless and Hollon (1998). Treatment approaches were classified as either (a) effective, (b) ineffective, (c) inconclusive, or (d) lacking sufficient evidence. A treatment approach was considered to be *effective* if there were at least three studies by

Table 9.1 Evidence Base for the Treatment of Sleep Problems

Treatment	Summary of evidence
Melatonin	Effective
Behavioral strategies	
Extinction	Effective
Graduated extinction	Lacks sufficient evidence
Bedtime fading	Effective
Differential reinforcement	Lacks sufficient evidence
Relaxation	Lacks sufficient evidence
Other strategies	
Sleep restriction	Lacks sufficient evidence
Alternative therapies	
Valerian	Lacks sufficient evidence

independent research teams showing that the treatment was successful in producing clinically significant reductions in sleep problems in at least nine individuals with ID. A treatment was considered *ineffective* if there were at least three studies by independent research teams showing that the treatment was unsuccessful in producing clinically significant reductions in sleep problems in at least nine individuals with ID. A treatment approach was considered *inconclusive* if there were at least three studies by independent research teams showing conflicting evidence regarding the success of the treatment. Finally, a treatment was considered as *lacking sufficient evidence* if there were fewer than three studies evaluating that treatment approach. Table 9.1 provides a summary of the evidence.

Search Strategy and Treatment Classification

We conducted a systematic search for studies that were focused on the treatment of sleep problems in individuals with ID. We conducted systematic searches in four electronic databases: Education Resources Information Center (ERIC), Medline, PsycINFO, and Web of Science. The terms *sleep, sleep problem, sleep disorder,* and *ID* (or *developmental disability* or *mental retardation*) were inserted into the keywords field. Abstracts returned from these electronic searches were reviewed to identify studies for inclusion in the review. The reference lists of the included studies were also reviewed to identify additional articles for possible inclusion.

To be included in this review, the article had to meet five inclusion criteria. First, the study was published in English and in a peer-reviewed journal. Second, the study reported an evaluation of one or more treatments for sleep problems. Treatment was defined as implementing one or more strategies aimed at reducing a sleep problem. Treatments involving the use of psychotropic medications were excluded from this review, except for melatonin. Third, the study presented data based on direct observation (e.g., sleep diary), rating scales, or actigraphy. Fourth, data were collected in an experimental $N = 1$ design (reversal design, multiple baseline design) or control group design. Fifth, the study was published between 1980 and 2013. Treatments meeting inclusion criteria were classified into one of four categories: (a) melatonin, (b) behavioral strategies (e.g., extinction), (c) other strategies (e.g., sleep restriction), and (d) alternative therapies (e.g., valerian).

Melatonin

Melatonin is a hormone synthesized and released by the pineal gland during darkness. It is a chronobiotic drug with hypnotic properties. Melatonin secretion is regulated by an endogenous pacemaker in the suprachiasmatic nuclei of the hypothalamus (biological clock). Information on the light/dark cycle through the retinohypothalamic tract is needed to synchronize the circadian melatonin rhythm to 24 hr (Braam, Didden, Smits, & Curfs, 2008a). Many conditions can disrupt this system which may lead to a circadian rhythm disorder of which the most common type is delayed sleep phase disorder. This condition results in an inability to fall asleep at an appropriate time in the evening, and because the child or adult has to get up in the morning, this condition results in sleep deprivation. The underlying cause is a disruption of the melatonin synthesis whereby melatonin levels needed to fall asleep remain too low and/or start to rise too late. Exogenous melatonin is indicated for the treatment of this type of circadian rhythm disorder and to establish a more appropriate sleep–wake rhythm (i.e., falling asleep at an earlier time in the evening). Exogenous melatonin causes a phase advance when administered in the late afternoon or early in the evening (Braam et al., 2008a).

Control group studies

Only few controlled group studies have been published on the effectiveness of exogenous melatonin for sleep problems in children and adults with ID. In most studies, a significant reduction in sleep latency and an increase in total sleep time were found. Wasdell et al. (2008) conducted a randomized double-blind crossover study on the effectiveness of melatonin in 50 children with neurodevelopmental disabilities who had a chronic (lasting >1.5 years) sleep problem. Their mean age in years was 7.4 (range 2–18 years). All children had more than one other diagnosis such as severe ID ($n = 32$), cerebral palsy ($n = 26$), epilepsy ($n = 23$), and ASD ($n = 16$). Twenty-six children had sleep onset (problems falling asleep at an appropriate bedtime) as well as sleep maintenance (night waking) problems, 16 had sleep onset problems only, and 8 suffered from sleep maintenance problems only. Before the trial, sleep hygiene advices had been given, and caregivers were supervised by a pediatric nurse trained in sleep medicine. Melatonin 5 mg (1-mg fast, 4-mg sustained release) was used. The trial consisted of 10 days of treatment (melatonin vs. placebo), followed by a placebo washout for 3–5 days, followed by 10 days of the alternate treatment (placebo vs. melatonin). The results of this study showed that compared to placebo, melatonin significantly advanced mean sleep onset time by little over half an hour and increased mean total sleep time also by half an hour. There was no significant reduction in the frequency of night waking.

Braam et al. (2008a) conducted a randomized double-blind parallel study on the effectiveness of melatonin in 51 individuals with profound to mild ID who had chronic (lasting >1 year) sleep problems. Their mean age in years was 23 (range 2–78 years). The most prevalent cause of the ID was genetic (e.g., Angelman, Down, and Prader–Willi syndrome), and 16 individuals had epilepsy. Twenty-one individuals had sleep onset as well as sleep maintenance problems, five individuals had sleep onset problems only, and three individuals suffered from sleep maintenance problems only. Somatic and psychiatric causes for the sleep problem were ruled out, and behavioral treatment and sleep hygiene had remained ineffective. The trial consisted of a 1-week baseline period and a 4-week intervention period during which participants were randomly allocated to placebo ($n = 22$) and melatonin ($n = 29$) conditions. Individuals aged 6 years and older were given 5 mg of melatonin (fast release) or an identically looking placebo at 7 p.m. Children aged under 6 years received 2.5 mg of melatonin at 6 p.m. To assess changes in circadian phase, salivary samples were collected hourly during five consecutive hours on the last night of baseline and on the last night of intervention when no melatonin was given. In this way, dim light melatonin onset (DLMO) was measured.

The results of this study showed that compared to placebo, melatonin significantly advanced mean sleep onset time by half an hour, increased mean total sleep time by almost 1 hr, and reduced frequency of night waking. Next to this, DLMO advanced almost 1.5 hr. There was no change in sleep offset time (i.e., time at which the child or adult wakes up in the morning) as a result of which total sleep time increased. Similar results were found in a randomized double-blind controlled study by Braam, Didden, Smits, and Curfs (2008b) on the effectiveness of melatonin in eight children with Angelman syndrome who had chronic sleep problems. Results of these studies and analysis of melatonin levels during baseline and after treatment suggested that their sleep problems were partly caused by a delayed sleep phase disorder. Parents and caregivers anecdotally reported an improvement in mood, vigilance, and/or daytime behavior and found that the participant was easier to manage with less settling problems and resistance at bedtime. This was not reported by caregivers in the placebo group.

Meta-analysis

Braam et al. (2009) conducted a meta-analysis of placebo-controlled randomized double-blind trials on melatonin in individuals with ID who have insomnia. They included studies that were published between 1990 and 2008. They found nine studies, including a total of 183 individuals. Although individuals' age ranged between 1 and 78 years, most studies included only or mainly children. Information on sleep parameters, such as sleep latency and total sleep time, was gathered through parental sleep diaries and/or actigraphy. Results of this meta-analysis showed that melatonin treatment decreased sleep latency by about 34 min on average, increased total sleep time by almost 1 hr on average, and decreased frequency of night waking. Because of the heterogeneity of sample as well as differences in timing of melatonin administration and dosage, no firm statements could be made about which time of administration and dosage of melatonin is most effective for particular groups of individuals with ID.

Conclusions

An increasing number of studies support the use of melatonin as treatment for sleep problems in individuals with ID. Melatonin is an effective treatment based on the Chambless and Hollon (1998) criteria. Melatonin is a safe treatment with almost no negative side effects (Braam et al., 2009). Long-term outcomes of melatonin treatment are still lacking. Braam et al. (2010) have observed that in some of their clients with ID, the initial good response to melatonin disappeared within several weeks after the start of treatment. Melatonin became effective only after considerable dose reduction. While the cause for the loss of response to melatonin is unknown, they have hypothesized that loss of response to melatonin may be caused by slow metabolization of exogenous melatonin as a result of decreased activity/inducibility of CYP1A2.

Behavioral Strategies

There are a number of behavioral strategies for the treatment of sleep problems in children and adults with ID. These are (graduated) extinction, bedtime fading (with response cost), differential reinforcement of appropriate sleep behavior, and relaxation. These approaches are often combined into treatment packages.

Extinction

N = 1 designs

A common behavioral strategy for promoting sleep in children with ID is extinction (see Didden, Sigafoos, & Lancioni, 2010). Extinction is indicated if sleep disruptive behavior is maintained (i.e., reinforced) by access to parental attention or activities (e.g., watching TV) or by avoidance of, and escape from, an unwanted situation (e.g., being put into bed). During extinction, the reward is withheld and the sleep disruptive behavior is no longer reinforced, and thus, it should decrease or extinguish. Didden, Curfs, van Driel, and de Moor (2002) showed that crying in a

4-year-old child with mild disability was functionally related to attention provided by her mother at bedtime. Anecdotal observations suggested that the child's crying and yelling were maintained by her mother's presence and provision of attention. Data that were collected in a reversal design showed that the child's sleep disruption was indeed related to the presence/absence of mother's attention and extinction (mother ignored crying and yelling) was effective in eliminating the child's sleep problem.

Thackeray and Richdale (2002) used extinction as the main component in a treatment package containing positive reinforcement, stimulus control, and extinction for sleep problems (cosleeping, settling problems, and night waking) in three children who functioned in the severe to mild range of ID. They were between 5 and 10 years old. Data were collected within a multiple baseline design with a 3-month follow-up. Sleep parameters were measured using actigraphy and sleep logs that were completed by parents. The intervention resulted in near-zero levels of bedtime disruptions and an increase to 100% of nights in which children fell asleep independently. Effects were maintained at follow-up, except in one child who showed baseline levels of bedtime disruptions. Improvement in sleep onset latency was found in two children, and total sleep time had increased in two children. Extinction for bedtime disruptions resulted in an extinction burst in two children (see Didden et al., 2010). Weiskop, Richdale, and Matthews (2005) investigated the effectiveness of a parent training program to address sleep problems in five children with autism or fragile X syndrome, some of whom functioned in the moderate to mild level of ID. The program included establishing stimulus control, positive reinforcement, and extinction. Parents were also taught how to provide support to each other to facilitate consistency in parenting, communication, and problem solving. Data were collected within a multiple baseline design, and results showed that the parent training program was effective in reducing children's settling problems, night waking, and cosleeping. These effects were maintained at the 3- to 12-month follow-ups.

Control group studies

Wiggs and Stores (1998) used a treatment package tailored to the needs of families of 15 children with severe ID who had a severe sleep problem. Next to extinction, the package included stimulus control procedures and positive reinforcement for appropriate sleep. The researchers made six home visits and discussed treatment options. Children in the treatment group were matched on gender and duration of sleep problems to those of a control group, and data were collected using sleep diaries. Mean age of children in the treatment group was about 8 years, and mean duration of their sleep problems was 6 years. Both mother and her child wore an actigraph for three nights. Actigraphs are wristwatch-sized sensors, worn on the nondominant wrist between getting into bed and getting out of bed the next morning. The amount of movement was calculated for every 30 s during recording and provided a measure for sleep and wakefulness. Parental reports showed that sleep problems had decreased following 1 month of treatment for children in the treatment group, but not for children in the control group. Effects were maintained at a 2-month follow-up. Mothers on children in the treatment group reported an increase in sleeping time themselves. Interestingly, objective changes (as measured by actigraphy) in the children's sleep quality and quantity were not seen after treatment.

Graduated Extinction

Some parents may find it difficult to implement a standard extinction procedure for their child's sleep problem, for example, when the extinction burst is intense. In these cases, parents may be more tolerant of using a graduated extinction strategy. During graduated extinction, the interval before checking the child is gradually increased while parental presence is gradually faded.

N = 1 *designs*

Durand, Gernert-Dott, and Mapstone (1996) used graduated extinction in the treatment of frequent night waking and bedtime disturbances of four children with developmental disabilities. Intervention consisted of establishing stimulus control and graduated extinction. For example, one of the participants was put to bed at 8 p.m., and her mother would read a story to her and spend 10–15 min of quiet time with her. Her mother then responded to any bedtime problem behavior using the graduated extinction strategy. She preferred a short initial interval (3 min) with 2-min increments on subsequent nights. Parents kept a sleep diary to monitor changes in children's sleep. Data were collected in a multiple baseline design across children. Overall, the results of this study showed that graduated extinction was highly effective in reducing percent of nights with night waking and settling problems.

Control group studies

Montgomery, Stores, and Wiggs (2004) used graduated extinction in the treatment of settling problems and night waking in a mixed sample consisting of 66 children with severe to mild ID and/or other developmental disabilities who were between 2 and 8 years old. Two approaches were compared to a wait-list control group. The intervention consisted of either a therapist-guided strategy using a written manual or providing parents with the written manual which covered information about their child's sleep, behavioral principles, and graduated extinction (plus stimulus control). The children were positively reinforced the next day for appropriate bedtime behavior. Results showed that both interventions were equally and significantly effective in reducing sleep problems in the children and effects were maintained at a 6-month follow-up.

Bedtime Fading

A behavioral strategy that has been shown effective in reducing bedtime disturbances and long sleep latency is bedtime fading, which may be implemented in combination with response cost and positive reinforcement.

$N = 1$ *designs*

Piazza and Fisher (1991) have used bedtime fading in four children (3–19 years old) with profound ID who were admitted to an inpatient unit for assessment and treatment of their self-injurious behavior. All children also had insomnia due to delayed sleep onset, frequent night waking, and/or early waking. The children exhibited various types of challenging behaviors when waking up during the night. Medication had remained unsuccessful in the treatment of their sleep problems. Percentage of being awake or asleep was measured through a 30-min momentary time sampling procedure. Data were collected within a multiple baseline across children design. Before intervention, mean bedtimes during a pretreatment baseline were calculated. Then, 30 min was added to that bedtime. If the child fell asleep within 15 min of bedtime, bedtime was then 30 min earlier on the next night (fading). If the child did not initiate sleep within this interval, the bedtime was moved 30 min later the subsequent night. Response cost consists of removing the child from the bed if she/he did not fall asleep within the interval and keeping the child awake for 1 hr after which the child was returned to the bed. This procedure was repeated throughout the night until the child was put to bed and fell asleep within 15 min. Daytime sleep was prevented and a consistent sleep and wake time was maintained. Through this procedure, the bedtime is gradually advanced until a desired time is attained. Results showed that following intervention, the frequency of night waking was reduced to near-zero levels and percentage of intervals with inappropriate sleep decreased to 0. Effects were maintained at follow-up for two children.

Piazza, Fisher, and Moser (1991) have used bedtime fading (and stimulus control) in the treatment of insomnia in three children with Rett syndrome who were between 4 and 8 years old. Their sleep problems consisted of sleep onset problems and night waking. Two of the girls also showed daytime sleepiness. Data were collected in a multiple baseline design. Results showed that bedtime fading was successful in increasing the amount of night sleep in two of the three girls and a reduction in settling problems in one child. Daytime napping was also reduced. No follow-up data were collected.

Control group studies

Piazza, Fisher, and Sherer (1997) evaluated the effectiveness of bedtime fading and response cost on insomnia in 14 children who functioned in the profound to severe range of ID and who were between 4 and 14 years old. Bedtime fading and response cost were compared to a control condition consisting of sleep scheduling. Statistical analyses showed that bedtime fading was significantly more effective in reducing the number of hours of disturbed sleep (i.e., night waking, sleep onset delay) than bedtime scheduling.

Differential Reinforcement

Differential positive reinforcement is often used in behavioral strategies for sleep problems in individuals with ID. This procedure consists of providing a reinforcer contingent on behavior that facilitates sleep. O'Reilly, Lancioni, and Sigafoos (2004) were the first to use an experimental functional analysis procedure in assessing the variable maintaining the sleep problems in a young child with severe ID. Her sleep problems consisted of frequently coming out of bed and leaving the bedroom. Using a paired-choice format, they found that parental reinforcement (cuddling) was a preferred stimulus that probably maintained the child's sleep onset problems. In the intervention condition, cuddling was used as a reinforcer for staying in bed. Data collected in a reversal design showed that the intervention was effective in eliminating the child's sleep problem.

Relaxation

Sleep problems may develop or be exacerbated if the individual has problems reaching a state of quietness while lying in bed. This may be due to, for example, intrusive thoughts, worrying, or an overactive mind (Gunning & Espie, 2003). Relaxation may be indicated as treatment. Gunning and Espie have used adapted progressive muscular relaxation and mental imagery for the treatment of delayed sleep phase syndrome in two individuals with ID. The first client had moderate ID and exhibited long sleep latency and cognitive overactivity upon retiring to bed. The second client had mild ID and showed an inability to fall asleep and cognitive overactivity. Data were collected in a multiple baseline design. The relaxation program resulted in a substantial reduction and normalization of the sleep onset latency: from an average of about 75 min during baseline to a mean of 25 min during intervention. Effects were maintained at a 36- and 50-week follow-up.

Conclusions

A wide range of behavioral strategies have been developed for the treatment of sleep problems among persons with ID. In almost all studies, different behavioral strategies were combined into a treatment package, precluding firm conclusions on the evidence base of each separate strategy (see Table 9.1). Despite this limitation, extinction meets the Chambless and Hollon criteria for evidence-based practice. Sufficient evidence was lacking for graduated extinction, bedtime fading, differential reinforcement, and relaxation. Two comments should be made concerning graduated extinction and bedtime fading. First, graduated extinction has been explored in only two studies, but in which more than 60 individuals with ID participated. Second, bedtime fading has been studied by researchers from the same research group but has been investigated in case studies and one randomized control group study including more than 20 participants.

Other Strategies

Sleep restriction

Many individuals with ID may have relatively low sleep efficiency (calculated as the time spent awake in bed divided by the total time spent in bed), and sleep problems may develop or exacerbate as a result of spending too much time in bed while awake. Sleep restriction involves restricting the amount of time in bed to the total amount of time asleep as a result of which reducing time spent awake in bed. Sleep restriction was used in two 4-year-old girls with developmental delay who lived at home with their parents (Durand & Christodulu, 2004). For example, one of the girls exhibited approximately one wakening per night that on average lasted more than 1 hr/episode. Attempts to return her to bed were often unsuccessful, and she slept in her parents' bed approximately four nights per week. She also occasionally displayed bedtime tantrums that lasted 2–4 hr. Medication (including 3-mg melatonin) had not resulted in better sleep. Baseline observations revealed that her sleep schedule was inconsistent. Her bedtime varied between 8 p.m. and 12 a.m., and her wake-up time varied between 3 a.m. and 9:30 a.m. She showed bedtime tantrums and frequent night waking (most often between 2:30 a.m. and 3:45 a.m.) after which she climbed into the parents' bed. Sleep restriction involved reducing the number of hours of sleep (to 90% of the total sleep time) while maintaining a consistent bedtime and awake time. The sleep restriction program for this child started with moving her bedtime to midnight and holding her wake-up time at 7 a.m. Once the strategy was successful, the amount of sleep was faded back to an age-appropriate level. Data were collected within a multiple baseline design across participants. Results showed that sleep restriction eliminated bedtime disturbances and markedly reduced night wakening in both girls.

Christodulu and Durand (2004) investigated effectiveness of sleep restriction on the sleep problems of four developmentally disabled children aged between 2 and

5 years of whom two had ASD. In two children, establishing stimulus control was evaluated in the treatment of their bedtime disturbances and night waking. Parents were instructed to follow a fixed routine 30 min prior to bedtime. They were also instructed to return the child in bed if the child were to come out of bed. Results showed that establishing stimulus control alone was ineffective in reducing sleep problems in both children. Then, sleep restriction was implemented for all four children, and intervention began by restricting the amount of time in bed to 90% of the total amount of time that the children slept. Sleep diaries were used to estimate this total sleep time, and data were collected within a multiple baseline design across children. Results showed that bedtime routines plus sleep restriction resulted in (near-)zero levels of bedtime disturbances and a reduced frequency in night waking in all children and the effects were maintained at a 6-week follow-up.

Conclusions

Several treatment approaches have been developed in which the sleep–wake pattern of the individual is addressed. Due to a small number of studies, sleep restriction lacks sufficient evidence.

Alternative Therapies

Effectiveness of valerian was evaluated by Francis and Dempster (2002) in five boys who were between 7 and 14 years old and who had ID. Medical causes for their severe sleep problems were ruled out. Following baseline, children were randomly assigned to valerian and placebo conditions. Valerian tablets contained 500 mg (100%) of dried and crushed whole root from *Valeriana edulis* plants. Each tablet contained 5.5 mg of valtrate/isovaltrate. During treatment, parents administered a dosage of 20 mg/kg body weight to their child, in a single nightly dose at least 1 hr before preferred bedtime. After 2 weeks, valerian resulted in a statistically significant decrease in sleep latency and nighttime waking as well as in an increase in total sleep time. No significant changes were found for placebo.

Conclusions

To date, only few studies have appeared on the effectiveness of alternative therapies for sleep problems in individuals with ID. Valerian lacks sufficient evidence.

Guidelines

Treatment of sleep problems should be tailored to the needs of the individual with ID, the type of sleep problem, and causal medical and environmental conditions. Treatment starts with a sleep history and recording of sleep–wake schedule and problematic behaviors. Sleep diaries and questionnaires provide much information on 24-hr sleep–wake schedule as well as on important sleep parameters such as sleep onset latency, frequency and time of night waking, and bedtime routines. To this purpose, Maas et al. (2011) used the Simonds and Parraga questionnaire (SQ-SP) that appears to be a reliable and valid tool in assessing sleep and different types of sleep disturbance in individuals with ID. Additional data may be collected through actigraphy, audiovisual recordings, and/or polysomnography (see Wiggs, 2007).

Sleep problems may be caused by a variety of medical and environmental conditions which should be assessed and treated. Common examples of medical conditions are epilepsy and gastroesophageal reflux. Also, melatonin synthesis should be assessed by measuring DLMO prior to prescribing exogenous melatonin, and dosage and timing of exogenous melatonin should be based on DLMO. Loss of response to melatonin may indicate poor metabolization of exogenous melatonin and should be dealt with accordingly (see Braam et al., 2010).

Assessing and changing sleep hygiene is an important step in the treatment of sleep problems in individuals with ID. Insufficient sleep hygiene may increase the likelihood of the development of a sleep problem. Jan et al. (2008) define sleep hygiene as "a set of sleep-related behaviors that expose persons to activities and cues that prepare them for and promote appropriately timed and effective sleep" (p. 1344). They distinguish between four groups of sleep hygiene activities and cues: (a) environmental (e.g., temperature, noise level), (b) scheduling (e.g., regular sleep–wake pattern), (c) sleep practice (e.g., bedtime routines), and (d) physiologic (e.g., exercise, caffeine use, medication). Appropriate sleep hygiene practice may function as stimulus control for appropriate sleep onset and may help the individual to entrain the circadian rhythm to the 24-hr light/dark cycle. Although sleep hygiene measures may be insufficiently effective in themselves in the treatment of a sleep problem, they should always be incorporated in an intervention for sleep disorders in individuals with ID. Jan et al. provide guidelines for implementing sleep hygiene practices in a variety of settings.

Behavioral strategies are effective in the treatment of sleep problems in individuals with ID. An important element in implementing behavioral strategies is conducting a pretreatment functional assessment of the (challenging) behaviors that are incompatible with sleep (see Didden & Sigafoos, 2001). During functional assessment, antecedent and consequent stimuli of problematic behaviors are recorded by caregivers and replaced by behaviors that facilitate sleep onset. In an experimental functional analysis, stimuli are manipulated to identify items that maintain problematic behaviors (see O'Reilly et al., 2004).

Extinction is probably the best studied approach for sleep problems in individuals with ID. It should be noted that this strategy is effective only if problematic sleep behaviors are maintained by attention from caregivers. Extinction is associated with the occurrence of an extinction burst, that is, temporary increase in the frequency of problematic behaviors such as crying, tantrums, calling out, and getting out of bed. An extinction burst means that the extinction procedure is effective, not ineffective.

Didden et al. (2010) have provided guidelines for the implementation of extinction as treatment for sleep problems in individuals with ID.

References

American Academy of Sleep Medicine. (2005). *International classification of sleep disorders: Diagnostic and coding manual* (2nd ed.). Westchester, IL: American Academy of Sleep Medicine.

Braam, W., Didden, R., Smits, M., & Curfs, L. (2008a). Melatonin treatment in individuals with intellectual disability and chronic insomnia: A randomized placebo-controlled study. *Journal of Intellectual Disability Research, 52*, 256–264.

Braam, W., Didden, R., Smits, M., & Curfs, L. (2008b). Melatonin for insomniac children with Angelman syndrome: A randomized placebo-controlled double-blind study. *Journal of Child Neurology, 23*, 649–654.

Braam, W., Smits, M., Didden, R., Korzilius, H., Van Geijlswijk, I., & Curfs, L. (2009). Exogenous melatonin for sleep problems in persons with intellectual disability: A meta-analysis. *Developmental Medicine and Child Neurology, 51*, 340–349.

Braam, W., Van Geijlswijk, I., Keijzer, H., Smits, M., Didden, R., & Curfs, L. (2010). Loss of response to melatonin treatment is associated with slow melatonin metabolism: A pilot study. *Journal of Intellectual Disability Research, 54*, 547–555.

Chambless, D. L., & Hollon, S. D. (1998). Defining empirically supported therapies. *Journal of Consulting and Clinical Psychology, 66*, 7–18.

Christodulu, K. V., & Durand, V. M. (2004). Reducing bedtime disturbance and night waking using positive bedtime routines and sleep restriction. *Focus on Autism and Other Developmental Disabilities, 19*, 130–139.

Cotton, S., & Richdale, A. (2010). Sleep patterns and behaviour in typically developing children and children with autism, Down syndrome, Prader-Willi syndrome and intellectual disability. *Research in Autism Spectrum Disorders, 4*, 490–500.

Didden, R., Curfs, L., van Driel, S., & de Moor, J. (2002). Sleep problems in children with developmental disabilities: Home-based functional assessment and treatment. *Journal of Behavior Therapy and Experimental Psychiatry, 33*, 49–58.

Didden, R., Korzilius, H., van Aperlo, B., van Overloop, C., & de Vries, M. (2002). Sleep problems and daytime problem behavior in children with developmental disabilities. *Journal of Intellectual Disability Research, 46*, 537–547.

Didden, R., & Sigafoos, J. (2001). A review of the nature and treatment of sleep problems in individuals with developmental disabilities. *Research in Developmental Disabilities, 22*, 255–272.

Didden, R., Sigafoos, J., & Lancioni, G. (2010). Unmodified extinction for childhood sleep disturbance. In M. Perlis, M. Aloia, & B. Kuhn (Eds.), *Behavioral treatments for sleep disorders: A comprehensive primer of behavioral sleep medicine treatment protocols* (pp. 257–263). London: Academic Press.

Durand, V. M., & Christodulu, K. V. (2004). Description of a sleep-restriction program to reduce bedtime disturbances and night waking. *Journal of Positive Behavior Interventions, 6*, 83–91.

Durand, V. M., Gernert-Dott, P., & Mapstone, E. (1996). Treatment of sleep disorders in children with developmental disabilities. *Journal of the Association for Persons with Severe Handicaps, 21*, 114–122.

Francis, A. J., & Dempster, R. J. (2002). Effects of valerian, *Valeriana edulis*, on sleep difficulties in children with intellectual deficits: Randomised trial. *Phytomedicine, 9*, 273–279.

Gunning, M., & Espie, C. (2003). Psychological treatment of reported sleep disorder in adults with intellectual disability using a multiple baseline design. *Journal of Intellectual Disability Research, 47*, 191–202.

Jan, J., Owens, J., Weiss, M., Johnson, K., Wasdell, M., Freeman, R., et al. (2008). Sleep hygiene for children with neurodevelopmental disabilities. *Pediatrics, 122*, 1343–1350.

Lenjavi, M., Ahuja, M., Touchette, P., & Sandman, C. (2010). Maladaptive behaviors are linked with inefficient sleep in individuals with developmental disabilities. *Journal of Neurodevelopmental Disorders, 2*, 174–180.

Maas, A., Didden, R., Korzilius, H., Braam, W., Collin, P., Smits, M., et al. (2011). Psychometric properties of a sleep questionnaire for use in individuals with intellectual disabilities. *Research in Developmental Disabilities, 32*, 2467–2479.

Montgomery, P., Stores, G., & Wiggs, L. (2004). The relative efficacy of two brief treatments for sleep problems in young learning disabled (mentally retarded) children: A randomised controlled trial. *Archives of Disease in Childhood, 89*, 125–130.

O'Reilly, M., Lancioni, G., & Sigafoos, J. (2004). Using paired-choice assessment to identify variables maintaining sleep problems in a child with severe disabilities. *Journal of Applied Behavior Analysis, 37*, 209–212.

Piazza, C., & Fisher, W. (1991). A faded bedtime with response cost protocol for treatment of multiple sleep problems in children. *Journal of Applied Behavior Analysis, 24*, 129–140.

Piazza, C., Fisher, W., & Moser, H. (1991). Behavioral treatment of sleep dysfunction in patients with the Rett syndrome. *Brain & Development, 13*, 232–237.

Piazza, C., Fisher, W., & Sherer, M. (1997). Treatment of multiple sleep problems in children with developmental disabilities: Faded bedtime with response cost versus bedtime scheduling. *Developmental Medicine and Child Neurology, 39*, 414–418.

Richdale, A., Gavidia-Payne, S., Francis, A., & Cotton, S. (2000). Stress, behaviour and sleep problems in children with an intellectual disability. *Journal of Intellectual and Developmental Disability, 25*, 147–161.

Richdale, A., & Wiggs, L. (2005). Behavioral approaches to the treatment of sleep problems in children with developmental disabilities: What is the state of the art? *International Journal of Behavioral and Consultation Therapy, 1*, 165–189.

Schreck, K., Mulick, J., & Smith, A. (2004). Sleep problems as possible predictors of intensified symptoms of autism. *Research in Developmental Disabilities, 25*, 57–66.

Thackeray, E. J., & Richdale, A. L. (2002). The behavioural treatment of sleep difficulties in children with an intellectual disability. *Behavioral Interventions, 17*, 211–231.

Van de Wouw, E., Evenhuis, H., & Echteld, M. (2012). Prevalence, associated factors and treatment of sleep problems in adults with intellectual disability: A systematic review. *Research in Developmental Disabilities, 33*, 1310–1332.

Wasdell, M. B., Jan, J. E., Bomben, M. M., Freeman, R. D., Rietveld, W. J., Tai, J., et al. (2008). A randomized, placebo controlled trial of controlled release melatonin treatment of delayed sleep phase syndrome and impaired sleep maintenance in children with neurodevelopmental disabilities. *Journal of Pineal Research, 44*, 57–64.

Weiskop, S., Richdale, A., & Matthews, J. (2005). Behavioural treatment to reduce sleep problems in children with autism or fragile X syndrome. *Developmental Medicine and Child Neurology, 47*, 94–104.

Wiggs, L. (2007). Sleep disorders. In A. Carr, G. O'Reilly, P. Noonan Walsh, & J. McEvoy (Eds.), *The handbook of intellectual disability and clinical psychology practice* (pp. 371–421). Hove, East Sussex: Routledge.

Wiggs, L., & Stores, G. (1998). Behavioural treatment for sleep problems in children with severe learning disabilities and challenging daytime behaviour: Effect on sleep pattern of mother and child. *Journal of Sleep Research, 7*, 119–126.

Wiggs, L., & Stores, G. (2001). Behavioural treatment for sleep problems in children with severe intellectual disabilities and daytime challenging behaviour: Effect on mothers and fathers. *British Journal of Health Psychology, 6*, 257–269.

10

Anxiety Disorders

Peter Sturmey, William R. Lindsay, Tricia Vause, and Nicole Neil

Overview

The Diagnostic and Statistical Manual of the American Psychiatric Associations (4th edition, text revision) (DSM-IV-TR; American Psychiatric Association [APA], 2000) lists the following anxiety disorders: panic disorder without agoraphobia, panic disorder with agoraphobia, agoraphobia without a history of agoraphobia, specific phobia, obsessive–compulsive disorder (OCD), posttraumatic stress disorder (PTSD), acute stress disorder, generalized anxiety disorder (GAD), anxiety disorder due to a medical condition, substance-induced anxiety disorder, and anxiety disorder not otherwise specified. Although DSM-IV-TR does not provide a general description of anxiety disorders, its descriptions of them often note anxiety symptoms such as palpitations; tremors; sweating; shortness of breath; feeling choking; chest pain or discomfort; nausea, gastrointestinal discomfort, or diarrhea; dizziness; derealization; fear of loss of control, going crazy, or dying; paresthesia, cold, and hot flushes (p. 395); muscle tension; blushing; and confusion (p. 412). Anxiety disorders are often also characterized by fear that is out of proportion to the objective threat and avoidance of feared situations. DSM-IV-TR's diagnostic criteria also note that the problem must be persistent, "clinically significant," often marked by insight as unreasonable and not better accounted for by other disorders, such as mood or pervasive developmental disorders. Broadly similar criteria for anxiety disorders can be found in the *International Classification of Diseases* (10th edition) (World Health Organisation, 2007).

Evidence-Based Practice and Intellectual Disabilities, First Edition.
Edited by Peter Sturmey and Robert Didden.
© 2014 John Wiley & Sons, Ltd. Published 2014 by John Wiley & Sons, Ltd.

Anxiety disorders are the most prevalent type of psychiatric disorders in general populations. For example, some studies have found a lifetime incidence of 29% and a 12-month incidence of around 18% (Hofman & Smits, 2008). Single anxiety disorders also have a high prevalence. For example, Wittchen, Zhao, Kessler, and Eaton (1994) found a lifetime prevalence of 5.1% and a 12-month prevalence of 3.1% for GAD; women were twice as likely to meet diagnostic criteria as men.

Cognitive behavioral therapy (CBT) is the prototypical psychological treatment for anxiety disorders which is characterized by teaching the so-called coping skills which include both cognitive and behavioral techniques that can counteract anxiety and are often related to relevant situations, such as those inducing anxiety. The person is encouraged to understand personal triggers and patterns of thought, behavior, and emotion (feelings) that may underpin the disorder and, subsequently, develop techniques for reacting to these triggers with appropriate cognitive, behavioral, and emotional techniques to cope with the incapacitating symptoms. For example, Beck and Emery (1979) developed a brief CBT for anxiety that included the exploration of underlying beliefs, examination and analysis of anxiety-related self-statements and automatic thoughts, challenging these cognitions and reviewing errors in thinking, rehearsal and imagination, homework assignments and reviewing the relationship between the underlying beliefs and self-statements to the patient's generalized anxiety and behavior. Two early evaluations of this treatment found that combined with relaxation, this approach was consistently more effective than relaxation approaches alone and a no-treatment control (Lindsay, Gamsu, McLaughlin, Hood, & Espie, 1987; Woodward & Jones, 1980).

Because there have been so many control group studies of CBT for anxiety disorders in nondisabled populations, there are a number of meta-analyses of CBT compared with a range of placebo, drug treatments, and no-treatment controls. Hofman and Smits (2008), for example, conducted a meta-analysis of randomized placebo control trials which included only studies with placebo psychotherapy and a randomization design. Twenty-seven studies fulfilled their criteria, of which 25 provided completer data for continuous measures of anxiety disorder severity with 1,496 participants. Anxiety disorders included social anxiety disorder, PTSD, panic disorder, acute stress disorder, OCD, and GAD. They found medium to large effect sizes (mean Hedges' $d = 0.73$ for anxiety measures). In a second meta-analysis of 11 studies combining pharmacology and CBT for anxiety disorders, Hofman, Sawyer, Korte, and Smits (2009) found that CBT plus pharmacology was generally more effective than CBT plus a placebo (Hedges' $g = 0.59$), although the enhanced effects of pharmacology were no longer evident at 6-month follow-up. With 27 studies fulfilling the criteria of randomized design and placebo control, this meta-analysis supports CBT as a *well-established* treatment for all disorders except panic disorder. Other meta-analyses have also supported the conclusion that CBT is a well-established treatment for a variety of anxiety disorders including GAD (Hunot et al., 2007) and when CBT was compared to other psychological treatments such as psychological placebo and psychodynamic therapy conditions (Borkovec & Ruscio,

2001). The extent of the evidence prompted the National Institute for Clinical Excellence (2011) in the United Kingdom to recommend CBT as a first-line treatment for anxiety disorders. Thus, there is now little doubt that CBT is effective in reducing anxiety symptoms in a range of related emotional disorders and fulfils the criteria for a well-established treatment.

Anxiety Disorders in People with Intellectual Disabilities

Epidemiology

Many of the early studies investigating mental health disorders in people with intellectual disabilities (ID) were conducted in large hospitals. For example, Penrose (1938), in a study of 1,280 people with ID living in an institution, reported a prevalence of 1.9% of affective disorders. Some contemporary research has separated specific anxiety diagnoses. For example, in a study of 101 adults, Deb, Thomas, and Bright (2001) used a number of structured psychiatric assessments and, depending on the assessment, found that up to 7.8% of participants showed an anxiety disorder. Cooper and Bailey (2001) reported on 207 individuals with ID and found a prevalence of 7.2% with anxiety disorder. In a third large-scale study of 1,023 individuals, Cooper, Smiley, Morrison, Williamson, and Allan (2007) found a point prevalence of 3.8% for anxiety disorders. Thus, these three studies are consistent with those reported in the general population at between 4% and 8%.

Assessment

Hagopian and Jennett (2008) suggested a number of approaches to assessing anxiety disorders in people with ID including direct observation, self-report of emotional and anxiety sensations, and physiological monitoring. In their studies on the effectiveness of relaxation treatments in reducing anxiety and agitation in people with severe ID, Lindsay and Baty (1986a, 1986b) assessed anxiety using behavioral observation checklist and physiological arousal by taking heart rate before and after treatment. Others have evaluated the results of relaxation treatment by monitoring the number of aggressive responses by participants (McPhail & Chamov, 1989; Steen & Zurrif, 1977). Since some people with ID have difficulty completing self-report assessments of anxiety as they have more impoverished comprehension and reading skills, it may be necessary to read items to participants and to simplify and otherwise modify items. These alterations mean that it may be necessary to conduct further standardization of the adaptive assessment to ensure that it continues to measure the relevant attribute in a reliable and valid fashion.

Fears and Phobias

Behavioral interventions

Definitions and characteristics of behavioral interventions

There are a wide range of behavioral interventions to treat anxiety and fear in people with developmental disabilities. One of the earliest and most commonly used behavioral interventions for anxiety disorders in people with developmental disabilities was various methods of relaxation training (Luiselli, 1980). One of the most common is Jacobsonian relaxation, in which the person tenses, holds, and relaxes major muscle group and focuses attention on the sensation of tension and relaxation. Other forms of relaxation used with people with developmental disabilities include abbreviated progressive muscle relaxation (APMR), EMG biofeedback (Schroeder, Peterson, Solomon, & Artley, 1977), and behavioral relaxation training (BRT) in which the therapist models relaxed and unrelaxed postures, instructs and manually prompts relaxed postures, and reinforces adoption of relaxed postures (Lindsay & Baty, 1986b; Schilling & Poppen, 1983).

Luiselli (1980) distinguished three ways relaxation can be used: First, it can be used as a setting event in which the client learns to relax before confronting an anxiety-provoking situation. Second, it can be used as response-independent cueing in which the client learns to relax in response to a covert self-instruction instruction, such as saying "relax," "quite," or "still" to oneself (Lindsay, Michie, Baty, & Smith, 1994). Finally, response-dependent cueing involves the client emitting a relaxation response following a change in behavior, such as the client's hands shaking.

Relaxation has usually been administered individually but has also been used in groups (Lindsay, Neilsen, & Lawrenson, 1999). Relaxation is a part of several important treatments for fears and phobias including systematic desensitization and covert sensitization and is sometimes used to treat problem behavior, such as agitation (Lindsay & Baty, 1986a), aggression (Lindsay et al., 1994), disruptive behavior (McPhail & Chamv, 1989), and self-injury (Steen & Zuriff, 1977), and psychophysiological problems, such as seizure disorders (Wells, Turner, Bellack, & Hersen, 1978), by interrupting response chains early or providing the opportunity for incompatible behavior. Thus, various forms of relaxation have been commonly used in behavioral interventions in a variety of manners for fear and anxiety in people with developmental disabilities.

Relaxation is not the only behavioral intervention used for fears and phobias. Jennett and Hagopian's (2008) systematic review of behavioral treatment of phobic avoidance noted that every paper they reviewed used treatment packages of 3–6 treatment components. All papers included in vivo exposure and reinforcement for exposure or some form of appropriate behavior. Other treatment components included prompting, modeling, a stimulus hierarchy, distraction, and extinction. Confusingly, each paper used their own idiosyncratic terminology, such as "participant modeling" or "operant-based procedures" which, by themselves, are imprecise. Jennett and Hagopian demonstrated that these imprecise labels could be analyzed into their component behavioral strategies, thereby facilitating comparisons across papers.

Search strategies
In order to identify randomized controlled trials (RCTs) of psychological treatment of anxiety disorders, the first author conducted 6 searches of PubMed© using the terms "mental retardation," "developmental disabilities," "intellectual disabilities," "mental deficiency," and "Autism," each crossed with the terms "(randomized controlled trial) AND (anxiety OR phobia)." These searches yielded 141 nonunique abstracts. Papers which evaluated nonpsychological treatments, such as psychotropic medications, hormone treatments, and other biomedical procedures, and papers which did not include people with developmental disabilities, such as those which evaluated treatment of anxiety and phobias in parents of people with developmental disabilities, were excluded. This yielded 13 unique potentially relevant papers. One was excluded because it was a description of a trial that had not yet been conducted (Hassiotis et al., 2011), and one was excluded because it only reported the effects on parental anxiety (Tonge et al., 2006). In order to update the results of Jennett and Hagopian (2007), an additional search of PubMed was conducted using the same search terms. This search yielded 2,676 abstracts. Since Hagopian and Jennett search until February 2007, we searched back to 2006, reviewing 1,220 abstracts of which 36 were potentially relevant. Of those 36 abstracts, 32 were excluded from the section on behavioral interventions because they used interventions other than BT, such as CBT, pharmacology, acceptance and commitment therapy (ACT), narrative therapy, and Tai massage, or were not experiments. (Some of these studies excluded from this section are discussed in other sections to follow.) Of the remaining four papers, only one was an experimental evaluation of behavioral treatment, although one paper used predominantly behavioral interventions as well as some cognitive treatments (Davis, Kurtz, Gardner, & Carman, 2007) and one reported a series of nonexperimental AB designs of behavioral treatment of compliance with encephalographic series (Slifer, Avis, & Frutchlet, 2008). An additional search of the abstracts of the *Journal of Applied Behavior Analysis* using the terms "fear" and "phobia" also revealed no relevant publications since 2006. Finally, a review of the references section of a recent review of anxiety disorders in people with developmental disabilities (Dagnan, 2001; Davis et al., 2007) did not yield any new references or systematic reviews. This, in combination with the updated searched, suggested that there was little or no new experimental studies or systematic reviews since Jennett and Hagopian (2008). Therefore, the following sections are based primarily on the two systematic reviews by Luiselli (1980) and Jennett and Hagopian (2008).

Systematic reviews
Luiselli (1980) reviewed relaxation training for people with developmental disabilities and identified 12 empirical studies. He then coded these studies to indicate which used experimental designs and confirmed that relaxation training

Table 10.1   A Summary of Evidence-Based Practice for
Behavioral Treatment of Fears and Phobias

Intervention	Status of evidence
Relaxation alone	Ineffective
Behavioral packages	Efficacious
ACT	Unevaluated
DSP	Ineffective
In vivo exposure > modeling	Possibly efficacious
APT > BRT	Possibly efficacious
Systematic desensitization	Unevaluated

resulted in relaxed behavior and whether participants had developmental disabilities. Additionally, he noted whether the experimental design was good enough to confirm that behavior change was due to relaxation and not other treatment elements or artifacts. For example, a relaxation procedure might include confounds, such as response interruption; changes of environment, such as going somewhere to relax that might function as time-out; and engaging in other behavior, such as closing one's eyes, which might also effect fearful or phobic behavior independently of relaxation itself.

Of the 12 studies, only two studies had adequate control procedures; however, Luiselli's Table 10.1 indicated that neither of these studies measured whether relaxation training resulted in relaxation occurring. Thus, this review did not find evidence that relaxation training alone was an evidence-based practice for people with developmental disabilities. It is also worth noting that Jennett and Hagopian (2008) did not identify any new reports of relaxation training for fears and phobias in people with developmental disabilities.

Luiselli's paper had a number of positive features that can guide other systematic reviews of treatment of anxiety. Namely, to conclude that relaxation caused a change in behavior, one must demonstrate that clients did indeed relax, that an experimental design was used, and that adequate controls were used to demonstrate that relaxation alone and no other confound was responsible for the observed change.

A second systematic review comes from Jennett and Hagopian (2008) who conducted a systematic search of PsycINFO and PubMed from 1970 through February 2007 using the terms "mental retardation," "intellectual disability" "developmental disability," "autism," or "autistic disorder," crossed with "avoidance behavior," "avoidance," "anxiety," "anxiety disorder," "anxious," "phobia," "phobic," or "fear." They included articles which evaluated psychological treatments of avoidance behavior and excluded medication studies. They also hand searched the references of articles that they initially selected. These searches yielded 38 articles, of which 4 were group studies, 13 were small *N* experiments, and 21 were nonexperiments. They then coded the articles for both participant and treatment characteristics. Coding reliability was 100% for group studies and 91% (range 83–97%) for small *N* experiments.

They retained 12 of the 13 small N experiments which all met minimum experimental design criteria including demonstration of experimental control, treatment superior to baseline with replication, attaining 90% of the treatment goal (e.g., completing 9 of 10 steps of an exposure hierarchy), treatment manual or equivalent treatment description, adequate description of participant characteristics, and interobserver agreement. These articles were published between 1981 and 2006. Half of participants were adults and half were children and adolescents. Sixty-eight percent of participants were male; 71% had a primary diagnosis of ID and 29% had a primary diagnosis of autism. Seven percent, 21%, 39%, 21%, and 11% had mild, moderate, severe, profound, and unspecified ID. Forty-two percent of studies were conducted in community settings, 25% took place in inpatient settings, 17% in home settings, and 17% in other settings. Intervention was most commonly provided by the authors of the articles (42%), only 25% were conducted by parents or teachers, and one third of the studies did not identify the change agent. The phobic stimuli addressed included water, dogs, strangers, animatronic figures, medical and dental procedures, riding escalators, and climbing stairs. There were a wide array of target behaviors including crying, screaming, physical resistance, and running away, which, in all but one case, were assessed with direct observation. No studies included physiological or verbal-cognitive-dependent variables, and only two studies used subjective ratings of fear. All studies used multiple treatment components (range 3–6 treatment components), but every study used in vivo exposure and reinforcement procedures. Other treatments included prompting (8 studies), modeling (7 studies), stimulus hierarchy (8 studies), distraction (4 studies), and extinction (2 studies). No interventions involved cognitions, psychodynamic concepts, or physiological states.

Of the four group designs, only Peck (1977) included a placebo control group with randomization. This study compared three types of desensitization with a placebo-attention control group with adults with rat or height phobia in adults with mild ID. There were no differences between the groups after treatment, perhaps due to the lack of experimental power, since there were only 20 participants in the entire study. Of the remaining three group studies, one failed to randomize participants (Altabet, 2002), but two (Matson, 1981; Obler & Terwillliger, 1970) did randomize, but only used no-treatment control groups. Thus, Jennett and Hagopian concluded that there was no evidence from RCTs relating to the effectiveness of behavioral treatment for phobias.

The 13 small N experiments contained 28 participants conducted by many independent researches. Twelve of 13 of the experiments had good experimental designs, and all 13 experiments demonstrated that treatment was superior to baseline. Further, this was a robust finding for many different kinds of phobias and participant characteristics. Thus, the authors concluded that "there is empirical sufficient support to characterize behavioural treatment as a well-established treatment for phobic avoidance displayed by in individuals with intellectual disabilities" (p. 158). Since, in contrast to the literature with other populations, there were no studies evaluating CBT and systematic desensitization, these were rated as "experimental treatments." Finally, they noted that all studies used in vivo exposure and reinforcement procedures and speculated that the two treatment components might be the effective components of behavioral packages to treat avoidance.

This study is impressive in that it systematically reviewed treatment of phobias in people with developmental disabilities; however, several limitations should be noted. For example, the authors did not calculate effect sizes, which perhaps may have shed light on the different effect sizes for different treatment procedures. A limitation that is worth noting is that this literature focused on simple phobias, rather than complex phobias, such as agoraphobia, panic disorder, and GAD. Thus, there is no evidence at this time that behavioral treatments are effective for these problems with people with developmental disabilities.

Heterosexual dating skills training.   The searches did identify one additional group design experiment using behavioral methods that included anxiety as a dependent variable. Valenti-Hein, Yarnold, and Mueser (1994) evaluated a heterosexual dating skills program (DSP) for 29 adults with "borderline" to moderate ID. The authors randomly assigned participants to either DSP or a wait list control (WLC). Twenty-six of 29 participants took part and completed the treatment. There were no differences between the groups on demographic variables, social anxiety, and social/sexual knowledge at baseline, and at posttraining, there was no statistically significant difference between the groups on social anxiety.

This trial had potential problems concerning treatment integrity since, although there was a treatment manual (Valenti-Hein & Muesser, 1990), the authors did not measure treatment integrity. There was some evidence of treatment nonadherence in that (a) one participant's data was dropped because this person attended less than half of the sessions, (b) no additional data on treatment attendance was provided for other participants, and (c) there were between 0 and 8 missing data points per participant, but further details were not provided. Hence, there is no evidence that DSP reduces social anxiety in people with developmental disabilities at this time.

Acceptance and commitment therapy.   The earlier searches identified one non-experimental case study on the application of ACT to anxious and obsessive thoughts in one person with ID (Brown & Hooper, 2009). Since there is no experimental evaluation of ACT for anxiety in people with developmental disabilities, ACT is not an evidence-based practice.

Treatment comparisons.   Only two studies compared two or more treatments. First, Lindsay, Baty, Michie, and Richardson (1989) compared BRT and APR in group and individual formats against a no-treatment control. Participants had a moderate and severe ID. Measures were taken before, midway, immediately after treatment, and at 3-week follow-up. There were 10 participants in each of the 5 groups who received 12 treatment sessions, 4 per week. They were assessed using a behavioral rating scale and pulse rate. There were improvements on the behavioral rating scale for all conditions when compared to the control group, but BRT produced significantly greater reductions in anxiety than APR, although this difference was not observed on pulse rate. There were no differences between group and individual treatment formats. Thus, this experiment provides some evidence that BRT is a more effective treatment than APR.

A second experiment that compared two treatments comes from Conyers et al. (2004) who compared in vivo desensitization with modeling in the treatment of dental phobias in six adults with severe and profound ID living in group homes. All participants required sedation before dental treatment, and four required mechanical restraints during dental treatment. All participated in in vivo desensitization, and three also participated in video modeling before in vivo desensitization. The authors used a multiple baseline design across participants to demonstrate experimental control. Modelling resulted in the participants completing all 18 steps of the task analysis in only 1 of 3 participants; however, in vivo desensitization resulted in 5 of 5 participants completing all 18 steps of the task analysis both in role-play treatment sessions and in generalization sessions with the actual dentist. Thus, this study provided some evidence that in vivo desensitization is superior to modeling. These findings are also consonant with Jennett and Hagopian's (2008) observation that all 13 experimental studies used in vivo exposure and reinforcement, whereas only 7 used modeling, again demonstrating that modeling is often not an essential component of effective treatment of fears and phobias.

These two studies suggest that BRT and in vivo exposure are more effective than some other behavioral treatments. Since these observations are only based on single studies in each case, these results require independent replication.

Evidence-based behavioral treatment for fear and phobias. Table 10.1 provides a summary of the evidence considered in this section. The first behavioral treatment considered was relaxation. Luiselli (1980) did not find two or more well-conducted group designs or 3 or more small *N* experiments with 9 or more participants. Further, Jennett and Hagopian (2008) and our own subsequent searches did not find any experimental evidence that relaxation alone was an effective treatment for fears and phobias. Therefore, we conclude that relaxation alone is *ineffective* for treatment of fears and phobias. In contrast, Jennett and Hagopian found that behavioral packages that all included in vivo exposure, reinforcement, and other treatment strategies were uniformly effective irrespective of the type of phobia, the client characteristics, the person who conducted the treatment (therapist, teacher, or parent), and the setting (community vs. institutional). Therefore, behavioral packages are an *efficacious* treatment for fears and phobias. Only one poor-quality RCT evaluated the effects of DSP on anxiety, and it found no effects on anxiety. Therefore, DSP is an *ineffective* treatment for anxiety. Likewise, since there was only one nonexperimental case study of ACT. ACT is also not an evidence-based practice for anxiety disorder for people with developmental disabilities. Finally, two experiments compared one behavioral treatment with another, and these studies reported evidence that in vivo exposure was superior to modeling and that BRT was superior to APR; however, since there was only one experiment for each of these comparisons, these differences must be considered only *possibly efficacious*.

Although this literature strongly supports the effectiveness of behavioral packages in treating phobias, several significant limitations should be noted that can usefully direct future research. First, the range of fears and phobias addressed was limited to specific phobias, but did not address panic disorder, agoraphobia, GAD, and PTSD. Thus, future research might usefully evaluate extending the application of behavioral packages that include in vivo exposure and reinforcement to other disorders. Second, although there were several papers that used teachers and parents to conduct behavioral packages, the paper did not operationalize how to train change agents and did not clearly show a functional relationship between the behavior of change agents and client behavior. Third, studies tended to report measures of reduction in phobic behavior, rather than increases in adaptive behavior. This, although some studies reported approach data, such as the number of steps completed on a task analysis (e.g., Conyers et al., 2004) on studies, reported data on assertive behavior, positive verbal behavior, and positive affect even though such behavioral changes are commonly observed. Finally, no studies reported pretreatment functional analyses of behavior. A few models for this exist. Indeed, pretreatment functional analyses have provided surprising and important information to guide treatment of phobias that may not be apparent from other assessment methods (e.g., Jones & Friman, 1999). Thus, given the effectiveness of functional assessment and analyses in enhancing treatment efficacy for a wide range of other problems (Didden, Ducker, & Korzelius, 1997), future research on this topic should also conduct functional assessment and analyses.

Cognitive and cognitive behavioral therapy

Overview
Much work has been done on adapting CBT for the treatment of anxiety disorders in people with ID including simplifying ones language and use of Socratic or inductive methods to guide therapist and client in the task of collaborative enquiry. Rather than presenting a large amount of didactic information to convey cognitive therapy concepts, Socratic dialogue allows the therapist to develop a series of questions that lead patients to the appropriate information. By helping to generate the information through guided discovery, clients may be more likely to consider that they have ownership of the content of the session thereby retaining the essential principles and components of CBT and procedures are maintained as far as possible (Jahoda, Dagnan, Stenfert Kroese, Pert, & Trower, 2009).

Several nonexperimental studies have been reported in the literature. For example, a book chapter by Lindsay, Neilson, and Lawrenson (1999) and Lindsay (1986) reported a case series of 15 individuals with anxiety all of whom were assessed on a revised version of the Beck Anxiety Inventory and the Zung Anxiety Scale (ZAS).

Treatment lasted an average of 23 sessions with a range of 15 to 47 sessions. CBT included cognitive strategies, such as isolating negative thoughts, eliciting underlying assumptions, testing the accuracy of cognitions, and generating alternate cognitions, as well as behavioral strategies, such as self-monitoring, role-playing anxiety-provoking situations (which also included rehearsal of alternate cognitions), and homework assignments to practice both cognitive and behavioral strategies in relevant settings. Lindsay transformed the Beck Anxiety Inventory and ZAS scores into percentages of the total scale. The total anxiety score fell from an average of 82% items at baseline to 39% of total items following treatment which was both statistically significant and maintained to 6-month follow-up. Thus, CBT can be adapted and applied to anxiety disorders.

Search strategies.   The terms (mental retardation OR intellectual disabilities) AND (cognitive therapy OR cognitive behavior therapy) AND (anxiety OR phobia OR fear) were used to search PubMed and Google Scholar on June 14, 2011. The first search returned 44 abstracts of which none were related to CBT and anxiety disorders in people with ID. A review of the first 200 abstracts of the search on Google Scholar revealed no experimental studies of CBT and anxiety disorders in people with ID.

The systematic searches conducted for behavioral treatments of anxiety disorders identified two systematic reviews of CBT and people with developmental disabilities. The first came from Lang, Regester, Lauderdale, Ashbaugh, and Haring (2010) who conducted a systematic review of CBT for anxiety in people with autism spectrum disorders (ASDs). A systematic search of PsycINFO, ERIC, and MEDLINE identified 164 potential studies. To be retained, studies had to evaluate CBT and include at least one participant with autism, Asperger syndrome, or pervasive developmental disorder not otherwise specified (PDD-NOS). Nine were retained. Studies that did not use CBT interventions, such as those that used only behavioral interventions, and that did not address anxiety, such as studies of self-injury, were excluded. These studies had 110 participants with ASD, 60% were male, and their ages ranged from 9 to 23 years. Most (67%) were diagnosed with Asperger syndrome; of the 20 (18%) diagnosed with autism, 9 were described as "high-functioning autism" and only 15% were diagnosed with PDD-NOS. Phobias included social phobias, OCD, and a range of other anxiety disorders. Dependent variables included self and other ratings and psychometric measures of psychopathology and adaptive behavior.

Lang et al. concluded that five studies were "suggestive" of treatment efficacy since they were nonexperimental. They classified three studies as providing evidence at the level of "preponderance level of certainty" since they were experiments but either were nonblind, did not randomize, or did not control for alternate explanations of change. Only one study was classified as providing "conclusive" evidence of treatment effects (Wood et al., 2009), since it was an experiment with blinding, random assignment, treatment fidelity measures, and interobserver agreement for the dependent variable and controlled for potential confounds. Based on these data, the authors concluded that "… CBT is an effective treatment for anxiety in individuals with Asperger's. However, data involving other A[utism] S[pectrum] D[isorders] sub-types is lacking" (p. 1).

Based on their descriptions of participants, the relevance of this meta-analysis to people with ID is limited. Some participants with PDD-NOS may have had some degree of intellectual impairment, but there was no direct evidence that CBT was an effective intervention for people with ID.

Lang, Mahonery, El Zein, Delaune, and Amidon (2011) conducted a similar updated systematic search and reached very similar conclusions. Their search identified four previous systematic reviews, no meta-analyses, and two RCTs. The two RCTs were Sofronoff, Attwood, and Hinton (2005) and Wood et al. (2009). Sofronoff et al.'s (2005) study only included participants with Asperger syndrome, but without ID. This led Lang et al. to conclude that "For individuals with an ASD and an anxiety disorder but no intellectual disability, CBT is supported by research when it is modified by direct instruction of social skills, increased family involvement, visual supports, individualized reinforcers, embedded perseverative interests in sessions, and reduced emphasis on abstract concepts and visualization. For individuals with an ASD and an anxiety disorder who do not have an intellectual disability, much less evidence is available. However, one systematic review (Hagopian & Jennett, 2008) suggests that behavioural approaches including contingent reinforcement and graduated exposure may be effective ...."

Summary. These searches and systematic reviews found no evidence that CBT is an evidence-based practice for anxiety disorders in people with ID at this time. Both systematic reviews by Lang et al. (2010) and Lang et al. (2011) concluded that CBT was an evidence-based practice for people with Asperger syndrome without ID, but the RCTs they reviewed often included behavioral procedures, such as social skills training, reinforcement procedures, and embedded perseverate interests. A notable gap in these systematic reviews is the absence of any meta-analysis and effect size calculations.

Other interventions

The hug machine

Temple Grandin, a well-known adult with ASD, developed a so-called hug machine to provide deep pressure to the torso to reduce anxiety in people with autism. Searches using the terms "hug machine" on PubMed and Google Scholar on June 14, 2011, yielded 4 and 65 abstracts, respectively, of which only 1 experimental study (Edelson, Edelson Kerr, & Grandin, 1999) was identified. A hand search of the reference section of this paper identified three additional nonexperimental papers which were excluded from this review. Unfortunately, Edelson et al. did not implement the randomization as planned and were not equivalent at baseline. Hence, there, the hug machine is not an evidence-based intervention for reduction of anxiety in people with intellectual or other developmental disabilities.

Traditional Tai massage

The earlier literature searches for behavioral and CBT also identified one RCT for Tai massage for anxiety in autistic children. Piravej, Tangtrongchitr, Chandarasiri, Paothong, and Sukprasong (2009) randomly assigned 60 children with autism to either sensory integration (SI) or SI plus traditional Tai massage (TTM). Both groups improved on behavior ratings on the Conners' Teacher Rating Scale and parent reports of sleep problems, but only the SI + TTM group improved on parent ratings of anxiety (*p* = .04).

This study has many limitations that preclude the conclusion that SI + TTM caused a reduction in anxiety in the children. First, the anxiety ratings were completed by parents who attended the TTM sessions and hence were not blind to treatment conditions. Second, the authors combined TTM with SI; hence, it is possible that changes were merely due to the increased quantity of any therapy, rather than specific effects of TTM. Finally, the authors analyzed their data using multiple Wilcoxon signed-rank and Mann–Whitney *U* tests rather than two-way ANOVAs and used many statistical tests without correcting the value of alpha. Therefore, there is no evidence that TTM is an effective treatment for anxiety in people with developmental disabilities.

Sensory-adapted dental environment

The searches for behavioral and cognitive behavioral interventions also identified two papers on Snoezelen sensory-adapted dental environment (SDE) for anxiety during dental procedures; the first author of these papers also provided a third paper. The intervention is described as based on Snoezelen and adapted for dental treatment. SDE includes (a) visual sensation, which includes removal of bright fluorescent lights, dimmed lighting, and slow-moving off-white netting patterns; (b) rhythmic music and bass vibrations connected to the dental chair; and (c) tactile "hugging" pressure, which in Shapiro, Sgan-Cohen, Eli, and Parush (2007) was provided by an X-ray vest and in Shapiro, Melmed, Sgan-Cohen, and Parush (2009) and Shapiro, Sgan-Cohen, Parush, and Melmed (2009) was provided by a "friendly butterfly" papoose that hugged the child tightly, which elsewhere is described as "physical restraint" to preemptively reduce disruptive movements (Shapiro, Sgan-Cohen et al., 2009, p. 547).

These three studies had several positive features, such as the use of random crossover design, in which each participant experienced SDE and the regular dental environment in randomized order and the use of standardized behavior ratings and psychophysiological measures of anxiety using electrodermal activity. Unfortunately, none of the data collectors were blind since it was apparent during observation which condition was in effect. Further, if behavior change did occur, it may simply have been due to the use of restraint, rather than SDE. Thus, since the design of these three experiments did not preclude the possibility that changes in dependent variables were due to nonblind raters, rather than true treatment effects, there is no evidence demonstrating that SDE is an evidence-based practice.

Other psychological treatments

The aforementioned searches and reviews did not identify any experimental studies of other psychological interventions, such as psychotherapy, counseling, or sensory interventions for anxiety disorders. Thus, none of these interventions are evidence-based practices for anxiety disorders in people with developmental disabilities.

Summary of evidence-based treatments for fears and phobias

The aforementioned systematic reviews only identified one evidence-based practice for fears and phobias, namely, a multicomponent behavioral package, that always included in vivo exposure and reinforcement for exposure or other appropriate behavior. There were no well-conducted experimental studies demonstrating that any other treatment was effective.

Obsessive–Compulsive Disorders

OCD is characterized by intrusive thoughts, images, or ideas (obsessions) and the engagement in repetitive, apparently nonfunctional overt and covert behavior to neutralize the obsessions or in response to rigid rules (*DSM-IV-TR*, APA, 2000). Researchers discuss the frequent occurrence of obsessions, compulsions, and rituals in individuals with ID of varying ages, especially given the high comorbidity of ID with ASD. Often, however, it is challenging for individuals with ID to vocalize their mental states, sometimes making it difficult to distinguish between OCD and repetitive and/or restrictive behaviors, and a definitive diagnosis of OCD is difficult (Gothelf et al., 2008; Hollander, Wang, Braun, & Marsh, 2009; Matson & Dempsey, 2009; Neil & Sturmey, in press). Therefore, in describing obsessions and compulsions in individuals with ID and related developmental disabilities, researchers often use broad terms such as obsessive–compulsive behavior (OCB). Currently, studies indicate a wide range of prevalence rates in individuals with ID. For example, Vitiello, Spreat, and Behar (1989) examined the prevalence of OCD in 283 adults with mild to profound ID; 3.5% of these individuals were reported to engage in compulsions.

Search strategies

A systematic review of published treatment studies for OCB in persons with ID was conducted using PsycINFO (1887 to June 8, 2011), Academic Search Premier (1965 to June 8, 2011), ERIC (1991 to June 8, 2011), and MEDLINE (1966 to June 8, 2011). Keywords were organized into three groups. Group A keywords were synonymous with ID or other disabilities comorbid with ID including intellectual disabilit*, mental retardation, learning disorder*, learning disabilit*, developmental disability*, pervasive developmental disorder*, and autism spectrum disorder*. Group B keywords were terms used to describe OCB including obsessive compulsive disorder, obsessive compulsive behavio*, obsess*, compulsi*, hoarding, repetitive, and ritual*. Group C keywords consisted of intervention, treatment, remediation, and therapy. The conjunction "or" was used to combine words within each group, and the conjunction "and" was used to search each possible combination of keywords in Groups A, B, and C. We also reviewed reference lists of all articles for pertinent citations.

Studies were included if they met the following criteria: (a) Participant(s) had a diagnosis of ID and also had OCD using the *DSM-IV-TR* (APA, 2000) diagnostic criteria; (b) participant(s) had a diagnosis of ID and reported obsessive–compulsive symptoms but did not have a formal diagnosis of OCD; and (c) the study involved psychosocial intervention to alleviate obsessive–compulsive symptoms. Treatment studies with a variety of methodological designs (e.g., case studies, single-subject designs) were included in the review. Studies that focused on the treatment of motor stereotypy and self-injury were excluded.

Nine studies met our inclusion/exclusion criteria. We examined participant characteristics, treatment, reliability/integrity measures, research design, and primary findings of each study. See Table 10.2 for an overview of participant and methodological characteristics across the 9 studies. These data will be discussed in sections to follow.

Participants ranged in age from 15 to 59 years, with studies focused on adolescents and adults. Eight of the nine studies involved male participants. Severity of ID ranged from mild to severe, but only 1 study (Klein-Tasman & Albano, 2007) noted standardized instruments to diagnose ID, and two studies (Prater & D'Addio, 2002; Sigafoos, Green, Payne, O'Reilly, & Lancioni, 2009) mentioned standardized tests of adaptive functioning. Three studies reported a diagnosis of OCD; assessment instruments ranged from "gold standard" OCD assessments (e.g., Child Yale–Brown Obsessive Compulsive Scale; Goodman, Price, Rasmussen, Riddle, & Rapoport, 1986) to compulsive behavior checklists to use of DSM-III or IV criteria (APA, 1980, 1994). Of the remaining six studies, compulsions were listed and four studies included operational definitions of these compulsions. Targeted compulsions included hoarding, following rigid routines, rearranging, checking, and "need-to-tell" compulsions. Only three studies included a description of related obsessions, but four other studies reported distress/agitation if participants were interrupted from performing compulsions.

Psychosocial treatment for OCB

Multicomponent behavioral packages
Matson (1982) used differential reinforcement (DRO), exposure and response prevention, overcorrection, modeling of appropriate behavior, and delivery of performance feedback to treat clothes and body checking in three adults with mild

Table 10.2   Participant Characteristics and Methodological
Considerations

Nine studies		
Age		
	Children (age <12)	0
	Adolescents (age 12–21)	3
	Adults	7
Gender		
	Male	8
	Female	1
ID		
	Mild	4
	Moderate	3
	Severe	1
	Unspecified	1
Research design		
	Multiple baseline	2
	Reversal	4
	Nonexperimental	3
Interobserver reliability		5
Treatment integrity		0

Adapted from Jennett and Hagopian (2008).

ID aged 18, 29, and 31 years. Participants engaged in a work task to provide exposure to feared stimuli (i.e., becoming wrinkled or dirty). Tokens were dispersed every minute contingent upon an absence of checking and could be exchanged for backup reinforcers. When a compulsion occurred, the participants were told to stop the behavior and were guided through a series of hand movements/positions for 2 min. Following this, a therapist modeled engagement in a work task and verbally described how this was incompatible with the target compulsions. The participant was then redirected to perform the work task. A multiple baseline across behaviors, settings, and participants showed that with the implementation of the treatment package, target behaviors decreased to near-zero or zero levels and results were maintained at 3-month follow-up.

More recently, Berry and Schell (2006) used a multiple baseline across participants to evaluate differential reinforcement of low rates of behavior (DRL) and differential reinforcement of other and incompatible behavior which included item return for decreasing hoarding in three adults (ages 49, 56, and 59 years) with severe ID. A systematic preference assessment including a single stimulus preference assessment (Pace, Ivancic, Edwards, Iwata, & Page, 1985) was used to identify individualized edible reinforcement. Following treatment, all participants showed a quick and clinically significant reduction in the number of items hoarded, and results were maintained when the treatment was applied by direct care staff. Both studies reported acceptable interobserver reliability of target behaviors but lacked a treatment integrity measure.

Using an ABCBC design, Kostinas, Scandlen, and Luiselli (2001) compared two DRL procedures, one involving response cost, to decrease "need-to-tell compulsions" surrounding washrooms, toileting behavior, and bodily functions in a 26-year-old male with moderate ID. Adding response cost (loss of a token) to DRL (access to a preferred snack contingent on fewer or equal to a set number of perseverative vocalizations) led to a greater decrease in "need-to-tell" compulsions compared to DRL alone; however, the authors mentioned the possibility of sequence effects associated with the research design. With implementation of DRL and response cost, perseverative vocalizations were initially reduced and then remained at zero levels.

Iqbal (2002) used an ABA experimental design to evaluate DRI and response cost for treating rituals in a 42-year-old male with moderate ID who engaged in repetitive behavior and checking rituals mainly in his bedroom but also during mealtimes; data indicated that prior to treatment, he spent over 50% of his day in his bedroom. DRI involved repeated prompts to complete his daily routine in his bedroom and at mealtimes in increasingly less time over days; if he met the criterion, he was reinforced by sensory activities with a clinical team member. Meals were removed at specific times, in an attempt to reduce prolonged engagement in rituals. The intervention proved effective, but due to ethical concerns (e.g., removal of meals), treatment was discontinued and rituals returned to pretreatment levels.

In 2009, two studies treated straightening behavior (Kuhn, Hardesty, & Sweeney, 2009) and object rearranging (Sigafoos et al., 2009) in two adolescent males (16 and 15 years, respectively) with ID and ASD. They used ABAB and ABCAC reversal designs, respectively. Upon implementation of the behavioral treatment packages, both behaviors decreased to near-zero or zero levels. Sigafoos et al. showed maintenance of the target behavior (i.e., rearranging objects) at 6 weeks but an increasing trend at 3-month follow-up.

Behavioral/pharmacological treatment package
A nonexperimental study by Prater and D'Addio (2002) reported using medication (e.g., paroxetine and mirtazapine) and introducing flexibility into daily routines to successfully treat rigidity, hoarding, and challenging behaviors (e.g., aggression) in a 29-year-old male with mild ID and Johanson–Blizzard syndrome. Flexibility was described as eating meals at different times, sitting in different seats, and varying choices of food options. This participant was on a number of medications prior to treatment, and it was unclear as to whether the dosages remained stable.

Cognitive behavioral treatment packages
Two nonexperimental case studies ($N = 1$) evaluated CBT packages for adults with OCB and mild ID (Klein-Tasman & Albano, 2007; Willner & Goody, 2006). Klein-Tasman and Albano treated an adult with Williams syndrome in his mid-20s who

displayed "need-to-tell" compulsions surrounding sexual behavior. With intensive CBT treatment, the participant displayed increased awareness of his behavior and exhibited good control; however, follow-up indicated that his gains were only partially maintained. In a second study by Willner and Goodey (2006), they treated checking/straightening/vocalizing to children related to a fear of harm to self and others in a 29-year-old woman. The authors reported using a manual on rational-emotive therapy that was individualized to the participant's cognitive developmental level. No standardized measures were used to evaluate the effects of treatment; however, this participant reportedly experienced a decrease in obsessions and compulsions, displayed by her accurate cognitions and reported behaviors.

Evidence-based practice for obsessive–compulsive behavior

Table 10.3 lists the treatments reviewed, target behaviors, and status of evidence. Given the wide array of behaviors categorized as OCB, we chose to include the target behavior(s) treated. Only two of nine treatments for checking (Matson, 1982) and hoarding (Berry & Schell, 2006) appear to meet criteria for "possibly efficacious." Note, however, that for both treatments, data on treatment integrity were not collected. Of the remaining treatments evaluated, four studies used experimental designs with one participant, and three reported acceptable interobserver reliability.

As discussed earlier, the majority of studies did not note the instruments used to diagnose ID and did not include information on adaptive functioning. Future research should include this information using standardized assessments. Also, assessment of anxiety, including OCB, in persons with ID is daunting. A suggested

Table 10.3 A Summary of Evidence-Based Practice for Treatment of OCBs

Intervention	Behavior	Status of evidence
Multicomponent behavioral package (DRO, exposure and response prevention (overcorrection), modeling of appropriate behavior, performance feedback)	Checking	Possibly efficacious
Differential reinforcement	Hoarding	Probably efficacious
Multicomponent behavioral packages	"Need to tell" Checking Rearranging Straightening	Insufficient evidence
Behavioral/pharmacological package	Rigid routines Hoarding	Insufficient evidence
Cognitive behavioral treatment packages	"Need to tell" Checking Straightening	Insufficient evidence

concentration of future research is on the development of assessments that are fitting for persons with cognitive challenges. Hagopian and Jennett (2008) mentioned informant report and observational assessments including function-based assessments to determine variables maintaining OCBs. Additionally, reviewed studies treated a wide range of OCBs in individuals with ID with and without identified syndromes. Research should continue to evaluate treatments for varying OCBs and for persons presenting with different syndromes to develop evidence-based treatment for persons with a wide range of presenting challenges. Last, in addition to replicating and extending upon successful behavioral and CBT treatments for OCB in individuals with ID, we should tap into research with similar populations, such as people with ASD (e.g., Reaven & Hepurn, 2003; Wood et al., 2009) whereby promising treatments have been adapted to fit participants' cognitive developmental levels and learning style.

Posttraumatic Stress Disorder

A systematic search of PubMed was conducted on June 18, 2011, using the search terms "((ment* AND retar*) OR (intellect* AND disabil*) OR (development* AND disabil*) OR (autis*) OR (down* AND syndrome)) AND (post traumatic stress disorder)." This search yielded 166 abstracts of which five reviews (McCreary & Thompson, 1999; Mevissen Lievegoed, & de Jongh, 2011; Mitchell, Clegg, & Furniss, 2011; Murphy, O'Callaghan, & Clare, 2007) and two treatment studies (Mevissen, Lievegoed, & de Jongh, 2011) appeared to contain potentially relevant treatment studies with experimental designs.

Mevissen and de Jongh (2010) identified a number of nonexperimental case studies of various therapies including eliminating "frightening cues," staff training, and five articles on various kinds of psychotherapy including CBT, exposure therapy, imagery rehearsal therapy for trauma-related nightmares, eye movement desensitization and reprocessing (EMDR), and psychodynamic psychotherapy. The search also identified a case series of four people with ID and PTSD treated with EMDR (Mevissen et al., 2011); however, the search revealed no experimental studies of psychological treatment of PTSD. The other reviews of PTSD (McCreary &

Table 10.4 A Summary of Evidence-Based Practice for
Behavioral Treatment of Posttraumatic Stress Disorder

Intervention	Status of evidence
Removal of cues	Unevaluated
Exposure	Unevaluated
CBT	Unevaluated
EMDR	Unevaluated
Imagery rehearsal therapy	Unevaluated
Psychodynamic psychotherapy	Unevaluated

Thompson, 1999; Mitchell et al., 2011; Murphy et al., 2007) also did not report any experimental evaluations of PTSD. Therefore, there is no evidence-based practice for PTSD at this time (see Table 10.4).

Summary and Conclusions

The evidence base for psychological treatment of anxiety disorders in people with ID is patchy. For fears and simple phobias, but not complex phobias, the multicomponent behavioral package that always contains exposure and reinforcement is *efficacious* (Chambless & Hollon, 1998). There was no evidence that other behavioral procedures alone, such as relaxation or systematic desensitization, or other forms of psychological treatment, such as CBT, were efficacious. In the case of CBT, this conclusion is justified by the absence of experimental studies and in the base of other psychological treatment by the absence of evidence. For OCD, there was evidence that differential reinforcement for hoarding and a multicomponent behavioral package for checking were *possible efficacious*, but there was a lot of evidence for checking, hoarding, rearranging, and "need to tell" and for CBT. Although there was evidence to support psychological treatment of fears and phobias and OCD, this was not the case for PTSD, where there were no experimental treatment studies of any psychological treatment. Thus, the current evidence supports the use of various behavioral packages for fears and simple phobias and perhaps OCD, but not for other anxiety disorders, but does not support the use of any psychological treatment for other anxiety disorders.

These findings have important implications for future research. At this time, behavioral packages appear to be the most promising treatments for anxiety disorders, but future research should extend the current literature by experimentally demonstrating their effectiveness for complex phobias including GAD, OCD, and PTSD. Although some research had demonstrated that routine caregivers, such as mothers of children with disabilities can implement treatment (Love, Matson, & West, 1990), there has been insufficient attention to dissemination of this efficacious treatment in routine settings. A second question related to behavioral packages is which of the components are effective. This is important practically in order to make delivering efficacious interventions as simple and efficient for practitioners to deliver. It is also important from a basic research perspective in understanding the mechanism(s) for change in efficacious treatments (Ward-Horner & Sturmey, 2010). A second broad set of research questions relate to CBT. For example, we need experimental studies to evaluate whether CBT is an efficacious treatment. All the case studies of CBT included treatment modifications such as elimination and simplification of certain procedures typically found in CBT and additional other procedures, such as Socratic questioning. There is no evidence to date to demonstrate that such modifications are effective. CBT packages often contain behavioral procedures, including those that may be the effective components of behavioral packages, such as exposure and reinforcement, among others. It is possible that these behavioral procedures alone may be the effective components of CBT (Sturmey,

2006); thus, future research should address this possibility by conducting a component analysis of the CBT package. Finally, there are a number of psychological treatments for anxiety disorders which practitioners may commonly use—this review identified EMDR, massage, and sensory treatments, among others, which have not been evaluated, and thus, future research should do so.

This chapter has a number of implications for practitioners. The interventions with strongest support for anxiety disorders are behavioral packages. Descriptions of these are available online in the method sections of journal articles reviewed here. Practitioners should use these procedures as first-line treatments and be competent to implement, evaluate, and modify such treatments. If practitioners prefer to use other treatments, they should incorporate exposure and reinforcement and perhaps other behavioral procedures to maximize the likelihood of treatment effectiveness. If practitioners decide not to use behavioral packages in the treatment of anxiety disorders, then there is an additional duty to demonstrate that the use of nonsupported treatments is effective for each client.

References

Altabet, S. (2002). Decreasing dental resistance among individuals with severe and profound mental retardation. *Journal of Developmental and Physical Disabilities, 14*, 297–305.

American Psychiatric Association [APA]. (1980). *Diagnostic and statistical manual of mental disorders DSM-III* (3rd ed.). Washington, DC: Author.

APA. (1994). *Diagnostic and statistical manual of mental disorders DSM-IV-TR* (4th ed.). Washington, DC: Author.

APA. (2000). *Diagnostic and statistical manual of mental disorders DSM-IV-TR* (4th ed., Text Revision). Washington, DC: Author.

Beck, A., & Emery, G. (1979). *Anxiety disorders and phobias: A cognitive perspective.* New York: Basic Books.

Berry, C. L., & Schell, R. M. (2006). Reducing hoarding behavior with individualized reinforcement and item return. *Behavioral Interventions, 21*, 123–135.

Brown, F. J., & Hooper, S. (2009). Acceptance and commitment therapy (ACT) with a learning disabled young person experiencing anxious and obsessive thoughts. *Journal of Intellect Disabilities, 13*, 195–201.

Chambless, D. L., & Hollon, S. D. (1998). Defining empirically supported therapies. *Journal of Consulting and Clinical Psychology, 66*, 7–18.

Conyers, C., Miltenberger, R. G., Peterson, B., Gubin, A., Jurgens, M. Selders, A., et al. (2004). An evaluation of in vivo desensitization and video modeling to increase compliance with dental procedures in persons with mental retardation. *Journal of Applied Behavior Analysis, 37*, 233–238.

Cooper, S.-A., & Bailey, N. M. (2001). Psychiatric disorders amongst adults with learning disabilities: Prevalence and relationship to ability level. *Irish Journal of Psychological Medicine, 18*, 45–53.

Cooper, S.-A., Smiley, E., Morrison, J., Williamson, A., & Allan, L. (2007). Mental ill-health in adults with intellectual disabilities: Prevalence and associated factors. *The British Journal of Psychiatry, 190*, 27–35.

Dagnan, D. (2001). Phobias and anxiety-related problems in mental retardation and developmental disabilities. In D. McKay & E. A. Storch (Eds.), *Handbook of child and adolescent anxiety disorders* (pp. 435–446). New York: Springer.

Davis, T. E., Kurtz, P. F., Gardner, A. W., & Carman, N. B. (2007). Cognitive-behavioral treatment for specific phobias with a child demonstrating severe problem behavior and developmental delays. *Research in Developmental Disabilities, 28,* 546–558.

Deb, S., Thomas, M., & Bright, C. (2001). Mental disorder in adults with intellectual disability. I: Prevalence of functional psychiatric illness among a community based population aged between 16 and 64 years. *Journal of Intellectual Disability Research, 45,* 295–505.

Didden, R., Duker, P. C., & Korzilius, H. (1997). Meta-analytic study on treatment effectiveness for problem behaviors with individuals who have mental retardation. *American Journal on Mental Retardation, 101,* 387–399.

Edelson, S. M., Edelson, M. G., Kerr, D. C., & Grandin, T. (1999). Behavioral and physiological effects of deep pressure on children with autism: A pilot study evaluating the efficacy of Grandin's hug machine. *American Journal of Occupational Therapy, 53,* 145–152.

Gothelf, D., Goraly, O., Avni, S., Stawski, M., Hartmann, I., Basel-Vanagaite, L., et al. (2008). Psychiatric morbidity with focus on obsessive-compulsive disorder in an Israeli cohort of adolescents with mild to moderate mental retardation. *Journal of Neural Transmission, 115,* 929–936.

Hagopian, L. P., & Jennett, H. K. (2008). Behavioral assessment and treatment of anxiety in individuals with intellectual disabilities and autism. *Journal of Developmental and Physical Disabilities, 20,* 467–483.

Hassiotis, A., Serfaty, M., Azam, K., Strydom, A., Martin, S., Parkes, C., et al. (2011). Cognitive behaviour therapy (CBT) for anxiety and depression in adults with mild intellectual disabilities (ID): A pilot randomised controlled trial. *Trials, 12,* 95.

Hofman, S. G., Sawyer, A. T., Korte, K. J., & Smits, J. A. (2009). Is it beneficial to add pharmacotherapy to cognitive-behavioral therapy when treating anxiety disorders? A meta-analytic review. *International Journal of Cognitive Therapy, 1,* 160–175.

Hofman, S. G., & Smits, J. A. J. (2008). Cognitive-behavioral therapy for adult anxiety disorders: A meta-analysis of randomized controlled trials. *Journal of Clinical Psychiatry, 69,* 621–632.

Hollander, E., Wang, A. T., Braun, A., & Marsh, L. (2009). Neurological considerations: Autism and Parkinson's disease. *Psychiatry Research, 170,* 43–51.

Hunot, V., Churchill, R., Teixeira, V., & Silva de Lima, M. (2007). *Psychological therapies for generalised anxiety disorder. Cochrane Database of Systematic Review,* (1), CD001848.

Hunot, V., Find all citations by this author (default).
Or filter your current search
Churchill, R., Find all citations by this **author** (default).
Or filter your current search
Silva de Lima, M. & Find all citations by this **author** (default).
Or filter your current search
Teixeira V. Psychological therapies for generalised anxiety disorder. Find all citations in this **journal** (default).Or filter your current search
Cochrane Database of Systematic Reviews (Online) [2007(1):CD001848] (PMID:17253466.)

Iqbal, Z. (2002). Ethical issues involved in the implementation of a differential reinforcement of inappropriate behaviour programme for the treatment of social isolation and ritualistic behaviour in an individual with intellectual disabilities. *Journal of Intellectual Disability Research, 46,* 82–93.

Jahoda, A., Dagnan, D., Stenfert Kroese, B., Pert, C., & Trower, P. (2009). Cognitive behavioural therapy: From face to face interaction to a broader contextual understanding of change. *Journal of Intellectual Disabilities Research, 53,* 759–771.

Jennett, H. K., & Hagopian, L. P. (2008). Identifying empirically supported treatments for phobic avoidance in individuals with intellectual disabilities. *Behavior Therapy, 39,* 151–161.

Jones, K. M., & Friman, P. C. (1999). A case study of behavioral assessment and treatment of insect phobia. *Journal of Applied Behavior Analysis, 32,* 95–98.

Klein-Tasman, B., & Albano, A. M. (2007). Intensive, short-term cognitive-behavioral treatment of OCD-like behavior with a young adult with Williams syndrome. *Clinical Case Studies, 6,* 483–492.

Kostinas, G., Scandlen, A., & Luiselli, J. K. (2001). Effects of DRL and DRL combined with response cost on perseverative verbal behavior of an adult with mental retardation and obsessive compulsive disorder. *Behavioral Interventions, 16,* 27–37.

Kuhn, D. E., Hardesty, S. L., & Sweeney, N. M. (2009). Assessment and treatment of excessive straightening and destructive behavior in an adolescent diagnosed with autism. *Journal of Applied Behavior Analysis, 42,* 355–360.

Lang, R., Mahoney, R., El Zein, F., Delaune, E., & Amidon, M. (2011). Evidence to practice: Treatment of anxiety in individuals with autism spectrum disorders. *Neuropsychiatric Disorders and Treatment, 25,* 27–30.

Lang, R., Regester, A., Lauderdale, S., Ashbaugh, K., & Haring, A. (2010). Treatment of anxiety in autism spectrum disorders using cognitive behaviour therapy: A systematic review. *Developmental Neurorehabilitation, 13,* 53–63.

Langdon, P. E., Clare, I. C., & Murphy, G. H. (2010). The impact of alleged abuse on behaviour in adults with severe intellectual disabilities. *Research in Developmental Disabilities, 31,* 1601–1608.

Lindsay, W. R. (1986). Cognitive changes after social skills training with young mildly mentally handicapped adults. *Journal of Mental Deficiency Research, 30,* 81–88.

Lindsay, W. R., & Baty, F. (1986a). Abbreviated progressive relaxation: Its use with adults who and mentally handicapped. *Mental Handicap, 14,* 123–126.

Lindsay, W. R., & Baty, F. (1986b). Behavioural relaxation training: Explorations with adults who are mentally handicapped. *Mental Handicap, 14,* 160–162.

Lindsay, W. R., Baty, F., Michie, A. M., & Richardson, I. (1989). A comparison of anxiety treatments with adults who have moderate and severe mental retardation. *Research in Developmental Disabilities, 10,* 129–140.

Lindsay, W. R., Gamsu, C., McLaughlin, E., Hood, E., & Espie, C. (1987). A controlled trial of treatments for generalised anxiety. *British Journal of Clinical Psychology, 26,* 3–15.

Lindsay, W. R., Michie, A. M., Baty, F. J., & Smith, A. W. H. (1994). The consistency of reports about feelings and emotions from people with intellectual disability. *Journal of Intellectual Disabilities Research, 31,* 61–66.

Lindsay, W. I., Neilsen, C., & Lawrenson, H. (1999). Cognitive-behaviour therapy for anxiety in people with learning disabilities. In B. Stenfert Kroese, D. Dagnan, & K. Loumidis (Eds.), *Cognitive-behaviour therapy for people with learning disabilities* (pp. 128–144). New York: Taylor & Francis.

Love, S. R., Matson, J. L., & West, D. (1990). Mothers as effective therapists for autistic children's phobias. *Journal of Applied Behavior Analysis, 23,* 379–385.

Luiselli, J. K. (1980). Relaxation training with a developmentally disabled: A reappraisal. *Behaviour Research and Severe Developmental Disability, 1*, 191–213.

Matson, J. L. (1981). A controlled outcome study of phobias in mentally retarded adults. *Behaviour, Research and Therapy, 19*, 101–107.

Matson, J. L. (1982). Treating obsessive-compulsive behavior in mentally retarded adults. *Behavior Modification, 6*, 551–568.

Matson, J. L., & Dempsey, T. (2009). The nature and treatment of compulsions, obsessions, and rituals in people with developmental disabilities. *Research in Developmental Disabilities, 30*, 603–611.

McCreary, B. D., & Thompson, J. (1999). Psychiatric aspects of sexual abuse involving persons with developmental disabilities. *Canadian Journal of Psychiatry, 44*, 350–355.

McPhail, C. H., & Chamove, A. S. (1989). Relaxation reduces disruption in mentally handicapped adults. *Journal of Mental Deficiency Research, 33*, 309–406.

Murphy, G. H., O'Callaghan, A. C., & Clare, I. C. H (2007). The impact of alleged abuse on behaviour in adults with severe intellectual disabilities. *Journal of intellectual Disabilities Research, 51*, 741–749.

National Institute of Clinical Excellence. (2011). *Quick reference guide generalised anxiety disorder and panic disorder (with or without agoraphobia) in adults. Management in Primary, Secondary and Community Care*. London: NICE.

Neil, N., & Sturmey, P. (2014). Assessment and treatment of obsessions and compulsions in individuals with autism spectrum disorders: A systematic review. *Review Journal of Autism Spectrum Disorders, in press*.

Obler, M., & Terwillger, R. F. (1970). Pilot study on the effectiveness of systematic desensitization with neurologically impaired children with phobic disorders. *Consulting and Clinical Psychology, 34*, 314–318.

Pace, G. M., Ivancic, M. T., Edwards, G. L., Iwata, B. A., & Page, T. J. (1985). Assessment of stimulus preference and reinforcer value with profoundly retarded individuals. *Psychiatric Quarterly, Journal of Applied Behavior Analysis, 18*, 249–255.

Peck, C. (1977). Desensitisation for the treatment of fear in the high-level adult retarded. *Behaviour, Research and Therapy, 13*, 137–148.

Penrose, L. (1938). *A clinical and genetic study of 1280 cases of mental defect*. London: HMO Stationary Office.

Piravej, K., Tangtrongchitr, P., Chandarasiri, P., Paothong, L., & Sukprasong, S. (2009). Effects of Thai traditional massage on autistic children's behavior. *Journal of Alternate and Complementary Medicine, 15*, 1355–1361.

Prater, J. F., & D'Addio. (2002). Johanson-Blizzard syndrome: A case study, behavioral manifestations, and successful treatment strategies. *Society of Biological Psychiatry, 51*, 515–517.

Reaven, J. A., & Hepburn, S. (2003). Cognitive-behavioral treatment of obsessive-compulsive disorder in a child with Asperger syndrome: A case report. *Autism, 7*, 145–164.

Schilling, D., & Poppen, R. (1983). Behavioural relaxation training and assessment. *Journal of Behaviour Therapy and Experimental Psychiatry, 14*, 99–107.

Schroeder, S. R., Peterson, C. R., Solomon, L. J., & Artley, J. J. (1977). EMG feedback and the contingent restraint of self-injurious behavior among the severely retarded: Two case illustrations. *Behavior Therapy, 8*, 738–741.

Shapiro, M., Melmed, R. N., Sgan-Cohen, H. D., Eli, I., & Parush, S. (2007). Behavioural and physiological effect of dental environment sensory adaptation on children's dental anxiety. *European Journal of Oral Science, 115*, 479–483.

Shapiro, M., Melmed, R. N., Sgan-Cohen, H. D., & Parush, S. (2009). Effect of sensory adaptation on anxiety of children with developmental disabilities: A new approach. *Pediatric Dentistry, 31*, 222–228.

Shapiro, M., Sgan-Cohen, H. D., Parush, S., & Melmed, R. N. (2009). Influence of adapted environment on the anxiety of medically treated children with developmental disability. *Journal of Pediatrics, 154*, 546–550.

Sigafoos, J., Green, V. A., Payne, D., O'Reilly, M. F., & Lancioni, G. E. (2009). A classroom-based antecedent intervention reduces obsessive-repetitive behavior in an adolescent with autism. *Clinical Case Studies, 8*, 3–13.

Slifer, K. J., Avis, K. T., & Frutchey, R. A. (2008). Behavioral intervention to increase compliance with electroencephalographic procedures in children with developmental disabilities. *Epilepsy and Behavior, 13*, 189–195.

Sofronoff, K., Attwood, T., & Hinton, S. (2005). A randomised controlled trial of a CBT intervention for anxiety in children with Asperger syndrome. *Journal of Child Psychology and Psychiatry, 46*, 1152–1160.

Steen, P. L., & Zuriff, G. E. (1977). The use of relaxation in the treatment of self-injurious behavior. *Journal of Behavior Therapy and Experimental Psychiatry, 8*, 447–448.

Sturmey, P. (2006). On some recent claims for the efficacy of cognitive therapy for people with intellectual disabilities. *Journal of Applied Research in Intellectual Disabilities, 19*, 109–118.

Tonge, B., Brereton, A., Kiomall, M., Mackinnon, A., King, N., & Rinehart, N. (2006). Effects on parental mental health of an education and skills training program for parents of young children with autism: A randomized controlled trial. *Journal of the American Academy of Child and Adolescent Psychiatry, 45*, 561–569.

Valenti-Hein, D. C., & Mueser, K. T. (1990). *The dating skills program: Teaching social-sexual skills to adults with mental retardation.* Champaign, IL: Research Press.

Valenti-Hein, D. C., Yarnold, P. R., & Mueser, K. T. (1994). Evaluation of the dating skills program for improving heterosocial interactions in people with mental retardation. *Behavior Modification, 18*, 32–46.

Vitiello, B., Spreat, S., & Behar, D. (1989). Obsessive-compulsive disorder in mentally retarded patients. *Journal of Nervous and Mental Disease, 177*, 256–263.

Ward-Horner, P., & Sturmey, P. (2010). Component analyses: A systematic review. *Journal of Applied Behavior Analysis, 43, 685–704.*

Wells, K. C., Turner, S. M., Bellack, A. S., & Hersen, M. (1978). Effects of cue-controlled relaxation on psychomotor seizures: An experimental analysis. *Behaviour, Research, & Therapy, 16*, 51–53.

Willner, P., & Goodey, R. (2006). Interaction of cognitive distortions and cognitive deficits in the formulation and treatment of obsessive-compulsive behaviours in a woman with an intellectual disability. *Journal of Applied Research in Intellectual Disabilities, 19*, 67–73.

Wittchen, H. U., Zhao, S., Kessler, R. C., & Eaton, W. W. (1994). DSM-III-R generalized anxiety disorder in the National Comorbidity Survey. *Archives of General Psychiatry, 51*, 355–364.

Wood, J., Drahota, A., Sze, K., Har, K., Chiu, A., & Langer, D. (2009). Cognitive behavioral therapy for anxiety in children with autism spectrum disorders: A randomized, controlled trial. *Journal of Child Psychology and Psychiatry, 50*, 224–234.

Woodward, R., & Jones, R. B. (1980). Cognitive restructuring treatment: A controlled trial with anxious patients. *Behaviour, Research and Therapy, 18*, 401–407.

World Health Organisation. (2007). *International classification of diseases* (10th. ed). Geneva, Switzerland: Author.

11

Mood Disorders

Peter Sturmey and Robert Didden

Introduction

Mood disorders are characterized by disturbances of affect that result in clinically significant impairment in daily functioning and that are not better accounted for by other psychiatric disorders and medical conditions and that are not culturally normative. DSM-IV (American Psychiatric Association [APA], 2000) distinguishes the following mood disorders: major depressive disorder (MDD), bipolar disorder type I and type II, cyclothymic disorder, atypical mood disorder, mood disorder due to a medical condition, and substance-induced mood disorder. Similar disorders are also to be found in ICD-10 (World Health Organization, 1992). DSM-5 is currently under development (APA, 2012). It includes many revisions to the DSM-IV classification of mood disorders, such as the addition of mixed anxiety/depression, and premenstrual dysphoric disorder and grading of severity of depression. It is unclear at this time what the final version of DSM-5 will include in the revision to mood disorders.

Mood disorders are relatively common. Depression, for example, is sometimes referred to as "the common cold" of mental health and is much more common than other mental health diagnoses. For example, the Epidemiologic Catchment Area study (Weissman, Bruce, Leaf, Florio, & Holzer, 1991) observed a 12-month prevalence of any affective disorder of 3.7% and a lifetime prevalence of any affective disorder of 7.8%. The 12-month prevalence of a major depressive episode was 2.7% and 0.6% for manic episode. A similar pattern of results has been reported by the National Comorbidity Survey (Kessler et al., 1994) which reported annual lifetime and annual prevalences of 16.2% and 6.6% for MDD, respectively (Kessler et al., 2003).

Evidence-Based Practice and Intellectual Disabilities, First Edition.
Edited by Peter Sturmey and Robert Didden.
© 2014 John Wiley & Sons, Ltd. Published 2014 by John Wiley & Sons, Ltd.

Mood disorders are both personally and economically costly. For the individual, they are personally distressing and cause much suffering, disrupt work, negatively influence personal and family life, and involve a risk of suicide and death. Episodes last 16 weeks on average; nearly 69% of people with MDD have major role impairment, such as inability to work; and over three-quarters have an additional DSM-IV disorder (Kessler et al., 2003). Mood disorders also disrupt and negatively influence the lives of people around the person with a mood disorder. Mood disorders are also costly to society. They are associated with direct costs such as consumption of mental and health services of the order of $4,100–$2,500 per year on average (Luppa, Heinrich, Angermeyer, Konig, & Rieder-Heller, 2007). Indirect morbidity and mortality costs, such as associated consumption of physical health services, loss of time at work, income and taxes, and death, may cost on average $2,000–$3,700 and $200–$400, respectively. Nationally, the direct costs of services and loss of employment amount to billions of dollars annually (National Institute of Clinical Excellence, 2009).

Mood disorders in people with intellectual disabilities

Mood disorders in people with intellectual disabilities (ID) were recognized long ago. For example, Penrose (1938) reported that affective psychosis was observed in 24 of 1,280 (1.9%) of all people with ID in the Colchester survey. The prevalences were 2.2%, 3.8%, 0.7%, and 0% for persons with mild, moderate, severe, and profound ID, respectively (Penrose, 1966). Mood disorders were perhaps underrecognized and neglected in the 1950s and 1960s. As the field of dual diagnosis developed, reviews of mood disorders were published (Matson, 1983, 1986; Matson, Barrett, & Helsel, 1988). Subsequently, the field has expanded considerably (see Dosen & Menolascino, 1990, and Sturmey, 2005, for comprehensive reviews). For example, many assessments of mood disorders were developed (Adams & Oliver, 2011; Deb & Iyer, 2005; Finlay, 2005; Hurley, 2008; Perez-Achiaga, Nelson, & Hassiotis, 2009; Ross & Oliver, 2003); a wide range of treatments were reported including behavior therapy and applied behavior analysis (Lindauer, DeLeon, & Fisher, 1999; Matson, Dettling, & Senatore, 1981), cognitive behavior therapy and cognitive therapy (Lindsay, Howells, & Pitcaithly, 1993; McCabe, McGillivray, & Newton, 2006; McGillivray, McCabe, & Kershaw, 2008), psychotherapy (Beail & Newman, 2005), pharmacotherapy (Janowsky & Davis, 2005), and electroconvulsive therapy (Reinblatt, Rifkin, & Freeman, 2004).

Recognition and diagnosis of mood disorders in people with ID comes with several challenges. Although it may be possible to apply unmodified standardized diagnostic criteria when diagnosing mood disorders with some people with mild ID, this may not be possible with all individuals. Evidence for this comes from a review that found that all studies reviewed had modified standard diagnostic criteria with people with ID (Sturmey, 1993) as well as other recent reviews reaching the similar conclusion (Fletcher, Loschen, Stavrakaki, & First, 2007a). The reasons for this are many (Sturmey, 2000) and include (a) problems in language limiting the ability to report mood symptoms; (b) atypical presentation of disorders; (c) accurately recognizing changes in functioning in people who already have an existing disability; and (d) interviewer errors, such as not understanding communication from the client or attributing unusual behavior to ID rather than a psychiatric disorder—so-called diagnostic overshadowing (Jopp & Keys, 2001). Some authors have used challenging behaviors as evidence of an underlying psychiatric disorder, termed "behavioral equivalents" (Charlot, 2005), although evidence for this is contradictory (Sturmey, Laud, Cooper, Matson, & Fodstad, 2010a, 2010b; Tsiouris, Mann, Patti, & Sturmey, 2004). Consequently, there have been at least two sets of modified standard diagnostic criteria—the *Diagnostic Manual-Intellectual Disability* (Fletcher, Loschen, Stavrakaki, & First, 2007b) and the *Diagnostic Criteria for Psychiatric Disorders for Use with Adults with Learning Disabilities/Mental Retardation (DC-LD)* (Royal College of Psychiatrists, 2001)—which have included modified criteria for mood disorders for people with ID.

Given the problems of accurately identifying mood disorders in people with ID and the methodological and practical problems of conducting epidemiological research with this population, it is unsurprising that the estimated prevalences of mood disorders have varied wildly from 0% to 10.9% (Rojahn & Esbensen, 2005). Some evidence of the high prevalence of mood disorders in people with ID also comes from surveys of drug prescription patterns. For example, Spreat, Conroy, and Jones (1997) found that 5.6% of people served by the Oklahoma state ID service were prescribed antidepressants.

While recognizing the limitations of the literature on mood disorders in people with ID, we may still make some cautious generalizations. These include that mood disorders may be relatively common in people with ID. Further, given that mood disorders are treatment responsive and that their effective treatment may have both economic and personal implications for both people with ID and their caregivers, we should be interested in identifying evidence-based psychosocial treatments for mood disorders in people with ID.

Search Strategies

A search was conducted in February 2012 of PubMed to identify abstracts from the 1960s to 2012 using the following terms: ((ment* AND retard*) OR (intellect* AND disabil*) OR (ment* AND handicap*) OR (down* AND syndrom*) OR (autis*) OR (Asperger*) OR (PDDNOS)) AND ((depression) OR (mood disorder) OR (mania) OR (dysthymia)). Inclusion criteria were that the study must include human participants with at least one of the following conditions: mental retardation, intellectual or learning disability, mentally handicap, Down syndrome, autism, Asperger syndrome, PDD-NOS, depression, mood disorder, mania, or dysthymia. We included abstracts on studies of individuals with ID experiencing depression with a disability. We excluded studies if (a) the disability mentioned in the study was not the main focus of the study; (b) the participants were parents or family members experiencing depression associated with caring for another person with a disability; (c) the treatment was not a psychosocial treatment, such as medication; or (d) the study was not a randomized controlled trial (RCT) or a small *N* experiment. The search yielded a preliminary database of 3,237 abstracts, of which 299 were retained for further review. Additional hand searches were made of the references sections of earlier reviews (Dosen & Menolascino, 1990; Sturmey, 2005).

The searches identified one RCT (McCabe et al., 2006) and two studies that included three small *N* experiments (Lindauer et al., 1999; Matson, 1982) on behavioral treatment of depression. We eliminated McGillivray et al. (2008) because this group design study did not randomly assign its participants to CBT and wait list control; rather, the authors assigned participants to CBT or wait list control based on geographical location. We also eliminated a second reference which was a registration of a pilot RCT for mixed anxiety and depression in adults with mild ID, but which has not yet been published (Hassiotis et al., in press). We eliminated Matson (1984) because, although it treated somatic complaints associated with depression, the participants were not diagnosed with depression. Finally, we eliminated Lindsay et al.'s (1993) study of CBT because it was a case series, rather than an experiment.

Review of the Evidence

Behavioral interventions

Randomized controlled trials
No RCTs of behavioral interventions were identified.

Small N experiments
Social skills   There were two small *N* experiments evaluating behavioral treatment for depression. Matson (1982) evaluated information, performance feedback, and token reinforcement to treat the behavioral characteristics of depression using two multiple baseline design experiments. The participants were four adults aged 32, 28, 26, and 48 years. Two had been diagnosed with mild and two with moderate ID, and all scored in the severely depressed range on three psychometric measures of depression (see succeeding text). They worked in a competitive employment center and lived in group homes. None took psychotropic medication, but two had previous failed trials of imipramine. All scored in the clinical range of depression on all three psychometric measures of depression—the *Self-Rating Depression Scale* (Zung, 1965), the *Beck Depression Inventory* (Beck, Ward, Mendelson, Mock, & Erbaugh, 1961), and the *Minnesota Multiphasic Personality Inventory* (Hathaway & McKinley, 1967). Additionally, at baseline, they were administered 20 interview questions related to negative self-statement (e.g., "Do you like the group home?") and somatic complaints (e.g., "Are you sick a lot?"). They were also observed on a

number of behaviors potentially related to depression, such as number of words spoken. Data were also collected on the eight target behaviors (see succeeding text) from eight additional adults with ID who did not score in the depressed range of the three psychometric measures and based on staff's clinical judgments. Baseline data from the four participants were all different from those 8 additional participants: the participants all showed more somatic complaints and less eye contact than the 8 nondepressed participants with ID.

The dependent variables were eight behaviors commonly considered to be behavioral manifestations of depression and included number of words spoken, somatic complaints, irritability, grooming, negative self-statements, flat affect, eye contact, and speech latency. Responses to questions were rated as "appropriate" or "inappropriate." For example, if the therapist asked the question "Do you like yourself?," the rater would score the response as "appropriate" if the participants said "It's okay" and as "inappropriate" if the participant said "I hate myself." The raters also collected data on depressed behaviors, again by scoring behavior dichotomously for each question. For example, speech latency was scored as correct if the participant responded within 3 s of the questions and as incorrect if they responded after 3 s. Thus, each question and behavioral item received a score out of 20 in each interview. To assess the social validity of change, the experimenter used pre- and postscores on the three depression measures listed earlier and staff's clinical judgments for each of the eight observable target behaviors. Data were collected without any programmatic reinforcement for answers.

Data were collected by live ratings for behavioral items and from audiotapes for responses to questions. Two undergraduates collected data on behavioral items from behind a one-way mirror. They had previously been trained to achieve at least 80% interobserver agreement (IOA) on all target behaviors. IOA was calculated as the number of exact agreements divided by the number of observations multiplied by 100%. IOA was high and ranged from 88% for irritability to 99% for grooming.

Treatment consisted of individual 40-min sessions administered by master-level psychologists and consisted of token reinforcement, instructions, performance feedback, modeling, and role-play. The therapist asked a question. If the participant made a correct response on all eight target behaviors being trained in that session, then the therapist gave the participant a token. The participant could exchange tokens approximately 5 cents of food per token at the end of the session. Participants always received at least 2 tokens. If the participant made an incorrect response, the therapist told the participant that the answer was incorrect. The therapist then modeled the correct response three times and asked the participant to imitate the correct answer. For example, if the question was "How do you feel?" and the participant said "Terrible, I should not have to work today," then the therapist said "That is not a good answer, so you do not earn a token. What you might say instead is 'I feel okay.' Now I will ask the question again and you say 'I feel okay.'" This was practiced three times.

In each session, the therapist and participant generally practiced 8 responses per session related to 2–3 questions. These were practiced in response to some somatic and negative self-statements in the first half of the session and in response to life events that had occurred since the last session during the second half of the session. The only variation from this procedure was intervention for grooming which was always done first. At the beginning of a session, the therapist gave feedback on each of the 6 items related to grooming and gave the participant a token if all 6 responses were correct.

In order to show experimental control, the experimenter used two multiple base-line designs. The first consisted of a multiple baseline design across responses and participants Ted and Ruth. The second consisted of multiple baseline design stag-gered across responses for Crystal and across the second participant Sheila. Thus, this paper reported two experiments with the second directly replicating the effects of the first on two new participants. Follow-up data were collected at 2-, 4-, and 6-month follow-up in experiment 1 and at 2-month follow-up only in experiment 2.

In both experiments, baseline data were outside the performance of the social validity data obtained from other nondepressed people with ID, that is, participants made many more somatic complaints and much less eye contact than nondepressed peers. In both experiments and for all participants, all 8 depressed behaviors improved upon introduction of the treatment such that target behaviors all changed to be similar to their peers' behavior. Thus, both experiments demonstrated clear experimental control of depressed behavior by the treatment. These treatment effects were maintained at follow-up for all four participants. Further, all partici-pants' scores on the three psychometric measures of depression changed from severe depression at pretest to no depression at posttest and follow-up. All participants' scores changed from "severely depressed" to "not depressed" on all three psycho-metric measures ($p < .05$ for all three measures).

This study had a number of positive features including the use of a multiple base-line experimental design and replication of the results in the second experiment. The study had reliable measures of depressed behavior similar to those recognized elsewhere as indicating depression (Lewinsohn, 1975) and included behaviors that differentiate depressed from nondepressed people with ID (Hartley & Birgenheir, 2009; Hartley, Lickel, & MacLean, 2008). Further, there was evidence that all four participants had clinical depression in baseline as shown by (a) psychometric scores in the clinical range, (b) a history of failed medication trials for two participants, and (c) depressed behaviors that were different from those of nondepressed peers. The treatment was described in fairly good detail in the method section so that it would probably be possible to replicate the treatment quite closely based on the available description. Additionally, the treatment implicitly incorporated multiple exemplar training in that the second half of the session included training related to life events since the last session, which presumably were varied from session to session; this strategy may well enhance generalization of skills (Stokes & Baer, 1977). There was a large, reliable, and replicable change in depressed behavior that was maintained at 4–6-month follow-up, which was also reflected in clinically meaningful changes from severely depressed to nondepressed scores on all three psychometric measures. Finally, the study evaluated treatment not merely by demonstrating the absence of problematic behavior but also by demonstrating improvements in appropriate, nondepressed behavior such as grooming, improvements in eye contact, and improvements in appropriate speech latency.

The study also had six main limitations. The first, and most important, limitation relates to the choice of dependent variables, namely, collecting data during clinical interviews in response to 20 set questions and when completing the psychometric measures. It is unclear how this behavior might relate to everyday behavior in naturalistic settings. Some might argue that the use of standardized psychometric measures attenuates this criticism since they may predict behavior in naturalistic settings; this is indeed the assumption of many psychological treatment studies that rely on such measures. This study, however, would have been stronger if it also had identified naturalistic situations in which depressed behavior was problematic and then showed that treatment resulted in improvements in depressed behavior and increases in positive behavior. Second, the study lacked a description of the baseline condition, perhaps because it consisted of treatment as usual. If so, this limits the ability of the study to clearly demonstrate that treatment caused the observed changes due to confounding of treatment with novelty and attention. Third, the study did not report data on treatment integrity. Fourth, the study did not include generalization probes, for example, to novel forms of questions, interviewers, and setting. Fifth, the study reported three *t*-tests and used a .05 significance level without correcting for multiple tests. Finally, there was no placebo condition in baseline.

Environmental enrichment   A second behavioral approach to treating depression is to use environmental enrichment (EE) with preferred activities that are associated with positive mood. Whereas other studies of providing enriched environments with stimuli associated with positive mood had participants without clinical mood disorders (Dillon & Carr, 2007), Lindauer et al. (1999) evaluated the effects of EE on SIB and mood-related behavior in Candy, a 23-year-old woman with severe ID, major depression, mild left hemiparesis, and autistic-like behavior. A functional analysis indicated that her SIB was negatively reinforced by escape from demands but was also present in all conditions. Candy took carbamazepine for her mood disorder and had responded well to medication combined with differential reinforcement of compliance and guiding her hands to her lap for 30 s contingent upon SIB. SIB and negative mood behavior, however, remained problematic when she was left alone.

To evaluate the effects of EE on depressed behavior and SIB, Lindauer et al. observed three target behaviors. SIB consisted of hitting her head with her hands, hitting her head against surfaces, and arm biting. Negative affect consisted of frowning, crying, and whining and stating "I'm sad." Positive affect included smiling, giggling, and laughing. Observers recorded SIB using frequency counts and affective behavior using 10-s interval time sampling. IOA was 99.7%, 95.1%, and 83.2% for SIB, positive affective behavior, and negative affective behavior, respectively. In baseline, Candy was alone with no items. In contrast, during treatment, Candy had 12 preferred items continuously available to her, which has been selected using a paired stimulus preference assessment. During all sessions, therapists implemented the quiet hands procedure contingent upon SIB. The experiment took place in a quiet 3 m × 3 m padded room and sessions lasted 20 minutes. The experimenters demonstrated experimental control using a reversal design.

Negative affective behavior occurred during 27% of intervals during the two baseline conditions and only during 0.1% of EE conditions. Candy showed positive affect during only 2% during baseline; positive affect increased during EE and occurred during 11% of intervals during the second EE phase. Finally, SIB only occurred during the baseline condition at a rate of 0.3 per min but never occurred during EE. SIB and negative affect were closely associated in that SIB occurred during 46% of the session in when she displayed negative affect but during only 1 session or 3% of intervals when she did not display negative affect.

This study is quite interesting in that it demonstrates that affective behavior could be modified using EE in a person with severe ID and depression. The study had reliable data and used an experimental design to show a clear relationship between treatment and affective behavior as well as SIB. The study is also important because it showed a clear association between negative affective behavior and SIB using reliable observational data, rather than clinical impressions. The treatment is also clearly described and is easy to replicate in clinical settings using the description in the method section. Thus, EE may be an effective treatment for mood-related SIB in a person with severe ID and a mood disorder.

Despite these strengths, this study has some limitations. The most notable of these is that the study took place in a treatment room rather than a natural setting using a therapist (no further description of that person was made) rather than a typical caregiver, such as a family member or direct care staff. Additionally, the study did not include data on treatment integrity, generalization, maintenance, or social validity. Finally, a limitation of the experimental design is that in the control condition there were no materials; in order to control for the presence of materials, it would have been better if the experimenters had included a control condition in which nonpreferred materials had been presented.

Conclusions

This systematic review identified only two papers containing three experiments with 5 adult participants with depression and mild through severe ID. They were successfully treated by social skills training that focused on answering questions appropriately (Matson, 1982) and noncontingent access to materials associated with positive affective behavior (Lindauer et al., 1999). Both studies had numerous limitations. Thus, the literature on behavioral treatment is both small and the experiments contained therein are imperfect. Thus, both interventions do not meet Chambless and Hollon's (1998) criteria for an evidence-based practice. Since behavioral treatment has proven effective in more than three participants in small *N* experiments (Chambless & Hollon, 1998, p. 13), we can conclude that it is a "possible efficacious" treatment.

Cognitive behavior therapy

Randomized controlled trials

McCabe et al. (2006) evaluated a CBT program for depression in adults with mild and moderate ID. The program consisted of 5 2-hr sessions delivered once per week over a 5-week period. In the first session, there were an introduction and a program outline and explanation of what depressed means and how looking after one's physical health can improve mood. In session 2, there was a discussion of having a strong supportive network, an activity scheduling and promotion of enjoyable activities, and a handout on community resources which the therapist encouraged group members to use. Session 3 taught that positive thinking resulted in positive mood and taught group members how to reduce negative thoughts and increase positive thoughts and explained the link between feeling depressed and one view of oneself Kendal et al. (1989). Members completed a list of positive self-attributes and positive qualities of other group members. Finally, they were taught strategies to increase positive and decrease negative self-talk. Session 4 taught strategies for dealing with problems, such as identifying recent problems, problem solving, assertiveness skills, role-playing effective solutions to problems, and discussing and giving feedback on these activities. The final session reviewed the program, encouraged group members to continue practicing skills, and assisted members in setting attainable goals. The program is available in a treatment manual available from the authors.

Sixteen men and 18 women with mild or moderate ID participated (total $N = 34$). Intervention was first delivered to a group of 19 participants, while the remaining 15 acted as a control group. The control group participants then received treatment. The authors recruited participants from supported employment settings. The mean ages of the intervention and control groups were approximately 34 and 40 years (range 22–58 years). Their mean BDI scores were approximately 15 and 14, respectively, and included "both people with clinical depression as well as those evidencing depressive symptoms who were at risk of developing depression ... potential participants were required to have sufficient language skills to participate ... " (p. 240). Dependent variables included scores on the *BDI*, the *Social Comparison Scale* (Allen & Gilbert, 1995), the *Rosenberg Self-esteem Scale* (Rosenberg, 1989), and the *Automatic Thoughts Questionnaire—Revised* (Hollon & Kendal, 1980). There were 8 treatment groups with 3–5 individuals in each group, and "the program ran ... on the premises of each group's workplace" (p. 243). The authors collected data at pretest, posttest, and at 3-month follow-up. Follow-up data were only collected for the first treatment group, but not the control group who subsequently received treatment.

At pretest, there were no statistically significant differences between the experimental and control groups on all measures. At posttreatment, the control group did not change, but the experimental group was less depressed, viewed themselves more positively, and reported fewer negative automatic thoughts than compared to their baseline scores and compared to the control group. There was no significant difference between the scores of the treatment group at follow-up and posttreatment indicating no regression at follow-up. The authors also reported the number and percentage of "responders" in the treatment and control groups (Johnson & Truax, 1991) and found that there was a greater proportion of the treatment group who made a substantial level of improvement than in the control group.

This study has a number of positive features. These include a treatment that can be delivered in groups with a manual that can be used to deliver treatment and train therapists. Further, this form of treatment is probably familiar to many therapists and hence may be easy to disseminate. Subsequently, McGillivray et al. (2008) demonstrated that this treatment could be delivered with similar results using routine therapists in multiple centers. The demonstration of maintenance of effects at a 3-month follow-up is also impressive. Finally, the use of multivariate statistics and Bonferroni corrections to correct for multiple tests guarded against false-positive results due to multiple statistical testing.

Despite these positive features, this study has some serious threats to internal validity, making it difficult to conclude that the treatment caused the change. First, the authors did not describe how or who randomized the participants to treatment and control groups. Second, the authors did not define or take data on treatment integrity. As noted elsewhere (Sturmey, 2004, 2006, 2006), such group treatments often fail to define if treatment integrity refers to whether the therapist delivered the treatment as planned, such as prompting clients to select preferred community activities, or whether the participants acquired certain therapeutic skills, such as making a schedule and participating in pleasurable community activities, that resulted in changes in problematic behavior (depressed behavior). Consider just one example. The authors described how "Group members were given a handout on community resources ... [were] encouraged to utilize these resources" (p. 242). Such an account does not describe what the therapist did to encourage the participants to use the handout on community resources. Perhaps more importantly, there were no data on whether some, all, or none of the participants used any of these community resources or indeed if use of community resources was a required or optional part of the treatment package. Thus, it is both unclear what the treatment was and whether the therapists delivered it. Third, the control group received treatment as usual rather than an active placebo treatment, thus confounding treatment with novelty, expectation, and nonspecific attention. For example, the authors reported that they wanted to create a warm atmosphere in the therapeutic group, but this was not done for the control group. Fourth, the authors did not describe the data collection in detail or who conducted the groups, but did not state that the data were collected blind. It is possible that the authors themselves both ran the groups and collected the data in nonblind fashion, thereby introducing possible expectation and other biases into the data. Fifth, all dependent variables were verbal self-reports and did not include any objective measures of depression or any measures that used responses other than verbal responses or social validity data from caregivers. Finally, there appears to be problem with the statistical analyses conducted. The data in Table 1 (p. 243) combined the pretest and posttest treatment data for both treatment and control groups. This procedure is unusual and, although it may increase the power of the statistical analyses, requires justification. Additionally, the data in Table 2 (p. 244) appears to be misset, and so, the data on clinical significance of findings appears not to be fully reported and appears to contain errors, such as data on follow-up for the control group when the control group did not provide any follow-up data. Thus, these data cannot be readily judged from the published journal article.

In addition to threats to internal validity, there were also two problems relating to external validity. First, the study did not include any measures of generalization. Thus, it is unclear if any of the verbal reports to therapists and researchers in the therapy setting generalized to other people, settings, or behavior. Second, the authors' description of participant eligibility could have been more clear in two respects: (a) the criteria for number of depressive symptoms were not clearly described—thus, the study may have included people with depressed mood, but not people who truly were at risk for depression—and (b) the decision as to whether someone had adequate verbal skills seems to have been left up to local service managers to decide and this was not clearly specified.

Small N experiments
No small *N* experiments evaluating CBT with persons with ID were identified.

Conclusions
Since there was only one RCT for CBT, it is possible (McCabe et al., 2006) for CBT to be a "possibly efficacious" treatment for depression in people with ID. This study, however, has so many methodological problems and alternate explanations for behavior change that it is unclear if CBT caused the changes in depression that may have occurred. Therefore, CBT is not yet an evidence-based practice for depression in people with ID.

Conclusions

What treatments are evidence-based practice?

The most striking feature of the literature on treatment of mood disorders in people with ID is its very small quantity. All studies were on depression and there were no treatment studies of other mood disorders, such as mania. There were three treatment papers: two of behavioral treatment and one of CBT. Even among the three experiments evaluating behavioral treatment, two were contained in one paper without any independent replication and with a dependent variable of limited validity. Hence, there is little evidence of the robustness of behavioral treatment effects. The RCT on CBT contained so many serious flaws that it is unclear if the treatment caused the change. Therefore, the only treatment with any empirical support for psychosocial treatment of depression is behavioral treatment; here, because of the small number of experiments, lack of independent replication, and methodological problems with the

Table 11.1 A Summary of the Experimental Evidence for Psychosocial Treatment of Depression in People with ID

Treatment	Status of evidence
Behavioral	Possibly efficacious
	Three experiments (Lindauer et al., 1999; Matson, 1982)
Mood induction	Insufficient evidence
	Studies in people with ID without depression (Carr et al., 2003; Green & Reid, 1996)
Behavioral activation	Insufficient evidence with people with ID and depression
	Nonexperimental case series (Jahoda et al., undated) and multiple studies in other populations (Cuijpers et al., 2012; Sturmey, 2009)
Cognitive behavior therapy	Insufficient evidence
	Nonexperimental case studies (Lindsay et al., 1993; McCabe et al., 2006; McGillivray et al., 2008)
Other treatment	Insufficient evidence
	Some narrative case studies (Beail & Newman, 2005)

available studies, we can only conclude that behavioral treatment is *possible efficacious* (Chambless & Hollon, 1998, p. 13). Because of the poor quality of the only available RCT for CBT and the absence of experimental evidence for other psychosocial therapies, we must conclude that CBT and other therapies are currently not evidence-based practices. See Table 11.1 for a summary of the evidence for psychosocial treatment of mood disorders in people with ID.

Practitioner Guidelines

Recommendations based on evidence
Practitioner recommendations are summarized in Table 11.2. Practitioners treating depression in people with ID can only take limited guidance from this literature. Since behavioral treatments have the best evidence to date, there should be a preference for behavioral treatments for depression. These two papers used a social skills training approach similar to Lewinsohn's (1975) work. To implement these treatments, there are adequate treatment descriptions of treatment in the journal articles for practitioners to implement treatment. The articles by Matson also used master-level therapists with some experience of working with people with ID. This indicates that these treatments can be implemented by practitioners with only a modest amount of experience in the field.

Lindauer et al.'s article contains a clear description of the use of preferred stimuli combined with a simple quiet hands procedure for SIB. As the authors themselves pointed out, this procedure requires little skill and effort to implement; however, the

Table 11.2   Summary of Practitioner Recommendations

1. Use behavioral interventions such as social skills training and EE based on a functional assessment of the stimuli selected. Do so with caution since this is only a "possible efficacious" treatment
2. Consider using CBT using existing manuals with materials modified for people with ID (LeJuez et al., 2011a, 2011b). Do so with caution since there is currently no good experimental evidence to support their use with people with ID
3. Consider using behavioral activation and mood induction procedures. Do so with caution since there is currently no evidence to support their use with people with ID
4. Do not use other treatment methods unless (a) behavioral, CBT, mood induction, and behavioral activation have been accurately implemented and failed and (b) there is clear evidence of benefits for this specific client. Do so with marked caution since there is currently no evidence to support their use with people with ID
5. When working with people with ID who have a high risk of suicidal, practitioners should consult general and local practice guidelines (e.g., Jacobs et al., 2003) and adapt them to working with people with ID

presentation of depression and SIB related to a lack of activity is a relatively specific and perhaps infrequent clinical problem, and so, this paper may have limited direct implications for practitioners.

For those practitioners who wish to use CBT, McCabe et al.'s procedure has some positive features. First, the procedure has been piloted out and, in a separate study (McGillivray & McCabe, 2006), evaluated using routine practitioners. Second, the procedure is quite brief—only five weekly 2-hr sessions—and was implemented in a group of 3–5 participants. These observations suggest that it could be an economic and practical treatment procedure, even if at this time it lacks evidence to support its use.

There are a number of nonexperimental case studies of CBT treatment of depression which the practitioner may find useful (Lindsay et al., 1993). These case studies included practical guidance on simplified CBT procedures and modified materials which have been piloted on people with ID and depression.

Unevaluated treatments to consider
It is not uncommon for practitioners to face problems with little or no evidence to guide practice (Strauss, Richardson, Glasziou, Haynes, & Strauss, 2009). Yet, they still can use evidence to guide treatment and avoid arbitrary selection of ineffective or harmful treatments. There are two related behavioral treatments for depression that have not been evaluated with people with ID which practitioners may consider: mood induction procedures and behavioral activation (see succeeding text).

Mood induction   There are several studies that have evaluated mood induction in people with ID without depression using activities to induce positive mood in a manner similar to Lindauer et al. (1999). For example, Green and Reid (1996) observed behavioral indices of happiness (smiling, laughing, and yelling while smiling) and unhappiness (frowning, grimacing, crying, and yelling without smiling). These behavioral indices of affect were validated by showing that staff and others agreed that the person was happy or unhappy when they displayed behavioral indices of happiness or unhappiness. Subsequently, they conducted a multiple baseline design across three participants with an additional reversal design embedded within the data for the first participant. In this experiment, they showed that when routine care staff presented stimuli associated with behavioral indices of happiness to three adults with profound ID and physical impairments, the proportion of time they exhibited happy behavior reliably increased. Dillon and Carr (2007) reviewed this literature and showed that the effects of mood induction are relatively robust.

One of the best experiments that exemplifies the clinical application of mood induction procedures comes from Carr, McLaughlin, Giacobbe-Grieco, and Smith (2003). They developed and evaluated a procedure to identify activities associated with positive, neutral, and negative mood and then evaluated the effects of inducing positive mood before presenting demands. Eight adults with mild through profound ID of whom 5 also had diagnoses of autism and who were aged 29–48 years participated. They selected them because staff rated them as having variable mood related to activities rather than biological variables, such as physical illness or bipolar disorder. They found that during naturalistic observation sessions, observers could rate mood very reliably on a 6-point Likert scale. Carr et al. then presented participants with a demand or preferred task during naturally occurring observed episodes of bad, neutral, or positive mood. They found that for all 8 participants their problem behavior was much more likely when demands were presented during bad mood sessions than any of the other six types of sessions. Carr et al. then conducted an intervention study over a 3-year period with the 3 participants whom staff judged to display the most severe problem behavior. During intervention, they taught staff to induce positive client mood by presenting activities associated with positive mood. Staff did this by presenting a preferred activity for up to 15 minutes. If the client did not display positive mood at the end of the session, then this procedure was repeated up to three times. Three mood induction sessions always resulted in induction of positive mood. The experiment used a multiple baseline design across participants and took place over 3 years. In baselines, participants almost always displayed problem behavior when demands were presented, resulting in termination of tasks in 100% of sessions. Following mood induction, clients almost always completed all task demands without problem behavior. There was good evidence of social validity. Twenty-three staff rated the procedure as producing highly desirable outcomes, reported using the procedure with other clients, and reported that the procedure was fun and appropriate. The only staff reservation was that the procedure was rated as being moderately effortful.

The results of this study suggest that mood induction with clients with severe behavior problems whose mood is labile and responsive to activities may be effectively treated with staff-mediated mood induction procedures. One limitation of this study for present purposes is that the authors did not report if the participants had any psychiatric disorders or took psychotropic medication. Nevertheless, this paper might provide a model for clinicians to use when managing mood disorders in people with ID. A second significant limitation was that the procedure was staff-mediated, that is, the staff selected and initiated activities associated with positive mood. Future research should develop this procedure further by teaching individuals with ID themselves to self-manage their own behavior, including arranging their own environment to make selecting activities associated with positive mood more likely (cf. Skinner, 1953).

Behavioral activation　A second procedure to consider is behavioral activation. Behavioral activation is a procedure in which people with depression first decide if the time is right to make a change, identify personally meaningful goals, engage in weekly assignments to work toward those goals, and record their own progress toward those goals (Martell, Dimidjian, & Herman-Dunn, 2010). There is good evidence from over 10 dismantling studies and studies of behavioral activation alone without cognitive restructuring, that behavioral activation is an evidence-based practice and that behavioral activation, rather than cognitive restructuring, is the effective component of CBT (Cuijpers et al., 2012; Sturmey, 2009).

Empirical support for behavioral activation comes from Jahoda et al. (undated) who reported a nonexperimental case series of the treatment of depression in 20 adults with mild ($N = 15$), moderate ($N = 3$), and severe ($N = 2$) ID who were currently experiencing depression using behavioral activation. The authors recruited participants from psychiatrists and psychologists, and participants had to have a family member or staff who knew them for at least 6 months available to participate. The authors developed a behavioral activation manual that targeted increasing purposeful, pleasurable domestic, daytime, and social/recreational activities. This version of behavioral activation was delivered by a nonlicensed psychology assistant over 10–12 weeks with regular supervision from a licensed psychologist. There was evidence from both self- and other-reports using standardized psychometric measures of depression that there was change from pre- to postintervention and some evidence of clinically significant changes.

These pilot data suggest that behavioral activation modified for use with people with ID may be another option for clinicians to consider, although there is no experimental evidence to support its use with people with ID at this time. Further, behavioral activation may have some specific advantages for populations with cognitive and linguistic limitations including the following: (a) the fact that behavioral activation focuses on engaging in activities rather than discriminating, modifying, and reporting one's own thoughts and feelings; (b) it may be easier than cognitive therapy for many people with ID; (c) there are treatment manuals available (LeJuez, Hopko, Acierno, Daughters, & Pagoto, 2011a, 2011b) including the manual used by Jahoda et al. (undated); and (d) routine practitioners including nonprofessionals could implement such treatments relatively easily using such modified manuals.

Acknowledgment

The authors would like to thank Dr. Anne Featherstone for assistance with literature searches related to this chapter.

References

Adams, D., & Oliver, C. (2011). The expression and assessment of emotions and internal states in individuals with severe or profound intellectual disabilities. *Clinical Psychology Review, 31*, 293–306.

Allen, S., & Gilbert, P. (1995). A social comparison scale: Psychometric properties and relationship to psychopathology. *Personality and Individual Differences, 19*, 293–299.

American Psychiatric Association [APA]. (2000). *Diagnostic and statistical manual of the American Psychiatric Association* (4th ed., Rev.). Washington, DC: Author.

APA. (2012). *DSM-5: The future of psychiatric diagnosis*. Retrieved 21 November, 2012, from http://www.dsm5.org/Pages/Default.aspx (accessed 21 October, 2013).

Beail, N., & Newman, D. (2005). Psychodynamic counseling and psychotherapy for mood disorders. In P. Sturmey (Ed.), *Mood disorders in people with mental retardation* (pp. 159–174). Kingston, NY: NADD Publishers.

Beck, A. T., Ward, C. H., Mendelson, M., Mock, J., & Erbaugh, J. (1961). An inventory for measuring depression. *Archives of General Psychiatry, 4*, 561–571.

Carr, E. G., McLaughlin, D. M., Giacobbe-Grieco, T., & Smith, C. E. (2003). Using mood ratings and mood induction in assessment and intervention for severe problem behavior. *American Journal on Mental Retardation, 108*, 32–55.

Chambless, D. L., & Hollon, S. D. (1998). Defining empirically supported therapies. *Journal of Consulting and Clinical Psychology, 66*, 7–18.

Charlot, L. (2005). Use of behavioral equivalents for symptoms of mood disorders. In P. Sturmey (Ed.), *Mood disorders in people with mental retardation* (pp. 17–47). Kingston, NY: NADD Publishers.

Cuijpers, P., van Straaten, A., Driessen, E., van Open, P., Bockting, C., & Andersson, A. (2012). Depression and dysthymic disorder. In P. Sturmey & M. Hersen (Eds.), *Handbook of evidence-based practice in clinical psychology. Vol: 1. Adults* (pp. 243–283). Hoboken, NJ: Wiley.

Deb, S., & Iyer, A. (2005). Clinical interviews. In P. Sturmey (Ed.), *Mood disorders in people with mental retardation* (pp. 159–174). Kingston, NY: NADD Publishers.

Dillon, C. M., & Carr, J. E. (2007). Assessing indices of happiness and unhappiness in individuals with developmental disabilities: A review. *Behavioral Interventions, 22*, 292–244.

Dosen, A., & Menolascino, F. J. (1990). *Depression in mentally retarded children and adults*. Leiden, the Netherlands: Logon Publishers.

Finlay, W. M. (2005). Psychometrics assessment of mood disorders in people with intellectual disabilities. In P. Sturmey (Ed.), *Mood disorders in people with mental retardation* (pp. 275–210). Kingston, NY: NADD Publishers.

Fletcher, R., Loschen, E., Stavrakaki, C., & First, M. (2007a). Introduction. In R. Fletcher, E. Loschen, C. Stavrakaki, & M. First (Eds.), *Diagnostic manual-intellectual disability: A clinical guide for diagnosis of mental disorders in persons with intellectual disability* (pp. 1–8). Kingston, NY: NADD Press.

Fletcher, R., Loschen, E., Stavrakaki, C., & First, M. (2007b). *Diagnostic manual-intellectual disability: A clinical guide for diagnosis of mental disorders in persons with intellectual disability*. Kingston, NY: NADD Press.

Green, C. W., & Reid, D. H. (1996). Defining, validating, and increasing indices of happiness among people with profound multiple disabilities. *Journal of Applied Behavior Analysis, 29*, 67–78.

Hartley, S. L., & Birgenheir, D. (2009). Nonverbal social skills of adults with mild intellectual disability diagnosed with depression. *Journal of Mental Health Research in Intellectual Disabilities, 1*, 11–28.

Hartley, S. L., Lickel, A. H., & MacLean, W. E., Jr. (2008). Reassurance seeking and depression in adults with mild intellectual disability. *Journal of Intellectual Disability Research, 52*, 917–929.

Hassiotis, A., Serfati, M., Azam, K., Strydom, A., Blizard, R., Romeo, R., et al. (in press). Manualised Individual Cognitive Behavioural Therapy for mood disorders in people with mild to moderate intellectual disability: A feasibility randomised controlled trial. *Journal of Affective Disorders, 151*, 186–195.

Hathaway, S. R., & McKinley, J. C. (1967). *Minnesota multiphasic personality inventory manual* (Rev. ed.). New York: Psychological Corporation.

Hollon, S. D., & Kendall, P. C. (1980). Cognitive self-statements in depression: Development of an automatic thoughts questionnaire. *Cognitive Therapy and Research, 4*, 383–395.

Hurley, A. D. (2008). Depression in adults with intellectual disability: Symptoms and challenging behaviour. *Journal of Intellectual Disabilities Research, 52*, 905–916.

Jacobs, D. G., Baldessarini, R. J., Conwell, Y., Fawcett, J. A., Horton, L., Meltzer, H., et al. (2003). American Psychiatric Association Work Group on Suicidal Behaviors. Practice guidelines for the assessment and treatment of patients with suicidal behaviors. *American Journal of Psychiatry (Supplement), 160*, 1–60.

Jahoda, A., Davisson, C., Melville, C., Pert, C., Cooper, A., Lynn, H., et al. (Undated). *A pilot study of behavioral activation for people with learning disabilities and depression: BEAT_IT*. Unpublished data available from Andrew Jahoda, Andrew.Jahoda@glasgow.ac.uk.

Janowsky, D. S., & Davis, J. M. (2005). Diagnosis and treatment of depression in patients with mental retardation. *Current Psychiatry Reports, 7*, 421–428.

Johnson, N. S., & Truax, P. (1991). Clinical significance: A statistical approach to defining a meaning change in psychotherapy research. *Journal of Clinical and Consulting Psychology, 59*, 12–19.

Jopp, D. A., & Keys, C. B. (2001). Diagnostic overshadowing reviewed and reconsidered. *American Journal on Mental Retardation, 106*, 416–433.

Kendal, P. C., Howard, B. L., & Hays, R.C. (1989). Self-referent speech and psychopathology: The balance of positive and negative thinking. *Cognitive Therapy and Research, 13*, 383–398.

Kessler, R., McGonagle, K., Nelson, C., Hughes, M., Swartz, M., & Blazer, D. (1994). Sex and depression in the National Comorbidity Survey 2: Cohort effects. *Journal of Affective Disorders, 30*, 15–26.

Kessler, R. C, Berglund, P., Demler, O., Jin, R., Koretz, D., Merikangas, K. R., et al. (2003). The epidemiology of major depressive disorder: Results from the national comorbidity survey replication (NCS-R). *Journal of the American Medical Association, 289*, 3095–3105.

Lejuez, C. W., Hopko, D. R., Acierno, R., Daughters, S. B., & Pagoto, S. L. (2011a). Ten year revision of the brief behavioral activation treatment for depression (BATD): Revised treatment manual (BATD-R). *Behavior Modification, 35*, 486–506.

Lejuez, C. W., Hopko, D. R., Acierno, R., Daughters, S. B., & Pagoto, S. L. (2011b). Ten year revision of the brief behavioral activation treatment for depression (BATD): Revised treatment manual (BATD-R). *Behavior Modification, 35*, 111–161.

Lewinsohn, P. M. (1975). Engagement in pleasant activities and depression level. *Journal of Abnormal Psychology, 84*, 729–731.

Lindauer, S. E., DeLeon, I. G., & Fisher, W. W. (1999). Decreasing signs of negative affect and correlated self-injury in an individual with mental retardation and mood disturbances. *Journal of Applied Behavior Analysis, 32*, 103–106.

Lindsay, W. R., Howells, L., & Pitcaithly, D. (1993). Cognitive therapy for depression with individuals with intellectual disabilities. *British Journal of Medical Psychology, 66*, 135–141.

Luppa, M., Heinrich, A., Angermeyer, M. C., Konig, H.-H., & Rieder-Heller, S. G. (2007). Cost-of-illness depression studies: A systematic review. *Journal of Affective Disorders, 98*, 29–43.

Martell, C. R., Dimidjian, S., & Herman-Dunn, R. (2010). *Behavioral activation for depression: A clinician's guide*. New York: Guilford.

McCabe, M. P., McGillivray, J. A., & Newton, D. C. (2006). Effectiveness of treatment programmes for depression among adults with mild/moderate intellectual disability. *Journal of Intellect Disabilities Research, 50*, 239–247.

McGillivray, J. A., & McCabe, M. P. (2006). Early detection and treatment of depression in adults with mild/moderate intellectual disability. *Australian Journal of Psychology, 58*, 164–165.

McGillivray, J. A., McCabe, M. P., & Kershaw, M. M. (2008). Depression in people with intellectual disability: An evaluation of a staff-administered treatment program. *Research in Developmental Disabilities, 29*, 524–536.

Matson, J. L. (1982). Treatment of the behavioral characteristics of depression in the mentally retarded. *Behavior Therapy, 13*, 209–218.

Matson, J. L. (1983). Depression in the mentally retarded: Toward a conceptual analysis of diagnosis. *Progress in Behavior Modification, 15*, 57–79.

Matson, J. L. (1984). Behavioral treatment of psychosomatic complaints of mentally retarded adults. *American Journal on Mental Retardation, 88*, 640–646.

Matson, J. L. (1986). Treatment outcome research for depression in mentally retarded children and youth: Methodological issues. *Psychopharmacology Bulletin, 22*, 1081–1085.

Matson, J. L., Barrett, R. P., & Helsel, W. J. (1988). Depression in mentally retarded children. *Research in Developmental Disabilities, 9*, 39–46.

Matson, J. L., Dettling, J., & Senatore, V. (1981). Treating depression of a mentally retarded adult. *British Journal of Mental Subnormality, 16*, 86–88.

National Institute of Clinical Excellent. (2009). *Costing statement: 'Depression: The treatment and management of depression in adults (update)' and 'Depression in adults with a chronic physical health problem: Treatment and management'*. London: Author. http://www.nice.org.uk/nicemedia/pdf/CG91CostStatement.pdf (accessed 21 October, 2013).

Penrose, L. S. (1938). *(Colchester survey). A clinic and genetic study of 1,280 cases of mental defect* (Special Report Series, No. 22). London: HMSO.

Penrose, L. S. (1966). *The biology of mental defect*. London: Sidgwick & Jackson.

Perez-Achiaga, N., Nelson, S., & Hassiotis A. J. (2009). Instruments for the detection of depressive symptoms in people with intellectual disabilities: A systematic review. *Intellectual Disabilities, 13*, 55–76.

Reinblatt, S. P., Rifkin, A., & Freeman, J. J. (2004). The efficacy of ECT in adults with mental retardation experiencing psychiatric disorders. *Journal of Electroconvulsive Therapy, 20*, 208–212.

Rojahn, J., & Esbensen, A. J. (2005). Epidemiology of mood disorders in people with mental retardation. In P. Sturmey (Ed.), *Mood disorders in individuals with mental retardation* (pp. 47–65). Kingston, NY: NADD Press.

Rosenberg, M. (1989). *Society and the adolescent self-image* (Rev. ed.). Middletown, CT: Wesleyan University Press.

Ross, E., & Oliver, C. (2003). The assessment of mood in adults who have severe or profound mental retardation. *Clinical Psychology Review, 23*, 225–245.

Royal College of Psychiatrists. (2001). *OP48 DC-LD: Diagnostic criteria for psychiatric disorders for use with adults with learning disabilities/mental retardation*. London: Gaskell.

Skinner, B. F. (1953). *Science and human behavior*. New York: MacMillan.

Spreat, S., Conroy, J. W., & Jones, J. C. (1997). Use of psychotropic medication in Oklahoma: A statewide survey. *American Journal on Mental Retardation, 102*, 80–85.

Stokes, T. F., & Baer, D. M. (1977). An implicit technology of generalization. *Journal of Applied Behavior Analysis, 10*, 349–367.

Strauss, S. E., Richardson, W. S., Glasziou, P., Haynes, R. B., & Strauss, S. E. (2009). *Evidence based medicine* (3rd ed.). London: Churchill Livingstone.

Sturmey, P. (1993). The use of ICD and DSM criteria in people with mental retardation: A review. *The Journal of Nervous and Mental Disease, 181*, 39–42.

Sturmey, P. (2000). Classification: Concepts, progress, and future. In N. Bouras (Ed.), *Psychiatric and behavioural disorders in mental retardation* (pp. 3–17). Cambridge, UK: Cambridge University Press.

Sturmey, P. (2004). Cognitive therapy with people with intellectual disabilities: A selective review and critique. *Clinical Psychology and Psychotherapy, 11*, 223–232.

Sturmey, P. (2005). *Mood disorders in people with mental retardation* (pp. 159–174). Kingston, NY: NADD Publishers.

Sturmey, P. (2006). On some recent claims for the efficacy of cognitive therapy for people with intellectual disabilities. *Journal of Applied Research in Intellectual Disabilities, 19*, 109–118.

Sturmey, P. (2009). Behavioral activation is an evidence-based treatment of depression. *Behavior Modification, 35*, 818–829.

Sturmey, P., Laud, R. B., Cooper, C. L., Matson, J. L., & Fodstad, C. L. (2010a). Challenging behaviors should not be considered depressive equivalents in individuals with intellectual disabilities. II. A replication study. *Research in Developmental Disabilities, 31*, 1002–1007.

Sturmey, P., Laud, R. B., Cooper, C. L., Matson, J. L., & Fodstad, C. L. (2010b). Mania and behavioral equivalents: A preliminary study. *Research in Developmental Disabilities, 31*, 1008–1014.

Tsiouris, J. A., Mann, R., Patti, P. J., & Sturmey, P. (2004). Symptoms of depression and challenging behaviors in people with intellectual disabilities: A Bayesian analysis. *Journal of Intellectual and Developmental Disabilities, 29*, 65–69.

Weissman, M. M., Bruce, M. L., Leaf, P. J., Florio, L. P., & Holzer, C. (1991). Affective disorders. In L. N. Robins & D. A. Regier (Eds.), *Psychiatric disorders in America: The epidemiological catchment area study* (pp. 53–80). New York: Free Press.

World Health Organization. (1992). *The ICD-10 classification of mental and behavioural disorders*. Geneva, Switzerland: WHO.

Zung, W. W. (1965). A self-rating depression scale. *Archives of General Psychiatry, 12*, 63–70.

12

Offenders with Developmental Disabilities

Peter Sturmey and Klaus Drieschner

Introduction

There is an extensive literature on offenders with ID (Chaplin, O'Hara, Holt, & Bouras, 2009; Lindsay, Taylor, & Sturmey, 2004; Luiselli, 2012; Mikkelsen & Stelk, 1999) including individuals with autism spectrum disorders (Debbaudt, 2001) and management of violence and aggression in offenders with ID (Taylor & Novaco, 2005) and sex offenders with ID (Craig, Lindsay, & Browne, 2010; Griffiths, Quinsey, & Hingsburger, 1989; Lindsay, 2009). This chapter will review the evidence from experiments evaluating the efficacy of treatments for offenders with ID. Because the relation between offence-like behavior and criminal conviction is complicated for individuals with ID (see the following text), we include experiments with individuals who had not been convicted of offences, but who were in forensic services because of illegal behavior similar to convicted offenders (Murphy et al., 2010).

Offenders with Intellectual and Developmental Disabilities

Definition

The definition of offenders with ID raises special problems. This is because the definition of *both* terms is challenging.

Most offenders have borderline or mild ID. This is difficult to define because of numerous problems in the accurate diagnosis of borderline and mild IQ. These include (a) problems with the reliability of measures of IQ and adaptive behavior;

Evidence-Based Practice and Intellectual Disabilities, First Edition.
Edited by Peter Sturmey and Robert Didden.
© 2014 John Wiley & Sons, Ltd. Published 2014 by John Wiley & Sons, Ltd.

(b) changes in IQ cutoffs over time within countries and differences between and within countries in the IQ cutoff used for ID; (c) drift in test norms, the so-called Flynn effect, in which IQ and other tests become progressively easier over time; (d) difficulty in accessing accurate developmental histories in some adults who may be offenders; and (e) motivation under certain circumstances to misrepresent oneself as having ID during the legal process.

Whether or not a person with ID who has engaged in potentially criminal behavior is convicted of an offence is an almost arbitrary process. One person with ID who approaches a child in a seeming lewd fashion may be dismissed as having odd or comical behavior without any legal repercussions. In another context, the same behavior may result in contact with the legal system and eventually treatment in forensic services without conviction. In a third context, the same behavior may result in conviction of a sexual offence.

Prevalence

There are no reliable data on the prevalence of offenders among individuals with ID. Several studies have reported prevalences of individuals with ID in forensic setting and prisons. The definitional difficulties outlined earlier and problems in sampling may account for the large differences across studies. For example, Fazel, Xenitidis, and Powell (2008) reported prevalences in the range between 0% and 11.2% from 12 primary studies conducted in prison populations between 1988 and 1998. Holland, Clare, and Mukhopadhyay (2002) found prevalences between 0% and 9.5% in eight prison studies published in 1971 and 1996. More recent studies from England, Norway, Australia, and Canada report higher prevalences, ranging between 1% and 18.9% for mild ID and between 11% and 29.9% for borderline ID (Cashin, Butler, Levy, and Potter, 2006; Crocker, Côté, Toupin, & St-Onge, 2007; Hayes, Shackell, Mottram, & Lancaster, 2007; Sondenaa, Rasmussen, Palmstierna, & Nottestad, 2008).

In a systematic review of the types of offences individuals with ID commit, Simpson and Hogg (2001) found that the proportion of offenders with ID who had been charged with or convicted of sexual offences were 20.5% (Ho, 1996), 17% (Klimecki, Jenkinson, & Wilson, 1994), and 16% (Mabile, 1982). Two studies provided data on the proportion of specific sexual offences. Ho found that 93 of 452 (20.5%) offenders with ID had been charged with a sex-related offence of which 27 (6.9%) involved a sexual assault on an adult, 44 (9.7%) sexual assault on a child, 7 (1.6%) a lewd act, and 15 (3.3%) a lewd act with a child. In a retrospective chart review, Day (1994) reported that of 191 offences and incidents committed by 47 inpatients, 56% were heterosexual offences, 25% involved indecent exposure, 12% were homosexual offences, and 7% involved stealing female underwear and cross-dressing. Fourteen percent of offences and incidents were considered serious and 4% involved violence.

Risk factors

Although prevention of reoffending is the ultimate purpose of offender treatment, this has to be achieved by influencing dynamic risk factors for offending (Andrews, Bonta, & Worminth, 2006), more specifically causal dynamic risk factors (Mann, Hanson, & Thornton, 2010). These are variables for which there is a plausible rationale that they could be a cause of offending and an empirically established association with offending (Mann et al., 2010).

There is a growing consensus concerning dynamic risk factors in violent offenders and sex offenders without ID (Andrews et al., 2006; Douglas & Skeem, 2005; Mann et al., 2010; Thornton, 2002). Among the most important factors are antisocial cognition, especially offence-supportive attitudes; impulsiveness and lifestyle impulsiveness; hostility and grievance; antisocial influences and lack of prosocial support; noncompliance with supervision and treatment, including medication; lack of problem-solving and coping skills; and problems in the areas of work or school. In addition, substance abuse and deviant sexual preferences are core dynamic risk factors for violent offenders and sex offenders, respectively.

There is less empirical evidence concerning dynamic risk factors in offenders with ID; however, the available evidence suggests that factors found in mainstream offender samples also often apply to offenders with ID. In several studies, dynamic risk measures predicted reoffending to a similar degree in samples of offenders with and without ID (Gray, Fitzgerald, Taylor, MacCulloch, & Snowden, 2007; Lindsay et al., 2008; Put, Asscher, Stams, & Moonen, 2013). Moreover, risk assessment measures developed for offenders with ID include the same or largely overlapping dynamic risk factors as measures for mainstream offenders (Boer, Tough, & Haaven, 2004; Quinsey, 2004; Steptoe, Lindsay, Murphy, & Young, 2008).

Offending and offending-related behavior refer to diverse behaviors including violence, fire setting, and a variety of illegal sexual behavior, such as pedophilia, rape, exposure, and stalking, among others. Moreover, the same offences can be committed by different groups, such as males versus females, adolescents versus adults, or individuals with diverse disorders such as autism or psychotic disorders. The same offending or offending-related behavior may reflect different criminogenic needs or serve different functions (Sturmey, 2007, 2008, 2008) which may be an essential aspect of forensic case formulation (Sturmey & McMurran, 2011). It is unknown to what extent the various dynamic risk factors apply to these subgroups, especially for offenders with ID.

Negative impacts and financial costs

Processing, treatment, and incarceration of offenders with ID undoubtedly result in significant costs to the person, to their victims, and to family members and society. These include preventable disability, loneliness, isolation, living in a restrictive environment with fewer opportunities to learn and enjoy life, and avoidance of others, ostracism by others, family stress, injury, financial costs and distress to victims, and the costs of treatment, additional staffing, higher program costs, and, in some cases, costs of extended incarceration. Unfortunately, there are no data that specifically address financial costs with offenders. It is also difficult to disentangle cause and consequence when comparing offenders with nonoffenders when comparing these groups on potential risk factors.

Treatment

Experiments on offending and reoffending

There are no experiments that report data on offending or reoffending. Two group studies and one case series on cognitive behavior therapy (CBT) with offenders with ID have reported data on reduction of reoffending. Lindsay and Smith (1998) reported reoffending among 14 adolescents convicted of sexual offences with 1- and 2-year probation sentences who had received CBT 2 years post treatment. They reported that two had been convicted of similar offences and two were strongly suspected by professionals of having reoffended. Lindsay, Michie, Haut, Steptoe, and Moore (2011) reported reoffending data on 30 men with ID who had committed sexual offences against women and children. They reported that when they followed up all participants "at least 6 years from referral," 23.3% had reoffended. The reoffences included three attempted sexual assaults against women talking to children and in breach of probation, a minor act of indecency with another male, indecent exposure in a public park, and photographing teenage girls. Lindsay, Olley, Baillie, and Smith (1999) reported reoffending data on four adolescent sex offenders with ID. At 2–4-year follow-up, there were no repeat offences.

Experiments on offending-related behavior and cognition

There were only three experiments evaluating treatment of convicted offenders and offending-like behavior in individuals with ID who had not been convicted. The first is an RCT comparing CBT with a wait list control group (Taylor, Novaco, Gillmer, Robertson, & Thorne, 2005), one multiple baseline experiment across participants on mindfulness (Singh et al., 2011), and one multiple baseline design across individual experiment on behavioral skills training (BST) (Travis & Sturmey, 2013). This section will consider each in detail.

Cognitive behavior therapy
CBT is an integrated treatment for a range of disorders that focuses on understanding the relationships between cognitions, feelings, behavior, and physiology that can result in emotional and behavioral problems. Cognitive strategies may include both procedures to remedy deficient processes, such as self-instruction, and procedures

to remedy cognitive content, such as modifying thoughts and schemas (Taylor, Novaco, Gillmer, & Thorne, 2002).

There are several versions of CBT available to treat violence, aggression, and anger in offenders with ID (Lindsay, Allan, Parry et al., 2004; Taylor & Novaco, 2005) which include education; behavioral strategies, such as relaxation training, problem solving, and role-play; and cognitive strategies, such as cognitive retraining. These interventions are typically delivered in groups which may or may not include participants' staff, but others have delivered treatment individually. These interventions also differ in the amount of individualization of content, such as the inclusion of standard, individualized, or both types of role-play. Therapy duration varies from 18 twice weekly 1-hr sessions over (Taylor et al., 2002, 2005, 2005) to 40 sessions scheduled for up to 2 years. Treatment is typically divided up into phases. The first example comes from Lindsay, Allan, Parry et al. (2004) that described CBT based on Novaco's work which included behavioral relaxation training; covert stress inoculation which involved imagining stress-provoking situations and relaxing; distinguishing between appropriate and inappropriate anger and linking behavior, physiology, and emotion; problem solving; and stress inoculation using role-play of standard and individualized anger-provoking situations, application of relaxation training during anger provocation, and individualized formulations of anger. The authors delivered this treatment in groups over approximately 40 40–60-min sessions over a 1-year period. The second example comes from Taylor and Novaco (2005) who divided treatment into an 8-week preparatory and 12-week treatment phase. The aim of the preparatory phase was to desensitize participants to participation by education, rapport building, encouragement to change, self-disclosure, self-monitoring and relaxation, and emphasis on the collaborative nature of therapy. The treatment phase included cognitive restructuring, arousal reduction, and BST, which included procedures such as advanced self-monitoring, analysis and case formulation, construction of an anger hierarchy, and various forms of relaxation, problem solving, and stress inoculation. Thus, both protocols share many common features.

There have been several nonexperimental studies evaluating CBT with violent offenders and sex offenders with ID. With respect to CBT for violent offenders with ID, there have been several narrative and data-based case studies (Black & Novaco, 1993; Novaco & Taylor, 2006) and case series (Allan, Lindsay, McLeod, & Smith, 2001; Burns, Bird, Leach, & Higgins, 2003; Lindsay, Allan, MacLeod, Smart, & Smith, 2003; Lindsay, Overend, Allen, Williams, & Black, 1998). In addition, there have been at least two studies with nonequivalent control group designs including one study of dialectic behavior therapy that have evaluated the use of CBT for violent offenders with ID (Lindsay, Allan, Parry et al., 2004; Sakdalan, Shaw, & Collier, 2010). These nonexperimental studies have reported reduction in ad hoc self-report and psychometric measures of anger, reduction in aggression, increase in social behavior, acquisition of social and problem-solving skills in role-play, reduction of dynamic risk factors, reduction of mental health needs, and, in one study (Lindsay, Allan, Parry et al., 2004), reduction in reoffending compared to a nonequivalent wait list contrast group.

There have been several case series of CBT for sex offenders with ID (Lindsay, Marshall, Neilson, Quinn, & Smith, 1998; Lindsay, Neilson, Morrison, & Smith, 1998; Lindsay, Olley, Baillie, & Smith, 1999; Rose, Jenkins, O'Connor, Jones, & Felce, 2002), uncontrolled repeated measures group studies (Craig, Stringer, & Moss, 2006; Keeling, Rose, & Beech, 2006, 2007, 2007; Lindsay et al., 2011; Murphy, Powell, Guzman, & Hays, 2007; Murphy et al., 2010; Rose, Rose, Hawkins, & Anderson, 2012), and one study with nonequivalent control group design (Lindsay & Smith, 1998). These studies reported changes in the intended direction concerning attitudes and beliefs consistent with sexual offending, victim empathy, and sex knowledge. A notable feature of Murphy et al. (2010) was that the study was a multisite study with positive 6-month follow-up data, indicating the feasibility of the approach across multiple sites.

There was one RCT for CBT for anger in offenders with mild/borderline ID (Taylor et al., 2002, 2005). Since the latter publication included data from the earlier publication, only the latter will be discussed here. Taylor et al. (2005) conducted a group design study comparing Taylor and Novaco's anger management protocol with a delayed wait list control. Participants had to be men aged 18–60 years with IQs of 55–80, detained under the British Mental Health Act with high scores on two self-report measures of anger. Forty participants entered the trial and 20 each entered anger management and wait list control, although four did not complete anger management. The groups did not differ on previous convictions, current staff reported levels of violence, and self-reported measures of anger, and 81% of them had had criminal convictions regarding physical violence, sexual aggression, or both and 61% had been physically violent after admission. There was a small but statistically significant difference between the groups in IQ (67 vs. 71 for anger treatment completers and routine care, respectively; $p < .05$). The experimenters administered measures at baseline screening, pretreatment, immediately post treatment, and at 4-month follow-up. There were two self-report measures and one staff rating of anger.

There was a statistically significant difference in the decline in anger between the anger treatment and the wait list control groups on two self-report measures with moderately large effect sizes. There were no statistically significant differences on four other self-report measures of anger and on staff ratings of anger, although there were nonsignificant trends in the expected direction. Generally, about twice as many participants in the experimental than the control group were likely to have change scores of 1 or more standard deviations on all measures in the direction of improvement, although no inferential statistics were reported for this difference. The authors also conducted post hoc tests comparing only pre- and posttreatment scores in the anger treatment and control groups and found statistically significant differences on two self-report measures, but not staff ratings.

Mindfulness

Singh et al. (2008) reported an experiment evaluating mindfulness training as an intervention for physical and verbal aggression for six offenders with unspecified degrees of ID in a forensic mental health facility. Participants had multiple psychiatric diagnoses and offending histories including sexual offences against minors. All had high rates of serious aggression that were uncontrolled by psychotropic medication and current behavioral programming. During baseline, the experimenters instructed the staff to implement current treatment programs. The experimenters taught participants the *Meditation on the soles of the feet* meditation which includes initial acquisition and subsequent practice and application of medication skills. In the acquisition training, the participants sit quietly with their eyes closed and their hands on their thighs in a comfortable chair, and the therapist instructs them through a task analysis of how to focus on the soles of their feet until they are calm and how to maintain a state of calmness while imagining different scenes that have evoked aggression in the past. The participants practiced the technique twice a day over the 27-month period of the experiment.

The authors reported that aggression was systematically reduced from 0 to 4 incidents per month in baseline to 0 incidents for the last 5 months of mindfulness training. Their Figure 1 demonstrated experimental control of physical aggression. In addition, the experimenters reported pre–post data on a range of relevant measures, such as PRN medication, restraints, staff and peer injuries, and behavioral incidents, all of which showed large reductions. In addition, they reported cost data, based on lost staff days and staff injuries, which indicated cost reductions from approximately \$52,000 per year to approximately \$2,000/year.

Behavioral skills training
Travis and Sturmey (2013) conduced a multiple baseline design across three participants on the effects of BST on aggression in three offenders with mild ID (IQs ranged from 58 to 63) and other mental health diagnoses, such as schizoaffective and bipolar disorder. All had been deemed incompetent to stand trial. The study took place in a locked inpatient forensic setting. Three staff also participated. The experimenters conducted functional assessment to identify similar pairs of discriminative stimuli for aggressive behavior, such as cancellation of a trip and work, one of which they used for training and one for generalization. Training took place in a therapy room, but the authors collected data on aggression and replacement behaviors in response to the systematic presentation of triggers in the participants' residential and work settings. Throughout the experiment, the experimenter presented five aggression-evoking stimuli five times over three 1-hr periods. Thus, the dependent variable was the proportion of occasions in that the triggers were followed by either an aggression or a replacement behavior.

In baseline, the experimenter instructed individuals with disabilities as to what replacement behavior they should engage in if a trigger was presented. Training included instructions, modeling, rehearsal, and feedback until the client met mastery criterion. The posttraining condition was the same as the baseline. There was a token economy in place throughout the experiment. All three participants emitted aggression approximately 45–80% and approximately 0–20% of opportunities in baseline and post-BST, respectively. They also emitted replacement behaviors during approximately 10–40% and approximately 70–90% of opportunities in baseline and post-BST, respectively. The results were very similar following presentation on generalization triggers that the experimenters did not use during training. Staff and family members informally made positive comments about the intervention, and there was an increase in community trips following BST for all three participants. Since client's behavior only changes after treatment and since there was a multiple baseline design across individuals, we can infer that treatment caused the change in client behavior.

Conclusions

Since no experiments were identified that reported data on reoffending, no interventions are evidence based for that outcome. There was only limited support for CBT, mindfulness, and BST for offenders. Support was limited because these studies addressed behavior such as self-reports and staff reports of anger (Taylor et al., 2005), staff reported of aggression, and other related outcomes (Singh et al., 2008) and observations of aggression (Travis & Sturmey, 2013) which may or may not be related to offending. Additionally, there are no independent replications of any of these three experiments at this time.

Practitioner guidelines

Practitioners often treat problems with little or no evidence to guide them. In the general absence of evidence for the effectiveness of treatments for offenders with ID, readers should regard these recommendations with caution and pay special attention to demonstrate positively that whichever treatment these use is effective for their client.

In the case of treatment of violence, aggression, and anger in offenders with ID:

1. Evaluate the outcome of treatment empirically on a case-by-case basis.
2. Consider the use of CBT using Taylor and Novaco's (2005) protocol.
3. Consider the use of mindfulness using Singh et al's (2011) protocol.
4. Consider the use of BST based on functional assessment using Travis and Sturmey's (2013) protocol.
5. Consider client preferences and skills that may match or mismatch treatments for the three treatment formats.
6. In order to evaluate if reoffending occurs, to take preventative action, and to reimplement treatment if necessary, collect data on long-term (minimum 2 years) follow-up.
7. Be cautious in implementing alternate treatments forms without attempting the current best three choices.
8. In the case of sexual offenders with ID, there is no experimental evidence to guide practitioners' choice of treatment. Based on nonexperimental evidence, practitioners should consider CBT and general principles of case formulation which should be evaluated on a case-by-case basis.

References

Allan, R., Lindsay, W. R., MacLeod, F., & Smith, A. H. W. (2001). Treatment of women with intellectual disabilities who have been involved with the criminal justice system for reasons of aggression. *Journal of Applied Research in Intellectual Disabilities, 14,* 340–347.

Andrews, D. A, Bonta, J., & Worminth, J. S. (2006). The recent past and near future of risk and/or need assessment. *Crime & Delinquency, 52,* 7–27.

Black, L., & Novaco, R. W. (1993). Treatment of anger with a developmentally disabled man. In R. A. Wells & V. J. Giannetti (Eds.), *Casebook of the brief psychotherapies* (pp. 143–158). New York: Plenum Press.

Boer, D. P., Tough, S., & Haaven, J. (2004). Assessment of risk manageability of intellectually disabled sex offenders. *Journal of Intellectual Disabilities Research, 17,* 275–283.

Burns, M., Bird, D., Leach, C., & Higgins, K. (2003). Anger management training: The effects of a structured programme on the self-reported anger experience of forensic inpatients with learning disability. *Journal of Psychiatric and Mental Health Nursing, 10,* 569–577.

Cashin, A., Butler, T., Levy, M., & Potter, E. (2006). Intellectual disability in the New South Wales inmate population. *International Journal of Prisoner Health, 2,* 115–120.

Chaplin, E., O'Hara, J., Holt, G., & Bouras, N. (2009). Mental health services for people with intellectual disability: Challenges to care delivery. *British Journal of Learning Disabilities, 37,* 157–164.

Craig, L. A., Lindsay, W. R., & Browne, K. D. (2010). *Assessment and treatment of sexual offenders with intellectual disabilities: A handbook.* Chichester, UK: Wiley.

Craig, L. A., Stringer, I., & Moss, T. (2006). Treating sexual offenders with learning disabilities in the community. *International Journal of Offender Therapy & Comparative Criminology, 50,* 111–122.

Crocker, A. G., Côté, G., Toupin, J., & St-Onge, B. (2007). Rate and characteristics of men with an intellectual disability in pre-trial detention. *Journal of Intellectual and Developmental Disability, 32,* 143–152.

Day, K. (1994). Male mentally handicapped sex offenders. *The British Journal of Psychiatry, 165,* 630–639.

Debbaudt, D. (2001). *Autism, advocates & law enforcement professionals: Recognizing and reducing risk situations for people with autism spectrum disorders.* London: Jessica Kingsley Publishers.

Douglas, K. S., & Skeem, J. L. (2005). Violence risk assessment: Getting specific about being dynamic. *Psychology, Public Policy, and Law, 11,* 347–383.

Fazel, S., Xenitidis, K., & Powell, J. (2008). The prevalence of intellectual disabilities among 12000 prisoners: A systematic review. *International Journal of Law and Psychiatry, 31,* 369–373.

Gray, N. S., Fitzgerald, S., Taylor, J., MacCulloch, M. J., & Snowden, R. J. (2007). Predicting future reconviction in offenders with intellectual disabilities: The predictive efficacy of VRAG, PCL-SV, and the HCR-20. *Psychological Assessment, 19,* 474–479.

Griffiths, D. M., Quinsey, V. L., & Hingsburger, D. (1989). *Changing inappropriate sexual behaviour: A community based approach for persons with developmental disabilities.* Baltimore: Paul Brooks Publishing.

Hayes, S., Shackell, P., Mottram, P., & Lancaster, R. (2007). The prevalence of intellectual disability in a major UK prison. *British Journal of Learning Disabilities, 35,* 162–167,

Ho, T. (1996). Assessment of retardation among mentally retarded criminal offenders: An examination of racial disparity. *Journal of Criminal Justice*, 24, 337–350.

Holland, T., Clare, I. C. H., & Mukhopadhyay, T. (2002). Prevalence of 'criminal offending' by men and women with intellectual disability and the characteristics of 'offenders': Implications for research and service development. *Journal of Intellectual Disability Research*, 46(Issue Suppl. s1), 6–20.

Keeling, J. A., Rose, J. L., & Beech, A. R. (2006). An investigation into the effectiveness of a custody-based cognitive-behavioural treatment for special needs sexual offenders. *Journal of Forensic Psychiatry & Psychology*, 17, 372–392.

Keeling, J. A., Rose, J. L., & Beech, A. R. (2007). Comparing sexual offender treatment efficacy: Mainstream sexual offenders and sexual offenders with special needs. *Journal of Intellectual & Developmental Disability*, 32, 117–124.

Klimecki, M. R., Jenkinson, K., & Wilson, L. (1994). A study of recidivism among offenders with an intellectual disability. *Journal of Intellectual and Developmental Disability*, 38, 209–219.

Lindsay, W. I., Taylor, J., & Sturmey, P. (Eds.). (2004a). *Offenders with developmental disabilities*. Chichester, UK: Wiley.

Lindsay, W. R. (2009). *The treatment of sex offenders with developmental disabilities: A practice workbook*. Chichester, UK: Wiley.

Lindsay, W. R., Allan, R., MacLeod, F., Smart, N., & Smith, A. H. W. (2003). Long term treatment and management of violent tendencies of men with intellectual disabilities convicted of assault. *Mental Retardation*, 41, 47–56.

Lindsay, W. R., Allan, R., Parry, C., MacLeod, F., Cottrell, J., Overend, H., et al. (2004b). Anger and aggression in people with intellectual disabilities: Treatment and follow-up of consecutive referrals and a waiting list comparison. *Clinical Psychology & Psychotherapy*, 11, 255–264.

Lindsay, W. R., Hogue, T. E., Taylor, J. L., Steptoe, L., Mooney, P., O'Brian, G., et al. (2008). Risk assessment in offenders with intellectual disability: A comparison across three levels of security. *International Journal of Offender Therapy and Comparative Criminology*, 52, 90–111.

Lindsay, W. R., Marshall, I., Neilson, C. Q., Quinn, K., & Smith, A. H. W. (1998a). The treatment of men with a learning disability convicted of exhibitionism. *Research on Developmental Disabilities*, 19, 295–316.

Lindsay, W. R., Michie, A. M., Haut, F., Steptoe, L., & Moore F. (2011). Comparing offenders against women and offenders against children on treatment outcome for offenders with intellectual disability. *Journal of Applied Research in Intellectual Disability*, 24, 361–369.

Lindsay, W. R., Neilson, C. Q., Morrison, F., & Smith, A. H. W. (1998b). The treatment of six men with a learning disability convicted of sex offences with children. *British Journal of Clinical Psychology*, 37, 83–98.

Lindsay, W. R., Olley, S., Baillie, N., & Smith, A. H. W. (1999). The treatment of adolescent sex offenders with intellectual disability. *Mental Retardation*, 37, 320–333.

Lindsay, W. R., Overend, H., Allan, R., Williams, C., & Black, L. (1998c). Using specific approaches for individual problems in the management of anger and aggression. *British Journal of Learning Disabilities*, 26, 44–45.

Lindsay, W. R., & Smith, A. H. W. (1998). Responses to treatment for sex offenders with intellectual disability: A comparison of men with 1 and 2 year probation sentences. *Journal of Intellectual Disability Research*, 42, 346–353.

Luiselli, J. (2012). *The handbook of high-risk challenging behaviors in people with intellectual and developmental disabilities*. Baltimore: Brooks.

Mabile, W. R. (1982) The mentally retarded defendant program. In M. Santamour & P. S. Watson (Eds.), *The retarded offender* (pp. 434–443). New York: Praeger.

Mann, R. W., Hanson, R. K., & Thornton, D. (2010). Assessing risk for sexual recidivism: Some proposals on the nature of psychologically meaningful risk factors. *Sex Abuse*, 22, 191–217.

Mikkelsen, E. J., & Stelk, W. J. (1999). *Criminal offenders with mental retardation: Risk assessment and the continuum of community based programs*. Kingston, NY: NADD Press.

Murphy, G., Powell, S., Guzman, A. M., & Hays, S. J. (2007). Cognitive-behavioural treatment for men with intellectual disabilities and sexually abusive behaviour: A pilot study. *Journal of Intellectual Disability Research*, 51, 902–912.

Murphy, G. H., Sinclair, N., Hays, S. J., Heaton, K., Powell, S., Langdon, P., et al. (SOTSEC – ID) (2010). Effectiveness of group cognitive behavioural treatment for men with intellectual disabilities at risk of sexual offending. *Journal of Applied Research in Intellectual Disabilities*, 23, 537–551.

Novaco, R. W., & Taylor, J. L. (2006). Cognitive-behavioural anger treatment. In M. McNulty & A. Carr (Eds.), *Handbook of adult clinical psychology: An evidence based practice approach* (pp. 978–1009). London: Routledge.

Put, C. E., Asscher, J. J., Stams, G. J. J. M., & Moonen, X. M. H. (2013). *Differences between juvenile offenders with and without intellectual disabilities in the importance of static and dynamic risk factors for recidivism*. Journal of Intellectual Disability Research.

Quinsey, V. L. (2004). Risk assessment and management in community settings. In W. R. Lindsay, J. L. Taylor, & P. Sturmey (Eds.), *Offenders with developmental disabilities* (pp. 132–142). Chichester, UK: Wiley.

Rose, J., Jenkins, R., O'Conner, C., Jones, C., & Felce, D. (2002). A group treatment for men with intellectual disabilities who sexually offend or abuse. *Journal of Applied Research in Intellectual Disabilities*, 15, 138–150.

Rose, J., Rose, D., Hawkins, C., & Anderson, C. (2012). A sex offender treatment group for men with intellectual disabilities in community settings. *Journal of Forensic Practice*, 14, 21–28.

Sakdalan, J. A., Shaw, J., & Collier, V. (2010). Staying in the here and now: A pilot study on the use of dialectical behaviour therapy group skills training for forensic clients with intellectual disability. *Journal of Intellectual Disability Research*, 54, 568–572.

Simpson, M. K., & Hogg, J. (2001). Patterns of offending among people with intellectual disability: A systematic review. *Part I: Methodology and prevalence data*. Journal of Intellectual Disabilities Research, 45, 384–396.

Singh, N. N., Lancioni, G., Winton, A. S. W., Singh, A., Adkins, A., & Singh, J. (2011). Can adult offenders with intellectual disabilities use mindfulness-based procedures to control and deviant sexual arousal? *Psychology, Crime and Law*, 17, 165–180.

Singh, N. N., Lancioni, G. E., Winton, A. S. W., Singh, A. N., Adkins, A. D., Singh, J. (2008). Clinical and benefit—cost outcomes of teaching a mindfulness-based procedure to adult offenders with intellectual disabilities. *Behavior Modification*, 32, 622–637.

Sondenaa, E., Rasmussen, K., Palmstierna, T., & Nottestad, J. (2008). The prevalence and nature of intellectual disability in Norwegian prisons. *Journal of Intellectual Disability Research*, 52, 1129–1137,

Steptoe, L. R., Lindsay, W. R., Murphy, L., & Young, S. J. (2008). Construct validity, reliability and predictive validity of the dynamic risk assessment and management system (DRAMS) in offenders with intellectual disability. *Legal and Criminological Psychology*, 13, 309–321.

Sturmey, P. (Ed.). (2007). *Functional analysis in clinical treatment*. New York: Academic Press.

Sturmey, P. (2008). *Behavioral case formulation and intervention. A functional analytic approach*. Chichester, UK: Wiley.

Sturmey, P., & McMurran, M. (Eds.). (2011). *Forensic case formulation*. Chichester, UK: Wiley.

Taylor, J. L., & Novaco, R. W. (2005). *Anger treatment for people with developmental disabilities: A theory, evidence and manual based approach*. Chichester, UK: Wiley.

Taylor, J. L., Novaco, R. W., Gillmer, B., & Thorne, I. (2002). Cognitive behavioural treatment of anger intensity among offenders with intellectual disabilities. *Journal of Applied Research in Intellectual Disabilities*, 15, 151–165.

Taylor, J. L., Novaco, R. W., Gillmer, B. T., Robertson, A., & Thorne, I. (2005). Individual cognitive behavioural anger treatment for people with mild-borderline intellectual disabilities and histories of aggression: A controlled trial. *British Journal of Clinical Psychology*, 44, 367–382.

Thornton, D. (2002). Constructing and testing a framework for dynamic risk assessment. *Sexual Abuse: A Journal of Research and Treatment*, 14, 139–153.

Travis, R., & Sturmey, P. (2013). Using behavioral skills training to teach anger management skills to adults with mild intellectual disability. *Journal of Applies Research in Intellectual Disability*, 26, 481–488.

Index